3

Sleep Disorders
SOURCEBOOK

FIFTH EDITION

Health Reference Series

Sleep Disorders
SOURCEBOOK

FIFTH EDITION

Basic Consumer Health Information about Sleep Disorders, Including Insomnia, Sleep Apnea and Snoring, Jet Lag and Other Circadian Rhythm Disorders, Narcolepsy, and Parasomnias, Such as Sleepwalking and Sleep Paralysis, and Featuring Facts about Other Health Problems That Affect Sleep, Why Sleep Is Necessary, How Much Sleep Is Needed, the Physical and Mental Effects of Sleep Deprivation, and Pediatric Sleep Issues

Along with Tips for Diagnosing and Treating Sleep Disorders, a Glossary of Related Terms, and a List of Resources for Additional Help and Information

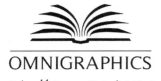

OMNIGRAPHICS

615 Griswold, Ste. 520, Detroit, MI 48226

Bibliographic Note
Because this page cannot legibly accommodate all the copyright notices, the Bibliographic
Note portion of the Preface constitutes an extension of the copyright notice.

* * *

OMNIGRAPHICS
Angela L. Williams, *Managing Editor*
* * *

Copyright © 2019 Omnigraphics

ISBN 978-0-7808-1713-5
E-ISBN 978-0-7808-1714-2

Library of Congress Cataloging-in-Publication Data

Names: Omnigraphics, Inc., issuing body.

Title: Sleep disorders sourcebook: basic consumer health information about sleep
disorders, including insomnia, sleep apnea and snoring, jet lag and other circadian
rhythm disorders, narcolepsy, and parasomnias, such as sleepwalking and sleep
paralysis, and featuring facts about other health problems that affect sleep, why
sleep is necessary, how much sleep is needed, the physical and mental effects of sleep
deprivation, and pediatric sleep issues; along with tips for diagnosing and treating
sleep disorders, a glossary of related terms, and a list of resources for additional help
and information.

Description: Fifth edition. | Detroit, MI: Omnigraphics, Inc., [2019] | Includes index.

Identifiers: LCCN 2019021356 (print) | LCCN 2019021862 (ebook) | ISBN
9780780817142 (ebook) | ISBN 9780780817135 (hard cover: alk. paper)

Subjects: LCSH: Sleep disorders. | Consumer education.

Classification: LCC RC547 (ebook) | LCC RC547.S536 2019 (print) | DDC 616.8/498-
-dc23

LC record available at https://lccn.loc.gov/2019021356

Table of Contents

Part II: The Causes and Consequences of Sleep Deprivation

Part III: Sleep Disorders

Part V: Preventing, Diagnosing, and Treating Sleep Disorders

Part VII: Research and Clinical Studies on Sleep and Sleep Disorders

Part VIII: Additional Help and Information

Preface

About This Book

Sleep is increasingly being recognized as important to public health. According to the Centers for Disease Control and Prevention (CDC), one-third of U.S. adults have reported that they usually get less than the recommended amount of sleep. It is estimated that 50 to 70 million Americans have sleep or wakefulness disorders. There is a general tendency among people to view sleep as merely a "down time" for their brains and rest for their bodies. People tend to cut back on sleep, thinking it will not be a problem. But, research shows otherwise. Not getting sufficient sleep has been linked with chronic diseases and conditions, such as type 2 diabetes, heart disease, obesity, and depression. Insufficient sleep can result in motor vehicle crashes, which can result in a lot of injury and disability each year.

Sleep Disorders Sourcebook, Fifth Edition offers basic consumer health information about common sleep disorders, including insomnia, sleep apnea, narcolepsy, circadian rhythm disorders, and parasomnias, and other health problems that affect sleep, such as cancer, pain, and respiratory disorders. It explains how much sleep is needed; the causes and consequences of sleep deprivation; and the methods used to prevent, diagnose, and treat sleep disorders. Pediatric sleep issues that impact children from infancy through the teen years are also discussed. A part on the latest from the field of research and clinical studies on sleep is included. A glossary of terms related to sleep disorders and a list of resources for further help and information are also included.

How to Use This Book

This book is divided into parts and chapters. Parts focus on broad areas of interest. Chapters are devoted to single topics within a part.

Part I: Sleep Basics presents facts about why and how people sleep, including an explanation of circadian rhythms, the physical characteristics of sleep, and the benefits of napping. It offers information on dreams and nightmares and explains how they affect sleep. It also describes sex differences in sleep, explains how aging affects sleep patterns, and discusses myths related to sleep.

Part II: The Causes and Consequences of Sleep Deprivation defines sleep deprivation and talks about the people most at risk for sleep deprivation. It provides information on why your brain and body need sleep. It also describes the molecular link between lack of sleep and weight gain. The part concludes with information on how sleep deprivation affects daily activities, such as learning and driving.

Part III: Sleep Disorders describes disorders that directly affect the ability to sleep. These include disorders such as sleep apnea, snoring, insomnia, circadian rhythm disorders, congenital central hypoventilation syndrome, and parasomnias. Narcolepsy and other disorders associated with excessive sleeping are also discussed.

Part IV: Other Health Problems That Often Affect Sleep provides information about disorders that often impact sleep quality, including cancer, fibromyalgia, headaches, and mental-health concerns. The symptoms that disrupt sleep are described and suggestions for lessening their impact are provided.

Part V: Preventing, Diagnosing, and Treating Sleep Disorders identifies common sleep disruptors and explains the importance of a proper sleep environment. It describes how sleep studies work and details treatment options, including medications, dietary supplements, continuous positive airway pressure, and other complementary and alternative medications.

Part VI: A Special Look at Pediatric Sleep Issues describes sleep disturbances in infancy, childhood, and adolescence. It discusses safe sleeping environments for infants and explains sudden infant death syndrome. It provides information on how to get children into bed and offers facts about bed-wetting, sleepwalking, and teeth grinding.

Part VII: Research and Clinical Studies on Sleep and Sleep Disorders offers information about various research studies and clinical trials that focus on the causes, diagnosis, treatment, and effects of sleep disorders.

Part VIII: Additional Help and Information includes a glossary of terms related to sleep and sleep disorders and directories of resources for additional help and support.

Bibliographic Note

This volume contains documents and excerpts from publications issued by the following U.S. government agencies: Centers for Disease Control and Prevention (CDC); *Eunice Kennedy Shriver* National Institute of Child Health and Human Development (NICHD); Genetic and Rare Diseases Information Center (GARD); Genetics Home Reference (GHR); National Cancer Institute (NCI); National Center for Complementary and Integrative Health (NCCIH); National Center for Posttraumatic Stress Disorder (NCPTSD); National Heart, Lung, and Blood Institute (NHLBI); National Highway Traffic Safety Administration (NHTSA); National Institute of Arthritis and Musculoskeletal and Skin Diseases (NIAMS); National Institute of Diabetes and Digestive and Kidney Diseases (NIDDK); National Institute of General Medical Sciences (NIGMS); National Institute of Justice (NIJ); National Institute of Mental Health (NIMH); National Institute of Neurological Disorders and Stroke (NINDS); National Institute on Aging (NIA); National Institute on Drug Abuse (NIDA); National Institutes of Health (NIH); *NIH News in Health*; Office of Disease Prevention and Health Promotion (ODPHP); Office on Women's Health (OWH); Rehabilitation Research & Development Service (RR&D); Substance Abuse and Mental Health Services Administration (SAMHSA); U.S. Department of Agriculture (USDA); U.S. Department of Health and Human Services (HHS); U.S. Department of Veterans Affairs (VA); and U.S. Food and Drug Administration (FDA).

It may also contain original material produced by Omnigraphics and reviewed by medical consultants.

About the Health Reference Series

The *Health Reference Series* is designed to provide basic medical information for patients, families, caregivers, and the general public. Each volume takes a particular topic and provides comprehensive coverage. This is especially important for people who may be dealing with a newly diagnosed disease or a chronic disorder in themselves or in a family member. People looking for preventive guidance, information about disease warning signs, medical statistics, and risk factors for health problems will also find answers to their questions in the *Health*

Reference Series. The *Series*, however, is not intended to serve as a tool for diagnosing illness, in prescribing treatments, or as a substitute for the physician/patient relationship. All people concerned about medical symptoms or the possibility of disease are encouraged to seek professional care from an appropriate healthcare provider.

A Note about Spelling and Style

Health Reference Series editors use *Stedman's Medical Dictionary* as an authority for questions related to the spelling of medical terms and the *Chicago Manual of Style* for questions related to grammatical structures, punctuation, and other editorial concerns. Consistent adherence is not always possible, however, because the individual volumes within the *Series* include many documents from a wide variety of different producers, and the editor's primary goal is to present material from each source as accurately as is possible. This sometimes means that information in different chapters or sections may follow other guidelines and alternate spelling authorities. For example, occasionally a copyright holder may require that eponymous terms be shown in possessive forms (Crohn's disease vs. Crohn disease) or that British spelling norms be retained (leukaemia vs. leukemia).

Medical Review

Omnigraphics contracts with a team of qualified, senior medical professionals who serve as medical consultants for the *Health Reference Series*. As necessary, medical consultants review reprinted and originally written material for currency and accuracy. Citations including the phrase "Reviewed (month, year)" indicate material reviewed by this team. Medical consultation services are provided to the *Health Reference Series* editors by:

Dr. Vijayalakshmi, MBBS, DGO, MD
Dr. Senthil Selvan, MBBS, DCH, MD
Dr. K. Sivanandham, MBBS, DCH, MS (Research), PhD

Our Advisory Board

We would like to thank the following board members for providing initial guidance on the development of this series:

- Dr. Lynda Baker, Associate Professor of Library and Information Science, Wayne State University, Detroit, MI

- Nancy Bulgarelli, William Beaumont Hospital Library, Royal Oak, MI

- Karen Imarisio, Bloomfield Township Public Library, Bloomfield Township, MI

- Karen Morgan, Mardigian Library, University of Michigan-Dearborn, Dearborn, MI

- Rosemary Orlando, St. Clair Shores Public Library, St. Clair Shores, MI

Health Reference Series *Update Policy*

The inaugural book in the *Health Reference Series* was the first edition of *Cancer Sourcebook* published in 1989. Since then, the *Series* has been enthusiastically received by librarians and in the medical community. In order to maintain the standard of providing high-quality health information for the layperson the editorial staff at Omnigraphics felt it was necessary to implement a policy of updating volumes when warranted.

Medical researchers have been making tremendous strides, and it is the purpose of the *Health Reference Series* to stay current with the most recent advances. Each decision to update a volume is made on an individual basis. Some of the considerations include how much new information is available and the feedback we receive from people who use the books. If there is a topic you would like to see added to the update list, or an area of medical concern you feel has not been adequately addressed, please write to:

Managing Editor
Health Reference Series
Omnigraphics
615 Griswold, Ste. 520
Detroit, MI 48226

Part One

Sleep Basics

Chapter 1

Understanding Sleep

Chapter Contents

Section 1.1

Sleep and Its Importance

This section contains text excerpted from the following sources:
Text in this section begins with excerpts from "About Sleep," *Eunice Kennedy Shriver* National Institute of Child Health and Human Development (NICHD), April 29, 2019; Text beginning with the heading "Get Enough Sleep" is excerpted from "Get Enough Sleep," Office of Disease Prevention and Health Promotion (ODPHP), U.S. Department of Health and Human Services (HHS), July 18, 2018; Text under the heading "What Are Some Tips for a Good Night's Sleep?" is excerpted from "Other Sleep FAQs," *Eunice Kennedy Shriver* National Institute of Child Health and Human Development (NICHD), April 29, 2019.

Sleep is a complex biological process that helps people process new information, stay healthy, and reenergize. Periods of sleep and wakefulness are part of how our bodies function.

Although you are resting while you sleep, your brain remains highly active. Sleep consists of different stages that repeat several times each night. During sleep, the brain cycles through two distinct phases: rapid eye movement (REM) sleep and non-REM sleep. Not completing the full sleep process can stress your body.

Why Is Sleep Important?

Each phase and stage of sleep is important to ensure that the mind and body are completely rested. Certain stages help you feel rested and energetic the next day, while other stages help you learn information and form memories. Sleep is important in the function of your body's other systems, such as your metabolism and immune system. Sleep may also help your body clear toxins from your brain that build up while you are awake.

Not getting enough or enough quality sleep contributes, in the short term, to problems with learning and processing information, and it can have a harmful effect on long-term health and well-being. According to the Centers for Disease Control and Prevention (CDC), many U.S. adults report that they do not get the recommended number of hours of sleep each night.

Sleep affects how well you do your daily tasks, your mood, and your health in the following ways:

- **Performance.** Cutting back on sleep by as little as one hour can make it difficult to focus the next day and can slow your response time. Insufficient sleep can also make you more likely to take risks and make poor decisions, according to the National Heart, Lung, and Blood Institute (NHLBI).

- **Mood.** Sleep affects your mood. Insufficient sleep can make you more easily annoyed or angry, and that can lead to trouble with relationships, particularly for children and teens. Also, people who do not get enough sleep are more likely to become depressed, according to the NHLBI.

- **Health.** Sleep is important for good health. Research in adults has shown that lack of sleep or lack of quality sleep increases a person's risk for high blood pressure, heart disease, and other medical conditions. Your environment can affect the quality of your sleep by causing disturbances that prevent you from sleeping through the night. Also, during sleep, the body produces hormones that help the body grow and, throughout life, build muscle, fight illnesses, and repair damage to the body. Growth hormone, for example, is produced during sleep, and it is essential for growth and development. Other hormones produced during sleep affect how the body uses energy, which may explain why lack of sleep contributes to obesity and diabetes.

Get Enough Sleep

It is important to get enough sleep. Sleep helps keep your mind and body healthy.

How Much Sleep Do I Need?

Most adults need seven to eight hours of good quality sleep on a regular schedule each night. Make changes to your routine if you cannot find enough time to sleep. Getting enough sleep is not only about total hours of sleep. It is also important to get good quality sleep on a regular schedule, so you feel rested when you wake up.

If you often have trouble sleeping—or if you often still feel tired after sleeping—talk with your doctor.

How Much Sleep Do Children Need?

Kids need even more sleep than adults.

- Teens need 8 to 10 hours of sleep each night.
- School-aged children need 9 to 12 hours of sleep each night.

- Preschoolers need to sleep between 10 and 13 hours a day (including naps).

- Toddlers need to sleep between 11 and 14 hours a day (including naps).

- Babies need to sleep between 12 and 16 hours a day (including naps).

Why Is Getting Enough Sleep Important?

Getting enough sleep has many benefits. It can help you:

- Get sick less often

- Stay at a healthy weight

- Lower your risk for serious health problems, such as diabetes and heart disease

- Reduce stress and improve your mood

- Think more clearly and do better in school and at work

- Get along better with people

- Make good decisions and avoid injuries—for example, sleepy drivers cause thousands of car accidents every year.

Does It Matter When I Sleep?

Yes. Your body sets your "biological clock" according to the pattern of daylight where you live. This helps you naturally get sleepy at night and stay alert during the day. If you have to work at night and sleep during the day, you may have trouble getting enough sleep. It can also be hard to sleep when you travel to a different time zone.

Why Cannot I Fall Asleep?

Many things can make it harder for you to sleep, including:

- Stress or anxiety

- Pain

- Certain health conditions, such as heartburn or asthma

- Some medicines
- Caffeine (usually from coffee, tea, and soda)
- Alcohol and other drugs
- Untreated sleep disorders, such as sleep apnea or insomnia

If you are having trouble sleeping, try making changes to your routine to get the sleep you need. You may want to:

- Change what you do during the day. For example, get your physical activity in the morning instead of at night.
- Create a comfortable sleep environment, and make sure your bedroom is dark and quiet.
- Set a bedtime routine, and go to bed at the same time every night.

How Can I Tell If I Have a Sleep Disorder?

Sleep disorders can cause many different problems. Keep in mind that it is normal to have trouble sleeping every now and then. People with sleep disorders generally experience these problems on a regular basis.

Common signs of sleep disorders include:

- Trouble falling or staying asleep
- Still feeling tired after a good night's sleep
- Sleepiness during the day that makes it difficult to do everyday activities, such as driving a car or concentrating at work
- Frequent loud snoring
- Pauses in breathing or gasping while sleeping
- Itchy feelings in your legs or arms at night that feel better when you move or massage the area
- Trouble moving your arms and legs when you wake up

If you have any of these signs, talk to a doctor or nurse. You may need to be tested or treated for a sleep disorder.

Take Action to Get Enough Sleep

Making small changes to your daily routine can help you get the sleep you need.

Change What You Do during the Day

- Try to spend some time outdoors every day.

- Plan your physical activity for earlier in the day, not right before you go to bed.

- Stay away from caffeine (including coffee, tea, and soda) late in the day.

- If you have trouble sleeping at night, limit daytime naps to 20 minutes or less.

- If you drink alcohol, drink only in moderation. This means no more than one drink a day for women and no more than two drinks a day for men. Alcohol can keep you from sleeping well.

- Do not eat a big meal close to bedtime.

- Quit smoking. The nicotine in cigarettes can make it harder for you to sleep.

Create a Good Sleep Environment

- Make sure your bedroom is dark. If there are street lights near your window, try putting up light-blocking curtains.

- Keep your bedroom quiet.

- Consider keeping electronic devices—such as TVs, computers, and smartphones—out of the bedroom.

Set a Bedtime Routine

- Go to bed at the same time every night.

- Get the same amount of sleep each night.

- Avoid eating, talking on the phone, or reading in bed.

- Avoid using computers or smartphones, watching TV, or playing video games at bedtime.

If you are still awake after staying in bed for more than 20 minutes, get up. Do something relaxing, such as reading or meditating, until you feel sleepy.

If You Are Concerned about Your Sleep, See a Doctor

Talk with a doctor or nurse if you have any of the following signs of a sleep disorder:

- Frequent, loud snoring
- Pauses in breathing during sleep
- Trouble waking up in the morning
- Pain or itchy feelings in your legs or arms at night that feel better when you move or massage the area
- Trouble staying awake during the day

Even if you are not aware of problems such as these, talk with a doctor if you feel as if you often have trouble sleeping.

Keep a sleep diary for a week and share it with your doctor. A doctor can suggest different sleep routines or medicines to treat sleep disorders. Talk with a doctor before trying over-the-counter (OTC) sleep medicine.

What Are Some Tips for a Good Night's Sleep?

Circadian rhythms are disrupted when people travel from one time zone to another. The feeling that you experience when your circadian rhythms (biological cycles) are disrupted is called "jet lag." The reason for jet lag is the change in time zones. For example, traveling from California to New York makes your body's biological clock "lose" three hours. When you are in New York and your alarm rings at 8:00 a.m., you will feel tired and groggy because your body is still on California time, which would be 5:00 a.m. It will take your body a few days to adjust to the new time zone, but the adjustment will eventually take place. After a couple of days, you will find that 8:00 a.m. feels like the correct time to wake up if that is part of your normal schedule and you have had adequate sleep.

Some studies have shown that supplements of melatonin, a hormone that is produced by the body and sold as a treatment for insomnia, can help treat jet lag. This supplement has been especially effective for people crossing five or more time zones and for those traveling east. However, additional studies are needed to test the safety and effectiveness of melatonin for insomnia and jet lag; few studies are available, and it has not been tested for long-term use. Before you take any kind of supplement, be sure to check with your healthcare provider.

9

Section 1.2

Anatomy of Sleep

This section includes text excerpted from "Brain Basics:
Understanding Sleep," National Institute of Neurological
Disorders and Stroke (NINDS), February 8, 2019.

Several structures within the brain are involved with sleep.

The **hypothalamus,** a peanut-sized structure deep inside the brain, contains groups of nerve cells that act as control centers affecting sleep and arousal. Within the hypothalamus is the suprachiasmatic nucleus (SCN)—clusters of thousands of cells that receive information about light exposure directly from the eyes and control your behavioral rhythm. Some people with damage to the SCN sleep erratically throughout the day because they are not able to match their circadian rhythms with the light–dark cycle. Most blind people maintain some ability to sense light and are able to modify their sleep–wake cycle.

The **brain stem,** at the base of the brain, communicates with the hypothalamus to control the transitions between wake and sleep. (The brain stem includes structures called the "pons," "medulla," and "midbrain.") Sleep-promoting cells within the hypothalamus and the brain stem produce a brain chemical called "gamma-aminobutyric acid" (GABA), which acts to reduce the activity of arousal centers in the hypothalamus and the brain stem. The brain stem (especially the pons and medulla) also plays a special role in rapid eye movement (REM) sleep; it sends signals to relax muscles essential for body posture and limb movements so that we do not act out our dreams.

The **thalamus** acts as a relay for information from the senses to the cerebral cortex (the covering of the brain that interprets and processes information from short- to long-term memory). During most stages of sleep, the thalamus becomes quiet, letting you tune out the external world. But during REM sleep, the thalamus is active, sending the cortex images, sounds, and other sensations that fill our dreams.

The pineal gland, located within the brain's two hemispheres, receives signals from the SCN and increases the production of the hormone melatonin, which helps put you to sleep once the lights go down. People who have lost their sight and cannot coordinate their natural sleep–wake cycle using natural light can stabilize their sleep patterns by taking small amounts of melatonin at the same time each day. Scientists believe that peaks and valleys of melatonin over time are important for matching the body's circadian rhythm to the external cycle of light and darkness.

The **basal forebrain,** near the front and bottom of the brain, also promotes sleep and wakefulness, while part of the midbrain acts as an arousal system. Release of adenosine (a chemical by-product of cellular energy consumption) from cells in the basal forebrain and probably other regions supports your sleep drive. Caffeine counteracts sleepiness by blocking the actions of adenosine.

The **amygdala,** an almond-shaped structure involved in processing emotions, becomes increasingly active during REM sleep.

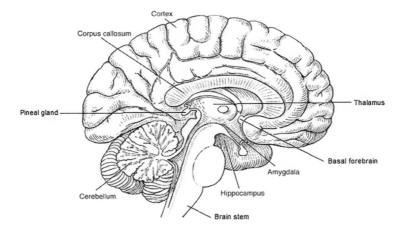

Figure 1.1. *The Human Brain* (Source: "Alcohol and the Adolescent Brain—Human Studies," National Institute on Alcohol Abuse and Alcoholism (NIAAA).)

Section 1.3

What Makes Us Sleep

This section includes text excerpted from "What Makes Us Sleep?"
Eunice Kennedy Shriver National Institute of Child Health and
Human Development (NICHD), April 29, 2019.

Sleep and wakefulness are generally regulated by your brain working with input from your senses and your circadian clock. This system pushes you to wake up and remain awake at certain times and pushes us to sleep at certain times.

Sleep Drive

The need for sleep is driven by the length of time you are awake. The longer you are awake, the greater your "drive" or need to sleep. The drive to sleep continues to build within your body until you are able to sleep.

Circadian Clock

Your body has a natural clock, called a "circadian clock," that helps you regulate your sleep. The word "circadian" refers to rhythmic biological cycles that repeat about every 24 hours. These cycles are also called "circadian rhythms." Your circadian clock is strongly influenced by light, which is the reason why people living in different regions have different sleeping schedules. This is also the reason why people who work night shifts can have difficulty falling asleep or staying awake.

At bedtime, when your drive to sleep is at its greatest, your sleep drive and circadian clock work together to allow you to fall asleep. After you have slept for some time, when your drive to sleep is lower, your circadian clock allows you to stay asleep until the end of the night.

Circadian Rhythms

Circadian rhythms regulate changes in the brain and body that occur over the course of a day. Your body's biological clock controls most circadian rhythms. This clock is found in a region of the brain called the "hypothalamus." The hypothalamus affects sleep and arousal.

Light detected by special neurons in the eye sends signals to many areas of the brain, including the hypothalamus. Signals from the hypothalamus travel to different regions of the brain, including the pineal gland. In response to light, such as sunlight, the pineal gland turns off the production of melatonin, a hormone that causes a feeling of drowsiness. The levels of melatonin in the body normally increase after darkness, which makes you feel drowsy.

The change in melatonin during the sleep–wake cycle reflects circadian rhythms. During sleep, the hypothalamus also controls changes in body temperature and blood pressure.

Because circadian rhythms are controlled by light, people who have some degree of blindness in both eyes may have trouble sleeping.

Section 1.4

Circadian Rhythms

This section contains text excerpted from the following sources:
Text in this section begins with excerpts from "Circadian Rhythms,"
National Institute of General Medical Sciences (NIGMS), August
2017; Text under the heading "Why Are Sleep Patterns Sometimes
Thrown off after Traveling across Time Zones?" from "Other Sleep
FAQs," *Eunice Kennedy Shriver*
National Institute of Child Health and Human
Development (NICHD), April 29, 2019.

Circadian rhythms are physical, mental, and behavioral changes that follow a daily cycle. They respond primarily to light and darkness in an organism's environment. Sleeping at night and being awake during the day is an example of a light-related circadian rhythm. Circadian rhythms are found in most living things, including animals, plants, and many tiny microbes. The study of circadian rhythms is called "chronobiology."

What Are Biological Clocks?

Biological clocks are an organism's innate timing device. They are composed of specific molecules (proteins) that interact in cells throughout the body. Biological clocks are found in nearly every tissue and organ. Researchers have identified similar genes in people, fruit flies, mice, fungi, and several other organisms that are responsible for making the clock's components.

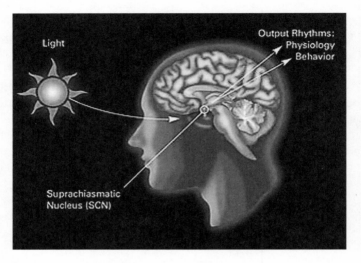

Figure 1.2. *Circadian Rhythms and the Brain*

Are Biological Clocks the Same Thing as Circadian Rhythms?

No, but they are related. Biological clocks produce circadian rhythms and regulate their timing.

What Is the Master Clock?

A master clock in the brain coordinates all the biological clocks in a living thing, keeping the clocks in sync. In vertebrate animals, including humans, the master clock is a group of about 20,000 nerve cells (neurons) that form a structure called the "suprachiasmatic nucleus," or "SCN." The SCN is located in a part of the brain called the "hypothalamus" and receives direct input from the eyes.

Does the Body Make and Keep Its Own Circadian Rhythms?

Natural factors within the body produce circadian rhythms. However, signals from the environment also affect them. The main cue influencing circadian rhythms is daylight. This light can turn on or turn off genes that control the molecular structure of biological clocks. Changing the light–dark cycles can speed up, slow down, or reset biological clocks, as well as circadian rhythms.

Do Circadian Rhythms Affect Body Function and Health?

Yes. Circadian rhythms can influence sleep–wake cycles, hormone release, eating habits and digestion, body temperature, and other important bodily functions. Biological clocks that run fast or slow can result in disrupted or abnormal circadian rhythms. Irregular rhythms have been linked to various chronic health conditions, such as sleep disorders, obesity, diabetes, depression, bipolar disorder, and seasonal affective disorder.

How Are Circadian Rhythms Related to Sleep?

Circadian rhythms help determine our sleep patterns. The SCN controls the production of melatonin, a hormone that makes you sleepy. It receives information about incoming light from the optic nerves, which relay information from the eyes to the brain. When there is less light—like at night—the SCN tells the brain to make more melatonin, so you get drowsy. Researchers are studying how shift work, as well as exposure to light from mobile devices, during the night may alter circadian rhythms and sleep–wake cycles.

How Do Researchers Study Circadian Rhythms?

Scientists learn about circadian rhythms by studying humans or by using organisms with similar biological clock genes, including fruit flies and mice. Researchers doing these experiments can control the subject's environment by altering light and dark periods. Then they look for changes in gene activity or other molecular signals. This research helps understand how biological clocks work and keep time.

Scientists also study organisms with irregular circadian rhythms to identify which genetic components of biological clocks may be broken.

How Does Circadian Rhythm Research Contribute to Human Health?

Understanding what makes biological clocks tick may lead to treatments for sleep disorders, obesity, mental-health disorders, jet lag, and other health problems. It can also improve ways for individuals to adjust to nighttime shift work. Learning more about the genes responsible for circadian rhythms will also help understand biological systems and the human body.

Why Are Sleep Patterns Sometimes Thrown off after Traveling across Time Zones?

Circadian rhythms are disrupted when people travel from one time zone to another. The feeling that you experience when your circadian rhythms (biological cycles) are disrupted is called "jet lag." The reason for jet lag is the change in time zones. For example, traveling from California to New York makes your body's biological clock "lose" three hours. When you are in New York and your alarm rings at 8:00 a.m., you will feel tired and groggy because your body is still on California time, which would be 5:00 a.m. It will take your body a few days to adjust to the new time zone, but the adjustment will eventually take place. After a couple of days, you will find that 8:00 a.m. feels like the correct time to wake up if that is part of your normal schedule and you have had adequate sleep.

Some studies have shown that supplements of melatonin, a hormone that is produced by the body and sold as a treatment for insomnia, can help treat jet lag. This supplement has been especially effective for people crossing five or more time zones and for those traveling east. However, additional studies are needed to test the safety and effectiveness of melatonin for insomnia and jet lag; few studies are available, and it has not been tested for long-term use. Before you take any kind of supplement, be sure to check with your healthcare provider.

Section 1.5

Sleep Myths

This section contains text excerpted from the following sources:
Text in this section begins with excerpts from "What Are Some
Myths about Sleep?" *Eunice Kennedy Shriver* National Institute of
Child Health and Human Development (NICHD), April 29, 2019;
Text under the heading "Myths and Facts about Sleep" is excerpted
from "Safety—Myths and Facts about Sleep," U.S. Department of
Agriculture (USDA), April 1, 2002. Reviewed May 2019.

There are several common myths about sleep, including the
following:

Myth: Snoring Is Not Harmful

The act of snoring, by itself, is often harmless. However, in some
people, it can signal a life-threatening disorder called "sleep apnea."
Sleep apnea causes pauses in your breathing that can last for seconds
or minutes, dozens of times each hour. These pauses disrupt your sleep
and cause you to wake up or sleep only lightly, which can make you
feel extremely tired during the day. The pauses also reduce the amount
of oxygen in your blood and can cause damage to the heart and blood
vessels, which increases the risk of heart disease. Sleep apnea also
increases the risk of high blood pressure, stroke, and diabetes.

Fortunately, sleep apnea is treatable. People who snore loudly, have
pauses in breathing during sleep, and feel very tired during the day
should speak with a healthcare provider.

Myth: You Can "Catch Up" on Sleep

Despite popular belief, you cannot regain or catch up on "lost"
sleep by sleeping more at another time. Being sleep deprived means
you accumulate a sleep debt that is impossible to "repay" as it gets
larger. In addition, long-term sleep deprivation puts you at risk for
health problems and may impair your safety and work performance.
Sleep deprivation has been linked to obesity; high blood pressure;
negative mood and behavior; decreased productivity at work; and
safety issues in the home, on the job, and on the road. Catching up
on sleep may help to reduce daytime sleepiness or drowsiness, but
it does not reverse the effects of not getting enough sleep or enough
quality sleep each night.

Myth: The Older You Get, the Fewer Hours of Sleep You Need

Sleep experts recommend seven to nine hours of sleep for most adults. While sleep patterns may change as we age, the amount of sleep the body needs does not usually change. Older people may wake up more frequently throughout the night and end up getting less sleep during the overnight hours. Older adults are more likely to be taking medicines that interfere with sleep. However, their need for sleep is not drastically less than that of younger adults. Older people may take more naps during the day because they get less sleep at night.

Other Myths and Facts about Sleep

Sleep is a basic necessity of life, as important to our health and well-being as air, food, and water. When we sleep well, we wake up feeling refreshed, alert, and ready to face daily challenges. When we do not, every part of our lives can suffer. Our jobs, relationships, productivity, health, and safety (and that of those around us) are all put at risk. There are many common myths about sleep. We hear them frequently, and may even experience them far too often. Sometimes they can be characterized as "old wives' tales," but there are other times the incorrect information can be serious and even dangerous. The National Sleep Foundation (NSF) has compiled this list of common myths about sleep and the facts that dispel them.

Turning Up the Radio, Opening the Window, or Turning On the Air Conditioner Are Effective Ways to Stay Awake When Driving

These "aids" are ineffective and can be dangerous to the person who is driving while feeling drowsy or sleepy. If you are feeling tired while driving, the best thing to do is to pull off the road in a safe rest area and take a nap for 15 to 45 minutes. Caffeinated beverages can help overcome drowsiness for a short period of time; however, it takes about 30 minutes before the effects are felt. The best prevention for drowsy driving is a good night's sleep the night before your trip.

Daytime Sleepiness Always Means a Person Is Not Getting Enough Sleep

Excessive daytime sleepiness is a condition in which an individual feels very drowsy during the day and has an urge to fall asleep when she or he should be fully alert and awake. The condition, which can occur even after getting enough nighttime sleep, can be a sign of an underlying medical condition or sleep disorder, such as narcolepsy or sleep apnea. These problems can often be treated, and symptoms should be discussed with a physician. Daytime sleepiness can be dangerous and puts a person at risk for drowsy driving, injury, and illness and can impair mental abilities, emotions, and performance.

You Can "Cheat" on the Amount of Sleep You Get

Sleep experts say most adults need between seven and nine hours of sleep each night for optimum performance, health, and safety. When we do not get adequate sleep, we accumulate a sleep debt that can be difficult to "pay back" if it becomes too big. The resulting sleep deprivation has been linked to health problems, such as obesity and high blood pressure; negative mood and behavior; decreased productivity; and safety issues in the home, on the job, and on the road.

During Sleep, Your Brain Rests

The body rests during sleep; however, the brain remains active, gets "recharged," and still controls many body functions, including breathing. When we sleep, we typically drift between 2 sleep states, rapid eye movement (REM) and non-REM, in 90-minute cycles. Non-REM sleep has 4 stages with distinct features, ranging from stage 1 drowsiness, when one can be easily awakened, to "deep sleep" stages 3 and 4, when awakenings are more difficult and where the most positive and restorative effects of sleep occur; however, even in the deepest non-REM sleep, our minds can still process information. REM sleep is an active sleep where dreams occur, breathing and heart rate increase and become irregular, muscles relax, and eyes move back and forth under the eyelids.

If You Wake Up in the Middle of the Night, It Is Best to Lie in Bed, Count Sheep, or Toss and Turn until You Eventually Fall Back Asleep

Waking up in the middle of the night and not being able to go back to sleep is a symptom of insomnia. Relaxing imagery or thoughts may help to induce sleep more than counting sheep, which some research suggests may be more distracting than relaxing. Whichever technique is used, most experts agree that if you do not fall back asleep within 15 to 20 minutes, you should get out of bed, go to another room and

19

engage in a relaxing activity, such as listening to music or reading. Return to bed when you feel sleepy. Avoid watching the clock.

Health Problems Such as Obesity, Diabetes, Hypertension, and Depression Are Unrelated to the Amount and Quality of a Person's Sleep

Studies have found a relationship between the quantity and quality of one's sleep and many health problems. For example, insufficient sleep affects growth hormone secretion that is linked to obesity; as the amount of hormone secretion decreases, the chance for weight gain increases. Blood pressure usually falls during the sleep cycle; however, interrupted sleep can adversely affect this normal decline, leading to hypertension and cardiovascular problems. Research has also shown that insufficient sleep impairs the body's ability to use insulin, which can lead to the onset of diabetes. More and more scientific studies are showing correlations between poor and insufficient sleep and disease.

Chapter 2

Phases of Sleep

Chapter Contents

Section 2.1

What Happens during Sleep

This section includes text excerpted from "What Happens during Sleep?" *Eunice Kennedy Shriver* National Institute of Child Health and Human Development (NICHD), April 29, 2019.

In broad terms, the brain of someone who is sleeping cycles through two basic phases: rapid eye movement (REM) sleep and non-REM sleep. Non-REM sleep includes three different stages. A person cycles through REM sleep and non-REM sleep several times a night.

Each phase of sleep helps the mind and body stay rested. Certain stages help you feel rested and energetic the next day, while both phases help you learn information and form memories.

Sleep progresses in a cycle: from non-REM sleep stage 1 to non-REM sleep stage 2, to non-REM sleep stage 3, to REM sleep. Then the process starts over again with non-REM sleep stage 1.

The length of sleep stages changes during a given night's sleep. For example, near the beginning of sleep, the body cycles through relatively short periods of REM sleep and long periods of deep sleep. As the night goes on, periods of REM sleep increase and those of deep sleep decrease. Near the end of a night of sleep, a person spends nearly all of their time in stages 1 and 2 and REM.

Characteristics of Sleep Phase
Nonrapid Eye Movement Sleep

As you begin to fall asleep, you enter non-REM sleep, which consists of stages 1 through 3, as follows:

Stage 1

- You are in between being awake and being asleep.

- Your heartbeat and breathing slow and your muscles relax.

Stage 2

- You are in a light sleep.

- Your brain waves slow down.

- Your body temperature lowers.

Stage 3

- Your deepest and most restorative sleep happens.

- Your heartbeat and breathing slow to their lowest levels.

- Your muscles relax.

- Your body increases the supply of blood to your muscles.

- Your body performs tissue growth and repair.

- Your energy is restored.

- Your body releases hormones.

Rapid Eye Movement Sleep

You first enter REM sleep about 90 minutes after you fall asleep. REM sleep becomes longer later into the night. REM is characterized as follows:

- Your brain and body are energized.

- Your breathing becomes fast and irregular.

- Your brain is active and dreaming occurs.

- Your eyes dart back and forth.

- Your body becomes immobile and relaxed, preventing you from acting out your dreams.

- Your body temperature is not as tightly regulated.

Rapid eye movement sleep begins in response to signals sent to and from different regions of the brain. Signals are sent to the brain's cerebral cortex, which is responsible for learning, thinking, and organizing information. Signals are also sent to the spinal cord to shut off the movement, creating a temporary inability to move the muscles ("paralysis") in the arms and legs. If this temporary paralysis is disrupted, people might move while they are dreaming ("sleepwalking"). A person who sleepwalks is at risk for injury.

Rapid eye movement sleep is thought to be involved in storing memories, learning, and balancing mood. REM sleep stimulates regions of the brain that are used for learning. Studies have shown that when people are deprived of REM sleep, they are not able to remember what they were taught before going to sleep. Lack of REM sleep has also been linked to certain health conditions, such as migraines. However, insufficient sleep, regardless of sleep stage, can interfere with learning, memory, and performance. If you have any concerns about your sleep quality and habits, speak with your healthcare provider.

Dreaming

Scientists are not sure why we dream. While some of the signals sent to the cortex during sleep are important for learning and memory, some signals seem to be random. Dreams are generally most vivid during REM sleep, but dreaming can also occur during non-REM sleep.

Through research, we are learning more about dreaming. One study, for example, found that a pattern of brain activity from a part of the cortex near the back of the brain is a good predictor of whether an individual is dreaming, and whether the individual was in the REM or non-REM sleep.

Section 2.2

How Sleep Resets the Brain

This section includes text excerpted from "How Sleep Resets the Brain," National Institutes of Health (NIH), February 14, 2017.

People spend about a third of their lives asleep. When we get too little shut-eye, it takes a toll on attention, learning and memory, not to mention our physical health. Virtually all animals with complex brains seem to have this same need for sleep. But exactly what is it about sleep that is so essential?

Two National Institutes of Health (NIH)-funded studies in mice now offer a possible answer. The two research teams used entirely different approaches to reach the same conclusion: the brain's neural connections grow stronger during waking hours but scale back during snooze time. This sleep-related phenomenon apparently keeps neural circuits from overloading, ensuring that mice (and, quite likely humans) awaken with brains that are refreshed and ready to tackle new challenges.

The idea that sleep is required to keep the brain wiring sharp goes back more than a decade. While a fair amount of evidence has emerged to support the hypothesis, its originators Chiara Cirelli and Giulio Tononi of the University of Wisconsin-Madison, set out in their new study to provide some of the first direct visual proof that it is indeed the case.

As published in the journal *Science*, the researchers used a painstaking, cutting-edge imaging technique to capture high-resolution pictures of two areas of the mouse's cerebral cortex, a part of the brain that coordinates incoming sensory and motor information. The technique, called "serial scanning 3-D electron microscopy," involves repeated scanning of small slices of the brain to produce many thousands of images, allowing the researchers to produce detailed 3-D reconstructions of individual neurons.

Their goal was to measure the size of the synapses, where the ends of two neurons connect. Synapses are critical for one neuron to pass signals on to the next, and the strength of those neural connections corresponds to their size.

The researchers measured close to 7,000 synapses in all. Their images show that synapses grew stronger and larger as these nocturnal mice scurried about at night. Then, after 6 to 8 hours of sleep during the day, those synapses shrank by about 18 percent as the brain reset for another night of activity. Importantly, the effects of sleep held when the researchers switched the mice's schedule, keeping them up and engaged with toys and other objects during the day.

In the second *Science* report, Richard Huganir and his colleagues at Johns Hopkins University School of Medicine, Baltimore measured changes in the levels of certain brain proteins associated with sleep to offer biochemical evidence for this weakening of synapses. Their findings show that levels of protein receptors found on the receiving ends of synapses dropped by 20 percent while their mice slept.

The researchers also show that the protein Homer1a—important in regulating sleep and wakefulness—rises in synapses during a long snooze, playing a critical role in the resetting process. When the protein was lacking, brains did not reset properly during sleep. This suggests that Homer1a responds to chemical cues in the brain that signal the need to sleep.

These studies add to prior work that suggests another function of sleep is to allow glial lymphatics in the brain to clear out proteins and other toxins that have deposited during the day. All of this goes to show that a good night's sleep really can bring clarity. So, the next time you are struggling to make a decision and someone tells you to "sleep on it"—that might be really good advice.

Section 2.3

The Brain May Flush Out Toxins during Sleep

This section includes text excerpted from "Brain May Flush Out Toxins during Sleep," News and Events, National Institutes of Health (NIH), October 17, 2013. Reviewed May 2019.

A good night's rest may literally clear the mind. Using mice, researchers showed for the first time that the space between brain cells may increase during sleep, allowing the brain to flush out toxins that build up during waking hours. These results suggest a new role for sleep in health and disease. The study was funded by the National Institute of Neurological Disorders and Stroke (NINDS), part of the National Institutes of Health (NIH).

"Sleep changes the cellular structure of the brain. It appears to be a completely different state," said Maiken Nedergaard, M.D., D.M.Sc., Co-Director of the Center for Translational Neuromedicine at the University of Rochester Medical Center in New York, and a leader of the study.

For centuries, scientists and philosophers have wondered why people sleep and how it affects the brain. Only recently have scientists shown that sleep is important for storing memories. In this study, Dr. Nedergaard and her colleagues unexpectedly found that sleep may also be the period when the brain cleanses itself of toxic molecules.

Their results, published in *Science*, show that during sleep a plumbing system called the "glymphatic system" may open, letting fluid flow rapidly through the brain. Dr. Nedergaard's lab discovered that the glymphatic system helps control the flow of cerebrospinal fluid (CSF), a clear liquid surrounding the brain and spinal cord.

"It is as if Dr. Nedergaard and her colleagues have uncovered a network of hidden caves and these exciting results highlight the potential importance of the network in normal brain function," said Roderick Corriveau, Ph.D., a Program Director at the NINDS.

Initially, the researchers studied the system by injecting dye into the CSF of mice and watching it flow through their brains while simultaneously monitoring electrical brain activity. The dye flowed rapidly when the mice were unconscious, either asleep or anesthetized. In contrast, the dye barely flowed when the same mice were awake.

"We were surprised by how little flow there was into the brain when the mice were awake," said Dr. Nedergaard. "It suggested that the space between brain cells changed greatly between conscious and unconscious states."

To test this idea, the researchers inserted electrodes into the brain to directly measure the space between brain cells. They found that the space inside the brains increased by 60 percent when the mice were asleep or anesthetized.

"These are some dramatic changes in extracellular space," said Charles Nicholson, Ph.D., a professor at New York University's Langone Medical Center and an expert in measuring the dynamics of brain fluid flow and how it influences nerve cell communication.

Certain brain cells, called "glia," control flow through the glymphatic system by shrinking or swelling. Noradrenaline is an arousing hormone that is also known to control cell volume. Similar to using anesthesia, treating awake mice with drugs that block noradrenaline-induced unconsciousness and increased brain fluid flow and the space between cells, further supporting the link between the glymphatic system and consciousness.

Previous studies suggest that toxic molecules involved in neurodegenerative disorders accumulate in the space between brain cells. In this study, the researchers tested whether the glymphatic system controls this by injecting mice with labeled beta-amyloid, a protein associated with Alzheimer disease (AD), and measuring how long it lasted in their brains when they were asleep or awake. Beta-amyloid disappeared faster in mice brains when the mice were asleep, suggesting that sleep normally clears toxic molecules from the brain.

"These results may have broad implications for multiple neurological disorders," said Jim Koenig, Ph.D., a Program Director at the NINDS. "This means the cells regulating the glymphatic system may be new targets for treating a range of disorders."

The results may also highlight the importance of sleep.

"We need sleep. It cleans up the brain," said Dr. Nedergaard.

Section 2.4

Sleep and Your Hormones

This section includes text excerpted from "Your Guide to Healthy Sleep," National Heart, Lung, and Blood Institute (NHLBI), August, 2011. Reviewed May 2019.

A number of aspects of your health and quality of life (QOL) are linked to sleep, and these aspects are impaired when you are sleep deprived.

When you were young, your mother may have told you that you need to get enough sleep to grow strong and tall. She may have been right. Deep sleep (stage 3 nonrapid eye movement (REM) sleep) triggers more release of growth hormone, which contributes to growth in children and boosts muscle mass and the repair of cells and tissues in children and adults. Sleep's effect on the release of sex hormones also contributes to puberty and fertility. Consequently, women who work at night and tend to lack sleep may be at an increased risk of miscarriage.

Your mother also probably was right if she told you that getting a good night's sleep on a regular basis would help keep you from getting sick and help you get better if you do get sick. During sleep, your body creates more cytokines—cellular hormones that help the immune system fight various infections. Lack of sleep can reduce your body's ability to fight off common infections. Research also reveals that a lack of sleep can reduce the body's response to the flu vaccine. For example, sleep deprived volunteers given the flu vaccine produced less than half as many flu antibodies as those who were well rested and given the same vaccine.

Although lack of exercise and other factors also contribute, diabetes and obesity seem to be related, at least in part, to chronically short or disrupted sleep or not sleeping during the night. Evidence is growing that sleep is a powerful regulator of appetite, energy use, and weight control. During sleep, the body's production of the appetite suppressor leptin increases, and the appetite stimulant ghrelin decreases. Studies find that the less people sleep, the more likely they are to be overweight or obese, and prefer eating foods that are higher in calories and carbohydrates. People who report an average total sleep time of five hours a night, for example, are much more likely to become obese when compared with people who sleep seven to eight hours a night.

A number of hormones released during sleep also control the body's use of energy. A distinct rise and fall of blood sugar levels during sleep appears to be linked to sleep stages. Not sleeping at the right time, not getting enough sleep overall, or not enough of each stage of sleep disrupts this pattern. One study found that, when healthy young men slept only four hours a night for six nights in a row, their insulin and blood sugar levels matched those seen in people who were developing diabetes. Another study found that women who slept less than seven hours a night were more likely to develop diabetes over time than those who slept between seven and eight hours a night.

Chapter 3

Napping: A Healthy Habit

Chapter Contents

Section 3.1

What Is Napping?

Most mammals are polyphasic sleepers, which means they sleep—or nap—multiple times during a 24-hour period. Humans, on the other hand, are monophasic sleepers since they have distinct, alternate phases of sleeping and waking. Whether this forms the natural sleep pattern for humans has not been clearly established; however, napping is an integral part of many cultures globally.

The United States is quickly becoming a nation of deprived sleepers, due primarily to a culture that often promotes a hectic lifestyle. Napping could be a solution, since sleeping for 20 to 30 minutes during normal waking hours has been shown to result in remarkable improvements in mood, alertness, and performance.

The Types of Napping

There are three different ways that we usually nap:

- **Planned napping,** also known as "preparatory napping," involves taking a nap before you are sleepy in anticipation of going to bed late. This helps you avoid feeling tired because of inadequate sleep later on.

- **Emergency napping.** You may take an emergency nap when you feel tired and unable to continue the task you were engaged in. This type of napping is very useful when you have been driving and are feeling drowsy or when you need to counter fatigue when operating dangerous machinery.

- **Habitual napping.** This is the practice of taking naps as a regular routine at a particular time of the day. Young children nap this way, and it is not uncommon in many cultures for adults to a nap after lunch.

Recommendations for Napping

A nap lasting for 20 to 30 minutes is optimal. It tends not to interfere with your regular sleep pattern and generally does not make you groggy.

Sleep in a comfortable place with moderate room temperature and without much noise or light filtering in. It is most beneficial to sleep rather than just lie in bed resting.

Do not take a nap too late in the day, because it will affect your regular sleep at night. Do not nap early in the day, either, since you may not be able to sleep well.

Seven Steps to Have the Perfect Nap

Just lying down, closing your eyes, and hoping for the best will not necessarily help you nap. You should think it out and employ a strategy to help you nap better. The following steps will help you get the perfect nap:

Step 1. Decide how long you want to nap. Different durations confer their own benefits.

- **6 minutes.** Provides improvement in memory functions.

- **10 to 15 minutes.** Improves focus and productivity.

- **20 to 30 minutes.** Optimum nap time, which results in alertness, concentration, and sharp motor skills.

- **40 to 60 minutes.** Boosts brain power, consolidates memory for facts, places, and faces, and improves learning ability.

- **90 to 120 minutes.** Improves creativity and emotional and procedural memory.

Step 2. Nap between 1 p.m. and 3 p.m. The body has an inherent biological clock, known as the "circadian rhythm," that controls the sleep–wake cycle. Humans experience intense sleep in 2 periods every 24 hours. One is between 1 and 3 p.m., and the other is from 2 to 4 a.m. Alertness, reaction time, coordination, and mood are decreased during these periods. The lethargy experienced after lunch is actually biological in nature. A nap around this time will put you back on track. Napping between 1 and 3 p.m. will generally not disturb regular sleep. If you work a night shift, the best time to take a nap would be 6 to 8 hours after waking.

Step 3. Create a conducive atmosphere. If you are unable to fall asleep during the day, you may not be approaching napping the right way. Lighting is an important factor because light inhibits melatonin, the sleep regulation hormone. Darken your room with window

33

shades or use an eye mask. Lie down, rather than sitting, when you take a nap. You will fall asleep 50 percent faster. Many people find that a hammock is the best place to nap because of the gentle swaying motion that promotes sleep.

Step 4. Use an alarm. You will need to wake up in time to get back to work after a snooze, so set an alarm to wake you up.

Step 5. Try a coffee nap. If you are concerned about becoming sleepy in the afternoon, try having a cup of coffee and taking a nap. Caffeine kicks into the body in 20 to 30 minutes. This should give you enough time to take a nap and get rejuvenated. Combining coffee and napping can be more beneficial than doing either of them alone.

Step 6. Avoid the blahs after napping. Make sure you avoid sleep inertia. If you take a long nap, you may feel groggy after waking up, because a full sleep cycle was not completed. Avoid this by having coffee, washing your face, or exposing yourself to bright light. An alternative is to complete a full sleep cycle by taking a nap for at least 90 minutes.

Step 7. Get adequate sleep at night. Nothing replaces a good night's sleep, and emergency napping cannot be a long-term substitute for regular, deep sleep. Inadequate sleep on a regular basis can result in hypertension, diabetes, weight gain, depression, and a general feeling of unease.

Pros of Napping

- Napping improves alertness and performance levels. It reduces mistakes and accidents. A NASA study conducted on military pilots showed that 40 minutes of napping increased alertness by 100 percent and performance by 34 percent.

- Naps improve alertness for some duration after the nap and often increase alertness to some extent over the entire day.

- Napping results in relaxation and rejuvenation. It is a luxurious and pleasant experience, something similar to a mini vacation.

- Taking a nap when you are feeling drowsy behind the wheel can help you regain alertness so that you can continue to drive safely.

- Night-shift workers who nap have been shown to experience improved alertness on the job.

- A 45-minute daytime nap improves memory functioning.
- Napping reduces blood pressure.
- It reduces the risk of cardiovascular diseases.
- Temporary sleep issues due to jet lag, stress, or illnesses can often be remedied by napping.
- A quick nap is very good for mental and physical stamina.
- Napping improves mental acuity and overall health.

Cons of Napping

- The stigma associated with napping is probably the biggest downside of napping.
- It may be equated with laziness.
- It is often associated with a lack of ambition and low standards.
- Napping may be seen as normal only for children, the sick, and the elderly.
- Napping can be counterproductive for people with sleep disorders or those with irregular sleep patterns.
- Naps are often not recommended for people with sleep apnea.

References

1. "Napping," National Sleep Foundation (NSF), n.d.

2. Belsky, Gail. "The Pros and Cons of Napping," Health.com, n.d.

3. Brown, Brendan. "A How-to Guide to the Perfect Nap [Infographic]," Art of Wellbeing, February 16, 2016.

Section 3.2

Benefits of Napping

This section includes text excerpted from "Sleep
Researchers Home in on the Benefits of Napping," Rehabilitation
Research & Development Service (RR&D), U.S. Department of
Veterans Affairs (VA), February 11, 2014. Reviewed May 2019.

Getting a good night's sleep is important for everyone. Good sleep refreshes people, helps them perform better, and contributes significantly to health and happiness. For many, however, getting a good night's sleep is extremely difficult.

Sleep disturbances are common in patients suffering from bipolar disorder, substance abuse, major depression, panic disorder, and chronic pain disorders. Sleep disorders following recent exposure to traumatic events can predict the later development of posttraumatic stress disorder (PTSD).

Disrupted sleep, or the inability to get a full night's sleep without interruption, is a very common negative consequence of PTSD. For some who simply cannot get a good night's sleep, there is a way to avoid many of the consequences of sleeplessness. "Napping has been shown to alleviate the negative physical and psychological symptoms of disrupted sleep," says Elizabeth A. McDevitt, a graduate student in the department of psychology at the University of California, Riverside. At the time the research was conducted, McDevitt was affiliated with the San Diego VA Medical Center and the University of California, San Diego (UCSD).

According to a study published online in the *Journal of Physiology and Behavior* by McDevitt and two colleagues from the San Diego VA and UCSD, napping is especially helpful to manage circadian disruption (problems related either from changes in a person's sleep–wake cycle, such as jet lag, daylight saving time, or between workweeks and weekends, or through the inability to get enough sleep in the time allotted for sleep.) In healthy, well-rested subjects, napping has also been shown to improve performance across a range of performance tasks.

Despite the benefits of napping, however, some people report that they simply cannot nap, or do not want to nap. In their study, McDevitt and her colleagues set out to determine why some people nap and others do not.

She and her colleagues asked 27 healthy, nonsmoking college students between the ages of 18 and 35 to participate in an experiment.

All of them spent between 7 and 9 hours in bed every night, and none of them had a sleep disorder. They were asked to keep a diary of their sleep habits for a week, including their daily naps if they took them, and they wore special actigraph wristwatches (small, wristwatch-shaped devices that record motion and are used to assess sleep by determining whether a person is active or inactive) to verify what they had put down in their diaries.

After a week of measurements, each participant reported to the Laboratory for Sleep and Behavioral Neuroscience at the San Diego VA Medical Center. Their level of sleepiness was measured at 9 a.m., 11 a.m., 4:30 p.m., and 6:30 p.m. At 1:30 p.m., they were all asked to take a nap and were allowed to sleep for a maximum of 90 minutes, but they were given no more than 120 minutes in bed whether they napped or not. While they napped, their brain waves were monitored through electrodes to see how deeply they were sleeping.

By correlating the information in the subjects' diaries, and analyzing the brain wave information they obtained, the team found that people who nap frequently sleep more lightly during their naps than those who usually never nap at all. In sleeping, the body progresses through a series of five stages, called the "sleep cycle," from light sleep through dreaming. (Sleep does not progress through these stages in order, however.)

Those who had taken three to four naps in the week before the brain wave tests took place had the least amount of slow wave sleep (scientist's term for stage 3, or deep sleep) and the most amount of stage 1, or light sleep; those who took one to two naps a week had the most amount of stage 2 sleep, which is somewhat deeper, and those who never napped at all had the highest amount of stage 3 sleep while in the laboratory, meaning that they slept the most deeply. The naps that people of all groups took did not measurably affect their sleep at night.

Using this data, the team developed two hypotheses. First, that some people avoid napping because of the high levels of deep sleep that they fall into when they do nap—meaning that, when they wake up, they feel groggy and tired instead of rested and refreshed. And second, people who choose to nap may just be sleepier people than those who do not.

"Individuals who frequently nap may generally be sleepier people who are self-treating their sleepiness with daytime naps," said McDevitt. "They might be predisposed to be good daytime nappers, or they have learned to become skilled nappers through practice."

The team suggested that future studies should consider the possibility of nap practice or nap training to maximize the benefits of napping and examine how differences in sleep associated with nap behavior may influence changes in performance following a nap.

Chapter 4

Benefits of Slumber

We have so many demands on our time—jobs, family, errands—not to mention finding some time to relax. To fit everything in, we often sacrifice sleep. But, sleep affects both mental and physical health. It is vital to your well-being. Of course, sleep helps you feel rested each day. However, while you are sleeping, your brain and body do not just shut down. Internal organs and processes are hard at work throughout the night.

"Sleep services all aspects of our body in one way or another: molecular, energy balance, as well as intellectual function, alertness, and mood," says Dr. Merrill Mitler, a sleep expert and neuroscientist at the National Institutes of Health (NIH).

When you are tired, you cannot function at your best. Sleep helps you think more clearly, have quicker reflexes and focus better. "The fact is, when we look at well-rested people, they are operating at a different level than people trying to get by on one or two hours less nightly sleep," says Mitler.

"Loss of sleep impairs your higher levels of reasoning, problem-solving and attention to detail," Mitler explains. Tired people tend to be less productive at work. They are at a much higher risk for

---

This chapter contains text excerpted from the following sources: Text in this chapter begins with excerpts from "The Benefits of Slumber," *NIH News in Health*, National Institutes of Health (NIH), April 2013. Reviewed May 2019; Text under the heading "Snoozing Strengthens Memory" is excerpted from "Sleep on It," *NIH News in Health*, National Institutes of Health (NIH), April 2013. Reviewed May 2019.

traffic accidents. Lack of sleep also influences your mood, which can affect how you interact with others. A sleep deficit over time can even put you at greater risk for developing depression.

But, sleep is not just essential for the brain. "Sleep affects almost every tissue in our bodies," says Dr. Michael Twery, a sleep expert at the NIH. "It affects growth and stress hormones, our immune system, appetite, breathing, blood pressure, and cardiovascular health."

Research shows that lack of sleep increases the risk for obesity, heart disease, and infections. Throughout the night, your heart rate, breathing rate, and blood pressure rise and fall, a process that may be important for cardiovascular health. Your body releases hormones during sleep that help repair cells and control the body's use of energy. These hormone changes can affect your body weight.

"Ongoing research shows a lack of sleep can produce diabetic-like conditions in otherwise healthy people," says Mitler.

Recent studies also reveal that sleep can affect the efficiency of vaccinations. Twery described research showing that well-rested people who received the flu vaccine developed stronger protection against the illness.

A good night's sleep consists of four to five sleep cycles. Each cycle includes periods of deep sleep and rapid eye movement (REM) sleep when we dream. "As the night goes on, the portion of that cycle that is in REM sleep increases. It turns out that this pattern of cycling and progression is critical to the biology of sleep," Twery says.

Although personal needs vary, on average, adults need 7 to 8 hours of sleep per night. Babies typically sleep about 16 hours a day. Young children need at least 10 hours of sleep, while teenagers need at least 9 hours. To attain the maximum restorative benefits of sleep, getting a full night of quality sleep is important, says Twery.

Sleep can be disrupted by many things. Stimulants, such as caffeine or certain medications, can keep you up. Distractions, such as electronics—especially the light from TVs, cell phones, tablets, and e-readers—can prevent you from falling asleep.

As people get older, they may not get enough sleep because of illness, medications, or sleep disorders. By some estimates, about 70 million Americans of all ages suffer from chronic sleep problems. The 2 most common sleep disorders are insomnia and sleep apnea.

People with insomnia have trouble falling or staying asleep. Anxiety about falling asleep often makes the condition worse. Most of us have occasional insomnia. But chronic insomnia—lasting at least three nights per week for more than a month—can trigger serious daytime problems, such as exhaustion, irritability, and difficulty concentrating.

Common therapies include relaxation and deep breathing techniques. Sometimes, medicine is prescribed. But, consult a doctor even before trying over-the-counter (OTC) sleep pills, as they may leave you feeling unrefreshed in the morning.

People with sleep apnea have a loud, uneven snore (although not everyone who snores has apnea). Breathing repeatedly stops or becomes shallow. If you have apnea, you are not getting enough oxygen, and your brain disturbs your sleep to open your windpipe.

Apnea is dangerous. "There is little air exchange for 10 seconds or more at a time," explains Dr. Phyllis Zee, a sleep apnea expert at Northwestern University. "The oxygen goes down and the body's fight or flight response is activated. Blood pressure spikes, your heart rate fluctuates, and the brain wakes you up partially to start your breathing again. This creates stress."

Apnea can leave you feeling tired and moody. You may have trouble thinking clearly. "Also, apnea affects the vessels that lead to the brain, so there is a higher risk of stroke associated with it," Zee adds.

If you have mild sleep apnea, you might try sleeping on your side, exercising, or losing weight to reduce symptoms. A continuous positive airway pressure (CPAP) machine, which pumps air into your throat to keep your airway open, can also help. Another treatment is a bite plate that moves the lower jaw forward. In some cases, however, people with sleep apnea need surgery.

"If you snore chronically and wake up choking or gasping for air, and feel that you are sleepy during the day, tell your doctor and get evaluated," Zee advises.

The National Institutes of Health is currently funding several studies to gain deeper insights into sleep apnea and other aspects of sleep. A 5-year study of 10,000 pregnant women is designed to gauge the effects of apnea on the mother's and fetus's health. Zee says this study will shed more light on apnea and the importance of treatment.

Good sleep is critical to your health. To make each day a safe, productive one, take steps to make sure you regularly get a good night's sleep.

Snoozing Strengthens Memory

When you learn something new, the best way to remember it is to sleep on it. That is because sleeping helps strengthen memories you have formed throughout the day. It also helps to link new memories to earlier ones. You might even come up with creative new ideas while you slumber.

What happens to memories in your brain while you sleep? And how does lack of sleep affect your ability to learn and remember? NIH-funded scientists have been gathering clues about the complex relationship between sleep and memory. Their findings might eventually lead to new approaches to help students learn or help older people hold onto memories as they age.

"We have learned that sleep before learning helps prepare your brain for the initial formation of memories," says Dr. Matthew Walker, a sleep scientist at the University of California, Berkeley. "And then, sleep after learning is essential to help save and cement that new information into the architecture of the brain, meaning that you are less likely to forget it."

While you snooze, your brain cycles through different phases of sleep, including light sleep, deep sleep, and REM sleep, when dreaming often occurs. The cycles repeat about every 90 minutes.

The non-REM stages of sleep seem to prime the brain for good learning the next day. If you have not slept, your ability to learn new things could drop up to 40 percent. "You cannot pull an all-nighter and still learn effectively," Walker says. Lack of sleep affects a part of the brain called the "hippocampus," which is key for making new memories.

You accumulate many memories, moment by moment, while you are awake. Most will be forgotten during the day. "When we first form memories, they are in a very raw and fragile form," says sleep expert Dr. Robert Stickgold of Harvard Medical School (HMS).

But when you doze off, "sleep seems to be a privileged time when the brain goes back through recent memories and decides both what to keep and what not to keep," Stickgold explains. "During a night of sleep, some memories are strengthened." Research has shown that memories of certain procedures, such as playing a melody on a piano, can actually improve while you sleep.

Memories seem to become more stable in the brain during the deep stages of sleep. After that, REM—the most active stage of sleep— seems to play a role in linking together related memories, sometimes in unexpected ways. That is why a full night of sleep may help with problem-solving. REM sleep also helps you process emotional memories, which can reduce the intensity of emotions.

It is well known that sleep patterns tend to change as we age. Unfortunately, the deep memory-strengthening stages of sleep start to decline in our late 30s. A study by Walker and colleagues found that adults older than 60 years of age had a 70 percent loss of deep sleep when compared to young adults between the ages of 18 and 25. Older adults had a harder time remembering things the next day, and memory impairment was linked to reductions in a deep sleep. The researchers are now exploring options for enhancing deep stages of sleep in this older age group.

"While we have limited medical treatments for memory impairment in aging, sleep actually is a potentially treatable target," Walker says. "By restoring sleep, it might be possible to improve memory in older people."

For younger people, especially students, Stickgold offers additional advice. "Realize that the sleep you get the night after you study is at least as important as the sleep you get the night before you study." When it comes to sleep and memory, he says, "you get very little benefit from cutting corners."

Chapter 5

Dreaming

Chapter Contents

Section 5.1

Dreaming and Rapid Eye Movement Sleep: The Science behind Dreams

This section includes text excerpted from "Brain Basics—Understanding Sleep," National Institute of Neurological Disorders and Stroke (NINDS), February 8, 2019.

We typically spend more than two hours each night dreaming. Scientists do not know much about how or why we dream. Sigmund Freud, who greatly influenced the field of psychology, believed dreaming was a "safety valve" for unconscious desires. Only after 1953, when researchers first described rapid eye movement (REM) in sleeping infants, did scientists begin to carefully study sleep and dreaming. They soon realized that the strange, illogical experiences we call "dreams" almost always occur during REM sleep. While most mammals and birds show signs of REM sleep, reptiles and other cold-blooded animals do not.

Rapid eye movement sleep begins with signals from an area at the base of the brain called the "pons" (see figure 5.1). These signals travel to a brain region called the "thalamus," which relays them to the cerebral cortex—the outer layer of the brain that is responsible for learning, thinking, and organizing information. The pons also sends signals that shut off neurons in the spinal cord, causing temporary paralysis of the limb muscles. If something interferes with this paralysis, people will begin to physically "act out" their dreams—a rare, dangerous problem called "REM sleep behavior disorder." A person dreaming about a ball game, for example, may run headlong into furniture or blindly strike someone sleeping nearby while trying to catch a ball in the dream.

Rapid eye movement sleep stimulates the brain regions used in learning. This may be important for normal brain development during infancy, which would explain why infants spend much more time in REM sleep than adults. As with deep sleep, REM sleep is associated with increased production of proteins. One study found that REM sleep affects the learning of certain mental skills. People taught a skill and then deprived of non-REM sleep could recall what they had learned after sleeping, while people deprived of REM sleep could not. Some scientists believe dreams are the cortex's attempt to find meaning in the random signals that it receives during REM sleep. The cortex is the part of the brain that interprets and organizes information from the environment during consciousness. It may be that given random signals from the pons during REM sleep, the cortex tries to interpret these signals as well, creating a "story" out of fragmented brain activity.

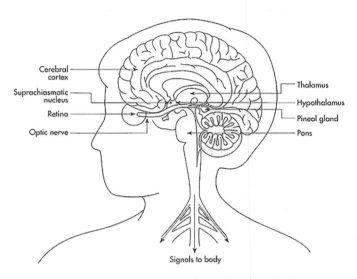

Figure 5.1. *Human Brain and It's Parts Associated with Dream and Sleep*

Section 5.2

Nightmares

This section contains text excerpted from the following sources: Text in this section begins with excerpts from "Nightmares and PTSD," National Center for Posttraumatic Stress Disorder (NCPTSD), U.S. Department of Veterans Affairs (VA), December 17, 2018; Text under the heading "Tips for Coping with Nightmare" is excerpted from "Sleep Problems and Nightmares," Mental Illness Research, Education and Clinical Centers (MIRECC), U.S. Department of Veterans Affairs (VA), May 10, 2017.

Nightmares are dreams that are threatening and scary. Nearly everyone has had a nightmare from time to time. For trauma survivors, though, nightmares are a common problem. Along with flashbacks and unwanted memories, nightmares are one of the ways in which a trauma survivor may relive the trauma for months or years after the event.

How Common Are Nightmares after Trauma?

Among the general public, about five percent of people complain of nightmares. Those who have gone through a trauma, though, are more likely to have distressing nightmares after the event. This is true no matter what type of trauma it is.

Those trauma survivors who get posttraumatic stress disorder (PTSD) are even more likely to complain of nightmares. Nightmares are one of the 17 symptoms of PTSD. For example, a study comparing Vietnam veterans to civilians showed that 52 percent of combat veterans with PTSD had nightmares fairly often. Only 3 percent of the civilians in the study reported that the same level of nightmares.

Other research has found even higher rates of nightmares. Of those with PTSD, 71 to 96 percent may have nightmares. People who have other mental-health problems, such as panic disorder, as well as PTSD are more likely to have nightmares than those with PTSD alone.

Not only are trauma survivors more likely to have nightmares, but those who do may also have them quite often. Some survivors may have nightmares several times a week.

Nightmares and Cultural Differences

Nightmares may be viewed differently in different cultures. For example, in some cultures, nightmares are thought to mean that the dreamer is open to physical or spiritual harm. In other cultures, it is believed that the dreams may contain messages from spirits or may forecast the future. These beliefs may lead those with nightmares to use certain practices in an effort to protect themselves.

Tips for Coping with Nightmare

It is not unusual to have nightmares during times of stress. If you have frequent and distressing nightmares, please talk to your medical or mental-health care provider. Frequent nightmares may be a sign of a more serious problem.

- The morning after a nightmare, spend some time thinking about what might be causing increased stress in your life. Even positive stress (such as getting married, a new job, moving) can cause anxiety that may result in nightmares.

- Practice some form of relaxation every night before bed. Try imagining yourself in a calming or relaxing place, practice deep slow breathing, or listen to soothing music or sounds.

- Make your bedroom as soothing and comfortable as possible. Think about leaving a dim light or nightlight on to help you recognize your surroundings more quickly if you wake up from a nightmare.

Section 5.3

Night Terrors

"Night Terrors," © 2019 Omnigraphics.
Reviewed May 2019.

Night terrors, also known as "sleep terrors," are sleep disorders that include episodes of screaming, flailing, or crying while being asleep. Night terrors are often paired with sleepwalking. It is most common in children between the ages of 3 and 12, and it affects very few adults. Night terrors in children resolve during the teenage years. Night terror episodes typically last from several seconds to minutes, but some may last longer.

Night terrors are not usually a cause for concern, but it may require medical attention if it causes problems with sleep.

Causes of Night Terrors

Night terrors are considered as parasomnia, which is an unusual behavior of the central nervous system during sleep. It happens during the deep nonrapid eye movement (non-REM) stage of sleep. There are various factors that contribute to night terrors such as:

- Extreme tiredness

- Sleep deprivation

- Sleep disruptions

- Fever

- Headache

A night terror can also be triggered by underlying conditions, such as:

- Restless legs syndrome (RLS)

- Sleep-disordered breathing

- Depression

- Anxiety

- Medication

A night terror can also occur in members of the same family, as it has a strong genetic link.

Symptoms of Night Terrors

The symptoms of night terrors are similar to a nightmare, but the person who has a night terror episode remains asleep. Night terrors typically occur in the first third to the first half of the sleep cycle. During a night terror episode, the person may:

- Suddenly sit up

- Have a wide-eyed stare

- Sweat

- Breathe heavily

- Kick and/or move their limbs forcefully

- Scream or shout

- Be hard to awaken

- Be inconsolable

Complications Associated with Night Terrors

Complications involved in experiencing night terrors include:

- Disrupted sleep

- Embarrassment about the condition
- Daytime sleepiness
- Injury to oneself or others rarely

When to See a Doctor

Night terrors are common in occurrence, however, consult your doctor if night terrors:

- Become more frequent
- Lead to accidental injury
- Periodically disrupt the sleep cycle
- Continue beyond teenage years

Diagnosis of Night Terrors

Diagnosis of night terrors begins with reviewing the symptoms and medical history of the patient. It is followed by:

- **A physical examination.** The doctor may perform a physical examination to identify any conditions that may contribute to the night terrors.

- **A discussion of your symptoms.** Night terrors are generally diagnosed based upon the description of events. Patients may be asked to complete a questionnaire about their sleep behavior.

- **Nocturnal sleep study (polysomnography).** The doctor may recommend an overnight sleep study in a lab. Sensors are placed on the patient's body, and their brain waves, heart rate, oxygen level, breathing, and eye and leg movements will be continuously monitored.

Treatment of Night Terrors

Treatment options for night terror include the following:

- **Treating an underlying condition.** If the night terrors are associated with any medical or mental-health condition, treatment is focused on that problem.

- **Resolving stress.** Relaxation therapy, biofeedback, hypnosis, and cognitive behavioral therapy may help in reducing stress or anxiety.

- **Anticipatory awakening.** This treatment option involves waking a person 15 minutes before she or he experiences a night terror episode.

- **Medication.** Medications are rarely used for night terrors. If necessary, antidepressants may be effective in treating the night terror.

Prevention of Night Terrors

Night terrors can be prevented by:

- **Getting adequate sleep** if you or your child is sleep deprived. Try to keep a sleep schedule, and follow an earlier bedtime.

- **Establishing a calm activity** before bedtime, such as reading a book, solving puzzles, taking a warm bath, meditating, or completing relaxing exercises.

- **Keeping a sleep diary** and taking note of your child's sleep pattern. If the night terror episodes are observed to consistent, it may be used for anticipatory awakening.

A night terror lasts only for a few minutes. During a night terror, try to calm the person down by using repeated soothing statements and providing physical comfort.

How to Help a Child during a Night Terror

When your child experiences a night terror episode, do the following:

- Try not to wake your child from sleep. Your child may feel disorientated and confused when you try to wake her or him.

- Guide your child safely to bed if she or he went left their bed during a night terror episode in order to avoid any injuries.

- Make the environment safe before going to bed by locking doors and windows, keeping fragile objects out of reach, etc.

References

1. "Sleep Terrors (Night Terrors)," Mayo Clinic, March 9, 2018.
2. "Night Terrors," The Nemours Foundation/KidsHealth®, June 2017.

3. "Sleep Disorders: Night Terrors," WebMD, November 16, 2018.

4. Newman, Tim. "What Are Night Terrors and Why Do They Happen?" Medical News Today (MNT), December 8, 2017.

5. "Night Terrors," Raising Children Network (Australia) Limited, June 12, 2018.

Chapter 6

What Are Sleep Disorders?

Chapter Contents

Section 6.1

Understanding Sleep Disorders

This section includes text excerpted from "Sleep Disorders,"
MedlinePlus, National Institutes of Health (NIH),
December 10, 2018.

Sleep is a complex biological process. While you are sleeping, you are unconscious, but your brain and body functions are still active. They are doing a number of important jobs that help you stay healthy and function at your best. So, when you do not get enough quality sleep, it does more than just make you feel tired. It can affect your physical and mental health, thinking, and daily functioning.

Sleep disorders are conditions that disturb your normal sleep patterns. There are more than 80 different sleep disorders. Some major types include:

- Insomnia
- Sleep apnea
- Restless legs syndrome (RLS)
- Hypersomnia
- Circadian rhythm disorders (CRD)
- Parasomnia

Some people who feel tired during the day have a true sleep disorder. But for others, the real problem is not allowing enough time for sleep. It is important to get enough sleep every night. The amount of sleep you need depends on several factors, including your age, lifestyle, health, and whether you have been getting enough sleep recently. Most adults need about seven to eight hours each night.

What Causes Sleep Disorders

There are different causes for different sleep disorders, including:

- Other conditions, such as heart disease, lung disease, nerve disorders, and pain
- Mental illnesses, including depression and anxiety
- Medicines
- Genetics

Sometimes, the cause is not known.

There are also some factors that can contribute to sleep problems, including:

- Caffeine and alcohol

- An irregular schedule, such as working the night shift

- Aging. As people age, they often get less sleep or spend less time in the deep, restful stage of sleep. They are also more easily awakened.

What Are the Symptoms of Sleep Disorders?

The symptoms of sleep disorders depend on the specific disorder. Some signs that you may have a sleep disorder include:

- You regularly take more than 30 minutes each night to fall asleep.

- You regularly wake up several times each night and then have trouble falling back to sleep, or you wake up too early in the morning.

- You often feel sleepy during the day, take frequent naps, or fall asleep at the wrong times during the day.

- Your bed partner says that when you sleep, you snore loudly, snort, gasp, make choking sounds, or stop breathing for short periods.

- You have creeping, tingling, or crawling feelings in your legs or arms that are relieved by moving or massaging them, especially in the evening and when trying to fall asleep.

- Your bed partner notices that your legs or arms jerk often during sleep.

- You have vivid, dream-like experiences while falling asleep or dozing.

- You have episodes of sudden muscle weakness when you are angry or fearful, or when you laugh.

- You feel as though you cannot move when you first wake up.

How Are Sleep Disorders Diagnosed?

To make a diagnosis, your healthcare provider will use your medical history, your sleep history, and a physical exam. You may also have a sleep study (polysomnogram). The most common types of sleep studies monitor and record data about your body during a full night of sleep. The data includes:

- Brain wave changes

- Eye movements

- Breathing rate

- Blood pressure

- Heart rate and electrical activity of the heart and other muscles

Other types of sleep studies may check how quickly you fall asleep during daytime naps or whether you are able to stay awake and alert during the day.

What Are the Treatments for Sleep Disorders?

Treatments for sleep disorders depend on which disorder you have. They may include:

- Good sleep habits and other lifestyle changes, such as a healthy diet and exercise

- Cognitive behavioral therapy or relaxation techniques to reduce anxiety about getting enough sleep

- Continuous positive airway pressure (CPAP) machine for sleep apnea

- Bright light therapy (in the morning)

- Medicines, including sleeping pills. Usually, providers recommend that you use sleeping pills for a short period of time.

- Natural products, such as melatonin. These products may help some people, but are generally for short-term use. Make sure to check with your healthcare provider before you take any of them.

Section 6.2

Key Sleep Disorders

This section includes text excerpted from "Key Sleep Disorders," Centers for Disease Control and Prevention (CDC), December 10, 2014. Reviewed May 2019.

Sleep-related difficulties affect many people. The following is a description of some of the major sleep disorders. If you, or someone you know, is experiencing any of the following, it is important to receive an evaluation by a healthcare provider or, if necessary, a provider specializing in sleep medicine.

Insomnia

Insomnia is characterized by an inability to initiate or maintain sleep. It may also take the form of early morning awakening in which the individual awakens several hours early and is unable to resume sleeping. Difficulty initiating or maintaining sleep may often manifest itself as excessive daytime sleepiness, which characteristically results in functional impairment throughout the day. Before arriving at a diagnosis of primary insomnia, the healthcare provider will rule out other potential causes, such as other sleep disorders, side effects of medications, substance abuse, depression, or other previously undetected illness. Chronic psychophysiological insomnia (or "learned" or "conditioned" insomnia) may result from a stressor combined with fear of being unable to sleep. Individuals with this condition may sleep better when not in their own beds. Healthcare providers may treat chronic insomnia with a combination of use of sedative-hypnotic or sedating antidepressant medications, along with behavioral techniques to promote regular sleep.

Narcolepsy

Excessive daytime sleepiness (including episodes of irresistible sleepiness) combined with sudden muscle weakness are the hallmark signs of narcolepsy. The sudden muscle weakness seen in narcolepsy may be elicited by strong emotion or surprise. Episodes of narcolepsy have been described as "sleep attacks" and may occur in unusual circumstances, such as walking and other forms of physical activity. The healthcare provider may treat narcolepsy with stimulant medications combined with behavioral interventions, such as regularly scheduled naps, to minimize the potential disruptiveness of narcolepsy on the individual's life.

Restless Legs Syndrome

Restless legs syndrome (RLS) is characterized by an unpleasant "creeping" sensation, often feeling like it is originating in the lower legs, but often associated with aches and pains throughout the legs. This often causes difficulty initiating sleep and is relieved by movement of the leg, such as walking or kicking. Abnormalities in the neurotransmitter dopamine have often been associated with RLS. Healthcare providers often combine a medication to help correct the underlying dopamine abnormality along with a medicine to promote sleep continuity in the treatment of RLS.

Sleep Apnea

Snoring may be more than just an annoying habit—It may be a sign of sleep apnea. Persons with sleep apnea characteristically make periodic gasping or "snorting" noises, during which their sleep is momentarily interrupted. Those with sleep apnea may also experience excessive daytime sleepiness, as their sleep is commonly interrupted and may not feel restorative. Treatment of sleep apnea is dependent on its cause. If other medical problems are present, such as congestive heart failure or nasal obstruction, sleep apnea may resolve with treatment of these conditions. Gentle air pressure administered during sleep (typically in the form of a nasal continuous positive airway pressure (CPAP) device) may also be effective in the treatment of sleep apnea. As interruption of regular breathing or obstruction of the airway during sleep can pose serious health complications, symptoms of sleep apnea should be taken seriously. Treatment should be sought from a healthcare provider.

Chapter 7

Sleep Disorders in Women

Sleep and Women

A healthy sleeping pattern is particularly important for women, as it has a direct bearing on the quality of their lives. Unlike their predecessors, today's women are faced with the challenge of balancing home and career, and getting adequate sleep—in terms of both quantity and quality—is particularly important in order to recharge depleted energy stores in the body and brain cells, and to lay the foundation for a productive day.

Studies have proved that the circadian rhythm, a 24-hour cycle that is internally generated in many organisms, including humans, has a deep impact on the sleep–wake cycle. Clinical evidence points to significant differences in the way men and women sleep, and in recent years, there has been growing interest in how gender influences sleep pathologies. While much is known about the mechanisms that link sleep and circadian rhythms, research on the way gender may affect sleep is still in its nascent stage but is vital to how we understand and treat sleep-related disorders.

Clinical studies across a broad range of ages have shown that women sleep longer but report poorer sleep quality than men. Women may also complain of sleep problems when there is no measurable evidence of sleep disturbance. This reflects a sleep state misperception (SSM), also known as "pseudo" or "paradoxical insomnia," a condition recognized as an intrinsic sleep disorder by the International Classification of Sleep Disorders (ICSD), which is a widely accepted tool for clinical practice and research in sleep-disorder medicine. The higher incidence of SSM in women may, in part, be attributed to the statistically higher incidence of anxiety, mood, and affective disorders in women.

Despite clinical evidence pointing to a higher incidence of SSM in women compared to men, there is also existing data that supports the fact that women are, in fact, more prone to sleep disorders than men. The risk ratio for sleep problems increases with age and is seen to be more apparent after puberty, indicating that reproductive hormones may affect sleep patterns and circadian rhythms in women. Changes in the ovarian hormonal milieu across the lifespan would also explain how age influences sleep patterns and circadian rhythms in women.

Menstrual Cycle and Sleep

A report suggests that more than two-thirds of women experience disrupted sleep patterns during their menstrual cycles. These changes in sleep patterns manifest as part of premenstrual syndrome (PMS), a group of symptoms that occur about a week to ten days before menstruation. Although PMS may affect individuals differently, it is generally associated with mood changes, depression, irritability, fatigue, and insomnia. For some, disturbed sleep patterns may continue even during periods, with abdominal cramping and other symptoms associated with menstruation affecting sleep quality. Studies show a reduction in REM sleep in the first few days of the menstrual cycle, while progesterone, the hormone whose levels spike in the latter half of the cycle, has a soporific effect and has been shown to help women sleep better.

Pregnancy and Sleep

It has been reported that more than three-quarters of women experience sleep problems during pregnancy. While insomnia is common, other sleep-related issues may include sleep apnea, restless leg syndrome, and periodic limb movement disorder. Pregnancy places considerable demands on the body, therefore, pregnant women may need a few extra hours of sleep, particularly during the last trimester. But during pregnancy, a number of conditions can impede a good night's sleep. These include increased heart rate, dyspnea (shortness of breath), anxiety, stress, and heartburn.

Women typically gain around 30 pounds of weight during pregnancy, and this puts extra pressure on the pelvis and spine. Consequently, pregnant women frequently experience aches in the legs and back, which often disrupt sleep. The kidneys also overwork during pregnancy since there is a marked increase in the filtration rate, and this results in frequent urination, meaning more trips to the bathroom at night. Unsurprisingly, sleep issues tend to continue for most women even after childbirth. The stress involved in caring for the newborn and waking up frequently to nurse the baby make it difficult to get through the night without sleep interruptions.

Menopause and Sleep

Many women face increased sleep issues during and after menopause. In fact, some women begin to experience sleep problems even during perimenopause, the natural transition from a woman's reproductive phase to the cessation of menstrual periods. Sleep issues in menopause are closely linked to altered levels of hormones. A drop in the estrogen level often causes hot flashes and night sweats, which can greatly disrupt sleep, depending on the severity and frequency of symptoms. Decrease in hormone levels can also lead to an increased heart rate and vaginal dryness, and these symptoms may exacerbate anxiety and stress, which may aggravate sleep problems further. There may also be other physical factors that could impact sleep in menopausal women. Arthritis and heartburn, for example, could keep women awake during the night, and the resulting sleep deprivation could lead to fatigue and further aggravate problems such as anxiety and depression.

Managing Sleep Disorders in Women

The protocol for treating insomnia and other sleep-related disorders is, by and large, the same for men and women and generally includes over-the-counter (OTC) and prescription medications, cognitive behavioral therapy (CBT), complementary and alternative treatments, and recommended lifestyle changes. That said, clinicians need to consider medical; social; and specific biological factors, such as pregnancy and menopause, to determine the type of treatment required for managing sleep disorders in women.

Healthy Sleep Tips for Women

Lifestyle changes may be particularly useful in dealing with insomnia and sleep issues during pregnancy and menopause. While a balanced diet, adequate physical activity, and effective coping strategies are key recommendations to deal with general sleep-related problems, specific medical conditions—such as osteoarthritis (OA), anxiety, and depression, which may co-occur with sleep disorders, particularly in older women—need to be addressed as well.

Following good nighttime practices can establish a regular wake-sleep pattern and help women deal with sleep issues. Avoiding heavy and spicy food just before bed can help reduce the chances of heartburn and sleep problems precipitated by it. Stimulants such as caffeine, alcohol, and nicotine can make it difficult to fall asleep, so those with sleep issues should avoid these stimulants in the late-afternoon and evening. Practicing relaxation techniques during menstruation could help deal with sleep problems associated with menstrual cycles. Exposure to daylight has been shown to release melatonin, a hormone that regulates the sleep and wake cycles and also enhances appetite and mood.

Failure to get a good night's sleep is a common enough problem today, and most people experience it at some time in their lives. These problems may hardly ever require medical attention and may be easily managed by lifestyle modifications. However, serious sleep disorders can have a detrimental effect on your physical, mental, and social well-being and do require medical attention. A sleep specialist can help diagnose sleep problems and develop a treatment plan best suited for you.

References

1. "Sleep and Women," UCLASleepCenter, n.d.

2. "Women and Sleep," National Sleep Foundation (NSF), n.d.

3. "Sleep, Rhythms, and the Endocrine Brain: Influence of Sex and Gonadal Hormones," *The Journal of Neuroscience,* November 9, 2011.

4. Hedaya, Robert J. "PMS and Insomnia: What to Do?" Psychology Today, May 4, 2010.

Chapter 8

Sleep Disorders in Men

Sleep and Men

Many men consider sleep to be just one more chore on a list of things to do during the course of a 24-hour period. Some may even consider it a waste of time that could be put to better use. But this attitude might be preventing them from harnessing the power of a well-rested mind and body.

Sleep should be considered to be one of the body's most valuable daily requirements. A sound investment in sleep provides valuable benefits to many other aspects of life. During sleep, the body recharges itself and prepares for another productive day. A good night's rest allows the human body to feel, think, and perform better, and a well-rested individual will find that he has more time and energy at his disposal during the day.

Causes of Sleeplessness in Men

A variety of factors may cause sleeplessness in men and prevent them from getting the amount of rest required for the body and mind to recharge.

Lack of Awareness

Many men simply are not aware of the importance of sleep. Some may even view it as an indication of not working enough and believe they have to fight the urge to sleep. Although the amount of sleep required varies from person to person, in general, adults need at least seven to eight hours of sleep per night. But, many people do not get enough sleep and consequently do not have optimal levels of energy and concentration to perform their daily activities.

Some signs that you are not sleeping enough:

- Feeling of tiredness and lack of energy throughout the day
- Difficulty concentrating
- Slow to get started in the morning
- Irritability
- Dozing off during the day

Sleeping late is not an option for people who have to be at work early, and most work policies do not allow for naps on the job. The only solution is to go to sleep earlier. Plan to get eight hours of sleep per night, and prioritize this to make it a goal.

Work Demands

Extra hours at work, the need to work during weekends, long commutes to work, and paperwork at home consume much of our time in the modern world. After checking emails and answering mobile phones, it is often past the ideal bedtime. Stress at the workplace and anxiety about the next day can also result in disturbed sleep. The body wants to sleep, but the mind remains awake, and you may toss and turn in bed.

Try to leave your work behind when you come home. Maintain boundaries between work and personal time. And working from home—as is common these days—can make the situation even worse. Talking to friends or coworkers about your work life may help relieve stress, as can meditation or physical exercise. Make your bed a place to relax and not to worry.

Full Schedules

Men have busy schedules these days, with many more planned activities in their lives than just work. After work, they might be playing sports or watching their favorite teams in action. They could be doing pet projects or be involved in clubs, civic groups, fraternities, or church activities. Single men could be going out on dates or spending time with friends. Married men might be picking their kids up from school or helping them with their homework.

The key is to prioritize the important things and balance time effectively. Not everything needs to be done each day. Scale back on the number of things you are doing, rearrange tasks, and eliminate less important ones. These can be done when you have free time on other days. When listing and prioritizing activities, make sure sleeping is ranked high on the list.

Life Changes

Changes in life have the potential to affect your sleep dramatically. These changes may come by surprise, or you might have been expecting them. Negative changes tend to be most disruptive to your sleep, but positive change could have this effect, as well, because of the excitement it causes. Some changes may bring new duties and responsibilities, which could increase stress and keep you up at night.

Some negative changes that could affect your sleep include:

- The death of a loved one
- Becoming unemployed
- Getting divorced
- Being involved in an accident
- Becoming aware of a major illness
- Having a lawsuit filed against you
- An investment that has turned bad

Some such positive changes include:

- Getting married
- Having a baby
- Getting a promotion or a new job
- Moving or relocating

Some changes may cause men to experience depression, which can have a major impact on sleep patterns. You could toss and turn in bed without sleeping much, or you could sleep longer with little motivation to get out of bed. Depression can also cause men to stop taking care of themselves. They may stop eating, grooming, and exercising. Abuse of alcohol and drugs is common with depression, and there could be a loss of interest in day to day activities.

Men often find it difficult to talk about depression and may find it preferable not to seek help from counselors. But, they need to be aware that their condition could be hazardous to their health and detrimental to their daily lives. They could begin by talking about the problem to a friend, spouse, doctor, or minister. These people could help them seek help from a counselor when they have made the decision to do so. It is advisable not to face the situation on your own.

Bad Habits

Poor sleep can be the result of bad habits or routines. These include the consumption of alcohol, nicotine, and coffee in the late afternoon, in the evening, or just before bedtime. Eating big meals or exercising before bedtime can also disturb your sleep. You might tend to have a big meal at night if you were busy during the evening. Instead, try and have a good lunch so that you are satisfied with a smaller dinner. Exercise before work or during your lunch break.

Going to sleep at irregular times and waking up at different times daily could disrupt your internal body clock and prevent you from sleeping soundly. To set your body's clock properly, try to wake up at a set time every day, including weekends and holidays. Avoid sleeping late on weekends to catch up on lost sleep. This does not work. Instead, go to bed earlier at night. Also, limit naps to an hour in order to avoid disrupting sleep at night.

Medical Conditions

Any number of medical conditions may result in poor sleep. The effects could be temporary, as with a sprained ankle, flu, or surgery, while others may be chronic and require long-term treatment. Some medical conditions become more common with increasing age, and they or their medications could begin to interfere with sleep.

The following are a few medical conditions could result in poor sleep patterns:

- Epilepsy

- Asthma

- Other respiratory diseases

- Heart disease

- Arthritis

Some medications may hinder sleep and keep you jittery through the night. Others may cause sleepiness during the day. Talk to your doctor about your medication; there may be alternatives that could eliminate these types of side-effects. The time at which you take your medicine and the dosage could also have a significant effect on the quality of your sleep.

Sleep Disorders That Affect Men

Many people spend enough time lying in bed but do not get quality sleep. Their sleep could be disturbed and broken, or they may sleep through the night but wake up tired. These are indications of an underlying sleep disorder. Sleep disorders are common, but many people who are afflicted with them remain unaware of the condition, and some may shy away from seeking help. But diagnosing and treating sleep disorders can result in a dramatic improvement in sleep, helping to establish healthy sleep patterns and allowing you to be at your best during the day.

The following are some sleep disorders commonly diagnosed among men:

Obstructive Sleep Apnea

During sleep, muscles in the throat become relaxed. Sometimes, the tissue in the mouth may collapse and prevent air from entering the lungs, or the tongue could fall back and block the airway. This is a disorder known as "obstructive sleep apnea" (OSA), a condition that affects one in four men. This blockage could occur a few times during the night or hundreds of times. Breathing pauses for a moment when this happens, and you tend to wake up. Someone with OSA often feels very tired during the day. Men are twice as likely as women to have OSA. Obesity and a larger neck girth increase the likelihood of having OSA because the larger amount of fatty tissue in the neck can block the airway.

In addition to sleepiness during the day, another sign of OSA is loud snoring, which is caused by a partially blocked airway passage. The intensity of snoring could range from mild to severe. Simple snoring is generally normal and harmless, but loud and severe snoring accompanied by gasping for air is a cause for concern. Men are often not aware that they snore. It usually becomes evident when a spouse or sleep partner notices it. Left untreated, sleep apnea carries with it the risk of lung disease, diabetes, and hypertension.

69

Talk to your doctor if you snore loudly in the night. She or he may refer you to a sleep specialist who can test for sleep apnea. Losing weight and sleeping on the side, rather than the back, are remedies that you can try on your own. But medical treatment is essential for more serious sleep apnea.

Continuous positive air pressure (CPAP) is one treatment that can be used to treat sleep apnea. A mask worn on the face during sleep delivers a steady flow of air through the nose. This keeps the airway open and prevents pauses in breathing. The use of an oral device, similar to a mouth guard, could bring relief to people with OSA. And in some cases, surgery may be recommended.

Narcolepsy

Narcolepsy is a chronic brain disorder that causes extreme sleepiness during day-to-day activities, such as while eating, walking, or driving. It causes people to fall asleep suddenly for a few seconds to several minutes. Narcolepsy commonly begins between the ages of 12 and 20; although, in some cases, it may begin later in life. The condition cannot be cured, but it can be controlled with treatment.

If you feel as if you could fall asleep at any time, talk to your doctor. She or he may refer you to a sleep specialist who will make a proper diagnosis. Narcolepsy can be treated using medication that will restore your sleep and wakefulness cycle to a normal pattern.

Delayed Sleep Phase Disorder

Delayed sleep phase disorder (DSPD)—also called "delayed sleep phase syndrome" (DSPS)—is a condition characterized by the tendency to go to sleep and wake up later than what is considered normal, usually by a couple of hours. Every person has an internal clock that prompts the body to sleep and wake up at a given time. Getting into the habit of going to sleep late at night can throw the body clock out of balance, preventing you from falling asleep at the right time.

To counteract delayed sleep phase disorder, stay away from bright lights during the late afternoon and evening. Use dim lighting in your house, and switch off the lights in the bedroom at when i is time to sleep. It is also important to get enough daylight in the morning and afternoon. This sends signals to the brain to set the body clock properly.

Jet-Lag Disorder and Shift Work Disorder

Jet-lag disorder is caused by traveling long distances by air. This disrupts your body clock, because you might reach your destination when your body expects you to sleep, but it could be daytime there, and you may need to be awake. Your body clock is not able to adjust itself because of the speed of travel involved, and this may make it hard for you to sleep.

Shift work disorder can occur in men who work late-night shifts or in rotating shifts and often need to work when the body senses that it is time to sleep. After work, these individuals feel that they want to sleep when it is actually the time for the body to remain awake. This results in tiredness and the inability to sleep properly.

Melatonin supplements have been shown to improve jet lag among travelers. Melatonin is a hormone that is released by the body at night and helps induce sleep. Light therapy has shown positive benefits on both jet-lag disorder and shift work disorder. In light therapy, the eyes are exposed to bright light at a regular time and for a specific duration. It mimics the effect of sunlight on the body's internal clock. Consult your doctor to see if melatonin or light therapy could be beneficial in your case.

How Can Men Sleep Better?

Developing good sleep practices is the first step in allowing men to sleep better. You can build these good habits by following some basic tips that will result in healthy sleep patterns and learning counter-productive practices to avoid.

One common misconception among men is that alcohol helps them sleep better. Alcohol might help you get to sleep, but it often causes you to wake up during the night. Many men who drink in the evening wake up very early in the morning and experience sleeplessness. To develop good sleep hygiene, refrain from drinking at least six hours before bedtime. Limit how much you drink and how frequently you drink. The heavy use of alcohol is detrimental to overall good health, as well as good sleep.

Men sometimes use prescription sleeping pills as a solution to sleep problems. These drugs help to an extent, but they should not be used as a long-term solution. Because of the danger of developing a dependency, doctors generally do not prescribe sleep medication beyond a few weeks at a time.

Over-the-counter (OTC) sleep medicines are readily available at drugstores. These formulations often use antihistamines to induce drowsiness. Even though they allow you to sleep, they can make you groggy during the day and may result in slow response times. They should be used sparingly and with caution.

If you have not been sleeping well for more than a month, it is a good idea to consult a doctor. Do not ignore the problem thinking it will disappear. Your physician will likely refer you to a sleep specialist who will diagnose the cause of the problem. Before visiting a sleep specialist, it can be useful to keep a sleep diary for two weeks. This will help the specialist understand your sleep patterns, provide clues about what is hindering your sleep, and assist her or him in suggesting remedies.

Sleep is crucial to your well-being, and it touches every other aspect of your life. Do not ignore signs of trouble when there is so much to gain from consulting a doctor for diagnosis and treatment.

References

1. "Sleep and Men," UCLA Health, n.d.

2. "Sleep Apnea and Insomnia in Men," BodyLogicMD.com, n.d.

3. "Sleep Disorders," Bon Secours for Men, n.d.

Chapter 9

Sleep and Aging

Older adults need about the same amount of sleep as all adults—seven to nine hours each night. But, older people tend to go to sleep earlier and get up earlier than they did when they were younger.

There are many reasons why older people may not get enough sleep at night. Feeling sick or being in pain can make it hard to sleep. Some medicines can keep you awake. No matter the reason, if you do not get a good night's sleep, the next day you may:

- Be irritable

- Have memory problems or be forgetful

- Feel depressed

- Have more falls or accidents

Get a Good Night's Sleep

Being older does not mean that you have to be tired all the time. You can do many things to get a good night's sleep. Here are some ideas:

- **Follow a regular sleep schedule.** Go to sleep and get up at the same time each day, even on weekends or when you are traveling.

This chapter includes text excerpted from "A Good Night's Sleep," National Institute on Aging (NIA), National Institutes of Health (NIH), May 1, 2016.

- **Avoid napping in the late afternoon or evening** if you can. Naps may keep you awake at night.

- **Develop a bedtime routine.** Take time to relax before bedtime each night. Some people read a book, listen to soothing music, or soak in a warm bath.

- **Try not to watch television or use your computer, cell phone, or tablet in the bedroom.** The light from these devices may make it difficult for you to fall asleep. Furthermore, alarming or unsettling shows or movies, such as horror movies, may keep you awake.

- **Keep your bedroom at a comfortable temperature,** not too hot or too cold, and as quiet as possible.

- **Use low lighting in the evenings** and as you prepare for bed.

- **Exercise at regular times each day** but not within three hours of your bedtime.

- **Avoid eating large meals close to bedtime**—they can keep you awake.

- **Stay away from caffeine late in the day.** Caffeine (found in coffee, tea, soda, and chocolate) can keep you awake.

- **Remember—alcohol will not help you sleep.** Even small amounts make it harder to stay asleep.

Insomnia Is Common in Older Adults

Insomnia is the most common sleep problem in adults 60 years of age and older. People with this condition have trouble falling asleep and staying asleep. Insomnia can last for days, months, and even years. Having trouble sleeping can mean you:

- Take a long time to fall asleep

- Wake up many times in the night

- Wake up early and are unable to get back to sleep

- Wake up tired

- Feel very sleepy during the day

Often, being unable to sleep becomes a habit. Some people worry about not sleeping even before they get into bed. This may make it harder to fall asleep and stay asleep.

Some older adults who have trouble sleeping may use over-the-counter (OTC) sleep aids. Others may use prescription medicines to help them sleep. These medicines may help when used for a short time. But remember, medicines are not a cure for insomnia.

Developing healthy habits at bedtime may help you get a good night's sleep.

Sleep Apnea

People with sleep apnea have short pauses in breathing while they are asleep. These pauses may happen many times during the night. If not treated, sleep apnea can lead to other problems, such as high blood pressure, stroke, or memory loss. You can have sleep apnea and not even know it. Feeling sleepy during the day and being told you are snoring loudly at night could be signs that you have sleep apnea.

If you think you have sleep apnea, see a doctor who can treat this sleep problem. You may need to learn to sleep in a position that keeps your airways open. Treatment using a continuous positive airway pressure (CPAP) device almost always helps people with sleep apnea. A dental device or surgery may also help.

Movement Disorders and Sleep

Restless legs syndrome (RLS), periodic limb movement disorder (PLMD), and rapid eye movement (REM) sleep behavior disorders are common in older adults. These movement disorders can rob you of needed sleep. People with RLS feel as if there is tingling, crawling, or pins and needles in one or both legs. This feeling is worse at night. See your doctor for more information about medicines to treat RLS. Periodic limb movement disorder causes people to jerk and kick their legs every 20 to 40 seconds during sleep. Medication, warm baths, exercise, and relaxation exercises can help.

Rapid eye movement sleep behavior disorder is another condition that may make it harder to get a good night's sleep. During normal REM sleep, your muscles cannot move, so your body stays still. But, if you have REM sleep behavior disorder, your muscles can move and your sleep is disrupted.

Alzheimer Disease and Sleep—A Special Problem

Alzheimer disease (AD) often changes a person's sleeping habits. Some people with AD sleep too much; others do not sleep enough.

Some people wake up many times during the night; others wander or yell at night. The person with AD is not the only one who loses sleep. Caregivers may have sleepless nights, leaving them tired for the challenges they face.

If you are caring for someone with AD, take these steps to make her or him safer and help you sleep better at night:

- Make sure the floor is clear of objects.

- Lock up any medicines.

- Attach grab bars in the bathroom.

- Place a gate across the stairs.

Safe Sleep for Older Adults

Try to set up a safe and restful place to sleep. Make sure you have smoke alarms on each floor of your home. Before going to bed, lock all windows and doors that lead outside. Other ideas for a safe night's sleep are:

- Keep a telephone with emergency phone numbers by your bed.

- Have a lamp within reach that is easy to turn on.

- Put a glass of water next to the bed in case you wake up thirsty.

- Do not smoke, especially in bed.

- Remove area rugs so you would not trip if you get out of bed during the night.

Tips to Help You Fall Asleep

You may have heard about some tricks to help you fall asleep. You do not really have to count sheep—you could try counting slowly to 100. Some people find that playing mental games makes them sleepy. For example, tell yourself it is 5 minutes before you have to get up, and you are just trying to get a little bit more sleep.

Some people find that relaxing their bodies puts them to sleep. One way to do this is to imagine your toes are completely relaxed, then your feet, and then your ankles are completely relaxed. Work your way up the rest of your body, section by section. You may drift off to sleep before getting to the top of your head.

Use your bedroom only for sleeping. After turning off the light, give yourself about 20 minutes to fall asleep. If you are still awake and not drowsy, get out of bed. When you feel sleepy, go back to bed. If you feel tired and unable to do your activities for more than two or three weeks, you may have a sleep problem. Talk with your doctor about changes you can make to get a better night's sleep.

Part Two

The Causes and Consequences of Sleep Deprivation

Chapter 10

Sleep Deprivation and Deficiency

What Are Sleep Deprivation and Deficiency?

Sleep deprivation is a condition that occurs if you do not get enough sleep. Sleep deficiency is a broader concept. It occurs if you have one or more of the following:

- You do not get enough sleep (sleep deprivation).

- You sleep at the wrong time of day (that is, you are out of sync with your body's natural clock).

- You do not sleep well or get all of the different types of sleep that your body needs.

- You have a sleep disorder that prevents you from getting enough sleep or causes poor quality sleep.

Sleeping is a basic human need, such as eating, drinking, and breathing. As with these other needs, sleeping is a vital part of the foundation for good health and well-being throughout your lifetime.

This chapter contains text excerpted from the following sources: Text beginning with the heading "What Are Sleep Deprivation and Deficiency?" is excerpted from "Sleep Deprivation and Deficiency," National Heart, Lung, and Blood Institute (NHLBI), April 22, 2019; Text beginning with the heading "Habits to Improve Your Sleep" is excerpted from "Are You Getting Enough Sleep?" Centers for Disease Control and Prevention (CDC), March 18, 2019.

Sleep deficiency can lead to physical and mental-health problems, injuries, loss of productivity, and even a greater risk of death.

How Much Sleep Is Enough?

The amount of sleep you need each day will change over the course of your life. Although sleep needs vary from person to person, the table below shows general recommendations for different age groups. This table reflects the American Academy of Sleep Medicine (AASM) recommendations that the American Academy of Pediatrics (AAP) has endorsed.

Table 10.1. Recommended Amount of Sleep for Various Age Groups

Age	Recommended Amount of Sleep
Infants aged 4 to 12 months	12 to 16 hours a day (including naps)
Children aged 1 to 2 years	11 to 14 hours a day (including naps)
Children aged 3 to 5 years	10 to 13 hours a day (including naps)
Children aged 6 to 12 years	9 to 12 hours a day
Teens aged 13 to 18 years	8 to 10 hours a day
Adults aged 18 years or older	7 to 8 hours a day

If you routinely lose sleep or choose to sleep less than needed, the sleep loss adds up. The total sleep lost is called your "sleep debt." For example, if you lose 2 hours of sleep each night, you will have a sleep debt of 14 hours after a week.

Some people nap as a way to deal with sleepiness. Naps may provide a short-term boost in alertness and performance. However, napping does not provide all of the other benefits of night-time sleep. Thus, you cannot really make up for lost sleep.

Some people sleep more on their days off than on work days. They also may go to bed later and get up later on days off.

Sleeping more on days off might be a sign that you are not getting enough sleep. Although extra sleep on days off might help you feel better, it can upset your body's sleep–wake rhythm.

Bad sleep habits and long-term sleep loss will affect your health. If you are worried about whether you are getting enough sleep, try using a sleep diary for a couple of weeks. Write down how much you sleep each night, how alert and rested you feel in the morning, and how sleepy you feel during the day. Show the results to your doctor and talk about how you can improve your sleep.

Sleeping when your body is ready to sleep also is very important. Sleep deficiency can affect people even when they sleep the total number of hours recommended for their age group. For example, people whose sleep is out of sync with their body clocks (such as shift workers) or routinely interrupted (such as caregivers or emergency responders) might need to pay special attention to their sleep needs.

If your job or daily routine limits your ability to get enough sleep or sleep at the right times, talk with your doctor. You also should talk with your doctor if you sleep more than eight hours a night but do not feel well rested. You may have a sleep disorder or other health problem.

Who Is at Risk for Sleep Deprivation and Deficiency?

Sleep deficiency, which includes sleep deprivation, affects people of all ages, races, and ethnicities. Certain groups of people may be more likely to be sleep deficient. Examples include people who:

- **Have limited time available for sleep,** such as caregivers or people working long hours or more than one job

- **Have schedules that conflict with their internal body clocks,** such as shift workers, first responders, teens who have early school schedules, or people who must travel for work

- **Make lifestyle choices that prevent them from getting enough sleep,** such as taking medicine to stay awake, abusing alcohol or drugs, or not leaving enough time for sleep

- **Have undiagnosed or untreated medical problems,** such as stress, anxiety, or sleep disorders

- **Have medical conditions or take medicines that interfere with sleep**

Certain medical conditions have been linked to sleep disorders. These conditions include heart failure, heart disease, obesity, diabetes, high blood pressure, stroke or transient ischemic attack (mini-stroke), depression, and attention deficit hyperactivity disorder (ADHD). If you have or have had one of these conditions, ask your doctor whether you might benefit from a sleep study. A sleep study allows your doctor to measure how much and how well you sleep. It also helps show whether you have sleep problems and how severe they are.

If you have a child who is overweight, talk with the doctor about your child's sleep habits.

Signs, Symptoms, and Complications of Sleep Deprivation and Deficiency

Sleep deficiency can cause you to feel very tired during the day. You may not feel refreshed and alert when you wake up. Sleep deficiency also can interfere with work, school, driving, and social functioning.

How sleepy you feel during the day can help you figure out whether you are having symptoms of problem sleepiness. You might be sleep deficient if you often feel as if you could doze off while:

- Sitting and reading or watching television (TV)

- Sitting still in a public place, such as a movie theater, meeting, or classroom

- Riding in a car for an hour without stopping

- Sitting and talking to someone

- Sitting quietly after lunch

- Sitting in traffic for a few minutes

Sleep deficiency can cause problems with learning, focusing, and reacting. You may have trouble making decisions, solving problems, remembering things, controlling your emotions and behavior, and coping with change. You may take longer to finish tasks, have a slower reaction time, and make more mistakes.

The signs and symptoms of sleep deficiency may differ between children and adults. Children who are sleep deficient might be overly active and have problems paying attention. They also might misbehave, and their school performance can suffer. Sleep-deficient children may feel angry and impulsive, have mood swings, feel sad or depressed, or lack motivation.

You may not notice how sleep deficiency affects your daily routine. A common myth is that people can learn to get by on little sleep with no negative effects. However, research shows that getting enough quality sleep at the right times is vital for mental health, physical health, quality of life (QOL), and safety.

To find out whether you are sleep deficient, try keeping a sleep diary for a couple of weeks. Write down how much you sleep each night, how alert and rested you feel in the morning, and how sleepy you feel during the day. Compare the amount of time you sleep each day with the average amount of sleep recommended for your age group, as shown in table 10.1. If you often feel very sleepy, and efforts to increase your sleep do not help, talk with your doctor.

Habits to Improve Your Sleep

There are some important habits that can improve your sleep health:

- **Be consistent.** Go to bed at the same time each night and get up at the same time each morning, including on the weekends.

- **Keep it dark.** Make sure your bedroom is quiet, dark, relaxing, and at a comfortable temperature.

- **Remove electronic devices,** such as televisions, computers, and smartphones, from the bedroom.

- **Food.** Avoid large meals, caffeine, and alcohol before bedtime.

- **No smoking.** Avoid tobacco/nicotine.

- **Get some exercise.** Being physically active during the day can help you fall asleep more easily at night.

What about Sleep Quality

Getting enough sleep is important, but good sleep quality is also essential. Signs of poor sleep quality include feeling sleepy or tired even after getting enough sleep, repeatedly waking up during the night, and having symptoms of sleep disorders (such as snoring or gasping for air). Better sleep habits may improve the quality of your sleep. If you have symptoms of a sleep disorder, such as snoring or being very sleepy during the day after a full night's sleep, make sure to tell your doctor.

Chapter 11

People at Risk of Sleep Deprivation

Chapter Contents

Section 11.1

One in Three Adults Do Not Get Enough Sleep

This section includes text excerpted from "1 in 3 Adults
Don't Get Enough Sleep," Centers for Disease Control
and Prevention (CDC), February 16, 2016.

A good night's sleep is critical for good health. More than a third of American adults are not getting enough sleep on a regular basis, according to a study in the Centers for Disease Control and Prevention's (CDC) Morbidity and Mortality Weekly Report. This is the first study to document estimates of self-reported healthy sleep duration (7 or more hours per day) for all 50 states and the District of Columbia.

The American Academy of Sleep Medicine (AASM) and the Sleep Research Society (SRS) recommend that adults between the ages of 18 and 60 sleep at least 7 hours each night to promote optimal health and well-being. Sleeping less than 7 hours per day is associated with an increased risk of developing chronic conditions, such as obesity, diabetes, high blood pressure, heart disease, stroke, and frequent mental distress.

"As a nation we are not getting enough sleep," said Wayne Giles, M.D., Director of the CDC's Division of Population Health (DPH). "Lifestyle changes, such as going to bed at the same time each night; rising at the same time each morning; and turning off or removing televisions, computers, mobile devices from the bedroom, can help people get the healthy sleep they need."

Prevalence of healthy sleep duration varies by geography, race/ethnicity, employment, marital status. The CDC researchers reviewed data from the 2014 Behavioral Risk Factor Surveillance System (BRFSS), a state-based, random-digit-dialed telephone survey conducted collaboratively by state health departments and the CDC. The key findings of this survey include:

- Healthy sleep duration was lower among Native Hawaiians/Pacific Islanders (54%), non-Hispanic Blacks (54%), multiracial non-Hispanics (54%) and American Indians/Alaska Natives (60%) compared with non-Hispanic Whites (67%), Hispanics (66%), and Asians (63%).

- The prevalence of healthy sleep duration varied among states and ranged from 56 percent in Hawaii to 72 percent in South Dakota.

- A lower proportion of adults reported getting at least seven hours of sleep per day in states clustered in the southeastern region of the United States and the Appalachian Mountains. Previous studies have shown that these regions also have the highest prevalence of obesity and other chronic conditions.

- People who reported they were unable to work or were unemployed had lower healthy sleep duration (51% and 60%, respectively) than did employed respondents (65%). The prevalence of healthy sleep duration was highest among people with a college degree or higher (72%).

- The percentage reporting a healthy sleep duration was higher among people who were married (67%) compared with those who were never married (62%) or divorced, widowed, or separated (56%).

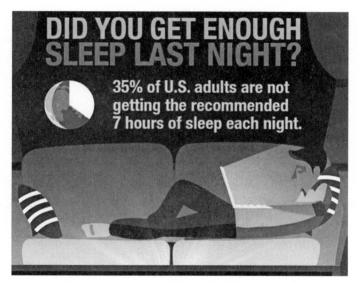

Figure 11.1. *Did You Get Enough Sleep?*

Healthy sleep tips:

- Healthcare providers should routinely assess patients' sleep patterns and discuss sleep-related problems, such as snoring and excessive daytime sleepiness.

- Healthcare providers should also educate patients about the importance of sleep to their health.

- Individuals should make getting enough sleep a priority and practice good sleep habits.

- Employers can consider adjusting work schedules to allow their workers time to get enough sleep.

- Employers can also educate their shift workers about how to improve their sleep.

Section 11.2

Short Sleep Duration among Adults and High-School Students in the United States

This section includes text excerpted from "Sleep and Sleep Disorders—Data and Statistics," Centers for Disease Control and Prevention (CDC), May 2, 2017.

Short Sleep Duration among Adults

Adults need 7 or more hours of sleep per night for the best health and well-being. Short sleep duration is defined as less than 7 hours of sleep per 24-hour period.

Geographic Variation in Short Sleep Duration

Figure 11.2 shows the age-adjusted percentage of adults who reported short sleep duration (less than 7 hours of sleep per 24-hour period), by state in the United States in 2014. The percentage varies considerably by state, from less than 30 percent in Colorado, South Dakota, and Minnesota to greater or equal to 40 percent in Kentucky and Hawaii. The highest percentages were in the southeastern United States and in states along the Appalachian Mountains. The lowest percentages were in the Great Plains states.

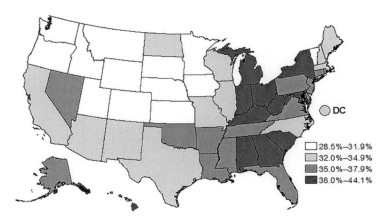

Figure 11.2. *Age-Adjusted Prevalence of Short Sleep Duration (Less Than 7 Hours) among Adults Aged Greater or Equal to 18 Years, by State, United States, 2014* (Source: Behavioral Risk Factor Surveillance System (BRFSS) 2014, Centers for Disease Control and Prevention (CDC).)

The Behavioral Risk Factor Surveillance System (BRFSS) provides data critical for monitoring national and state population health. However, the BRFSS surveys do not have sufficient samples to produce direct survey estimates for most counties or subcounty areas.

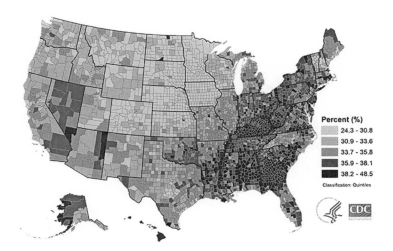

Figure 11.3. *Prevalence of Short Sleep Duration (Less Than 7 Hours) for Adults Aged Greater or Equal to 18 Years, by County, United States, 2014* (Source: Behavioral Risk Factor Surveillance System (BRFSS) 2014, Centers for Disease Control and Prevention (CDC).)

The BRFSS data was used to estimate short sleep duration prevalence at different geographic levels, including counties, congressional districts, and census tracts. These estimates could be used in a variety of contexts and meet the diverse small-area health data needs of local policymakers, program planners, and communities for public-health program planning and evaluation.

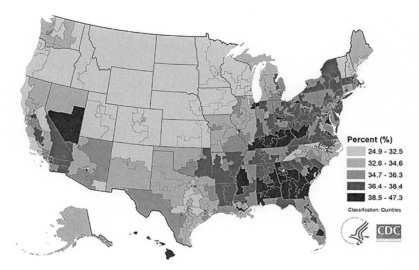

Figure 11.4. *Prevalence of Short Sleep Duration (Less Than 7 Hours) for Adults Aged Greater or Equal to 18 Years, by Congressional District, United States, 2014* (Source: Behavioral Risk Factor Surveillance System (BRFSS) 2014, Centers for Disease Control and Prevention (CDC).)

Short Sleep Duration by Sex, Age, and Race/Ethnicity

In 2014, short sleep duration (less than 7 hours) was less common among respondents 65 years of age or older (26.3%) compared with other age groups (see Table 11.1). The age-adjusted prevalence of short sleep duration was higher among Native Hawaiians/ Pacific Islanders (46.3%), non-Hispanic Blacks (45.8%), multiracial non-Hispanics (44.3%), and American Indians/Alaska Natives (40.4%) compared with non-Hispanic Whites (33.4%), Hispanics (34.5%), and Asians (37.5%). Short sleep prevalence did not differ between men and women.

Table 11.1. Short Sleep Duration (Less Than 7 Hours) by Sex, Age, and Race/Ethnicity—Behavioral Risk Factor Surveillance System (BRFSS), United States, 2014

Characteristic	Percentage	95 Percent Confidence Interval
All Adults*	35.2	(34.9 to 35.5)
Sex*		
Men	35.5	(35.1 to 36.0)
Women	34.8	(34.4 to 35.2)
Age (Years)		
18 to 24	32.2	(31.3 to 33.2)
25 to 34	37.9	(37.1 to 38.7)
35 to 44	38.3	(37.5 to 39.1)
45 to 54	39	(38.3 to 39.6)
55 to 64	35.6	(34.9 to 36.2)
≥65	26.3	(25.8 to 26.8)
Race/Ethnicity*		
White	33.4	(33.0 to 33.7)
Hispanic	34.5	(33.6 to 35.5)
Black	45.8	(44.9 to 46.8)
Asian	37.5	(35.2 to 39.7)
American Indian/Alaska Native	40.4	(37.9 to 43.0)
Native Hawaiian/Pacific Islander	46.3	(39.9 to 52.8)
Other/Multiracial	44.3	(42.4 to 46.2)

* Age-adjusted to the 2000 U.S. standard population.

Health Risk Factors by Sleep Duration

Adults who were short sleepers (less than 7 hours of sleep per 24-hour period) were more likely to report being obese, physically inactive, and current smokers compared to people who got enough sleep (7 or more hours per 24-hour period) (see Table 11.2).

Table 11.2. Age-Adjusted Percentage Reporting Health Risk Factors by Sleep Duration—Behavioral Risk Factor Surveillance System, United States, 2014

Health Risk Factor	Definition	Short Sleep (Less Than 7 Hours)		Sufficient Sleep (Greater Than 7 Hours)	
		Percentage	95 Percentage CI	Percentage	95 Percentage CI
Obese	Body Mass Index ≥30 kg/m2	33	(32.5 to 33.5)	26.5	(26.2 to 26.9)
Physically inactive	No leisure-time physical activity in past 30 days	27.2	(26.8 to 27.7)	20.9	(20.6 to 21.2)
Current smoker	Currently, smoke cigarettes every day or some days	22.9	(22.4 to 23.4)	14.9	(14.6 to 15.2)
Excessive alcohol	Underage drinker, binge drinker, or heavy drinker*	19.4	(18.9 to 19.8)	19.1	(18.7 to 19.4)

Abbreviations: CI = confidence interval.

Age-adjusted to the 2000 U.S. standard population.

"* Underage drinker is defined as any alcohol use among those aged 18 to 20 yrs. Binge drinker is defined as greater or equal to 4 drinks for women and greater or equal to 5 drinks for men during a single occasion. Heavy drinker is defined as greater or equal to 8 drinks for women and greater or equal to 15 drinks for men per week. All differences statistically significant at p<0.05 except excessive alcohol."

Chronic Health Conditions by Sleep Duration

Adults who were short sleepers (less than 7 hours per 24-hour period) were more likely to report 10 chronic health conditions compared to those who got enough sleep (7 or more hours per 24-hour period) (see Table 11.3).

Table 11.3. Age-Adjusted Percentage Reporting Chronic Health Conditions by Sleep Duration—Behavioral Risk Factor Surveillance System, United States, 2014

Chronic condition	Short Sleep (Less Than 7 Hours)		Sufficient Sleep (Greater Than 7 Hours)	
	Percentage	95 Percentage CI	Percentage	95 Percentage CI
Heart attack	4.8	(4.6 to 5.0)	3.4	(3.3 to 3.5)
Coronary heart disease	4.7	(4.5 to 4.9)	3.4	(3.3 to 3.5)
Stroke	3.6	(3.4 to 3.8)	2.4	(2.3 to 2.5)
Asthma	16.5	(16.1 to 16.9)	11.8	(11.5 to 12.0)
Chronic obstructive pulmonary disease (COPD)	8.6	(8.3 to 8.9)	4.7	(4.6 to 4.8)
Cancer	10.2	(10.0 to 10.5)	9.8	(9.7 to 10.0)
Arthritis	28.8	(28.4 to 29.2)	20.5	(20.2 to 20.7)
Depression	22.9	(22.5 to 23.3)	14.6	(14.3 to 14.8)
Chronic kidney disease	3.3	(3.1 to 3.5)	2.2	(2.1 to 2.3)
Diabetes	11.1	(10.8 to 11.4)	8.6	(8.4 to 8.8)

Abbreviations: CI = confidence interval.
Age-adjusted to the 2000 U.S. standard population.
The prevalence of each condition is significantly higher (p<0.05) for persons reporting short sleep compared with those reporting sufficient sleep.

Short Sleep Duration among High-School Students

Adolescents need 8 to 10 hours of sleep per night. But, more than two-thirds of U.S. high-school students report getting less than 8 hours of sleep on school nights (see Table 11.4). Female students are more likely to report not getting enough sleep than male students. Short sleep duration (less than 8 hours) is lowest among ninth graders and highest among twelfth graders. Prevalence of short sleep duration also varies by race/ethnicity, with the lowest prevalence among American Indian/Alaska Native students and the highest among Asian students.

Table 11.4. Short Sleep Duration by Selected Characteristics— Youth Risk Behavior Survey, United States, 2007 to 2013

Characteristic	Short Sleep Duration (Less Than 8 Hours)	
	Percentage (Weighted Percentages)	95 Percentage Confidence Interval
Total	68.8	(68.0 to 69.6)
Survey year		
2007	69	(67.0 to 70.9)
2009	69.1	(67.5 to 70.6)
2011	68.6	(67.2 to 69.9)
2013	68.4	(66.9 to 69.9)
Sex		
Female	71.3	(70.4 to 72.1)
Male	66.4	(65.4 to 67.4)
Grade		
9th	59.7	(58.6 to 60.8)
10th	67.4	(66.1 to 68.8)
11th	73.3	(72.0 to 74.5)
12th	76.6	(75.4 to 77.8)
Race/ethnicity		
White*	68.3	(67.3 to 69.4)
Black*	71.2	(69.9 to 72.5)
Hispanic	67	(65.5 to 68.5)
American Indian/Alaska Native*	60.3	(52.4 to 67.6)
Asian*	75.7	(72.7 to 78.5)
Native Hawaiian/Pacific Islander*	68.3	(62.1 to 73.9)
Multiracial*	72	(69.2 to 74.7)

* Non-Hispanic

Section 11.3

Sleep Deprivation: What Does It Mean for Public Safety Officers?

This section includes text excerpted from "Sleep Deprivation: What Does It Mean for Public Safety Officers?," National Institute of Justice (NIJ), U.S. Department of Justice (DOJ), March 27, 2009. Reviewed May 2019.

Scheduling and staffing around the clock requires finding a way to balance each organization's unique needs with those of its officers. Questions such as "How many hours in a row should officers work?" and "How many officers are needed on which shift?" need to be balanced against "How much time off do officers need to rest and recuperate properly?" and "What is the best way to schedule those hours to keep employees safe and performing well?" After all, shift work interferes with normal sleep and forces people to work at unnatural times of the day when their bodies are programmed to sleep. Sleep-loss-related fatigue degrades performance, productivity, and safety, as well as health and well-being. Fatigue costs the U.S. economy $136 billion per year in health-related lost productivity alone.

Many managers in policing and corrections have begun to acknowledge—such as their counterparts in other industries—that rotating shift work is inherently dangerous, especially when one works the graveyard shift. Managers in aviation, railroading and trucking, for example, have had mandated hours-of-work laws for decades. They have begun to use complex mathematical models to manage fatigue-related risks.

All of us experience the everyday stress associated with family life, health, and finances. Most of us also feel work-related stress associated with bad supervisors, long commutes, inadequate equipment and difficult assignments. But, police and corrections officers also must deal with the stresses of working shifts, witnessing or experiencing trauma, and managing dangerous confrontations.

John Violanti, Ph.D., is a 23-year veteran of the New York State Police, a professor in the Department of Social and Preventive Medicine at the University at Buffalo, and an instructor with the Law Enforcement Wellness Association. His research shows that law enforcement officers are dying earlier than they should. The average age of death for police officers in his 40-year study was 66 years of age—a full 10 years sooner than the norm. He and other researchers also found that police officers were much more likely than the general public to have higher-than-recommended cholesterol levels, higher-than-average pulse rates and diastolic blood pressure, and much higher prevalence of sleep disorders.

So, what can be done to make police work healthier?

Many things. One of the most effective strategies is to get enough sleep. More than half of police officers fail to get adequate rest, and they have 44 percent higher levels of obstructive sleep apnea (OSA) than the general public. More than 90 percent report being routinely fatigued, and 85 percent report driving while drowsy.

Sleep deprivation is dangerous. Researchers have shown that being awake for 19 hours produces impairments that are comparable to having a blood alcohol concentration (BAC) of .05 percent. Being awake for 24 hours is comparable to having a BAC of roughly 10 percent. This means that in just 5 hours—the difference between going without sleep for 19 hours versus 24 hours—the impact essentially doubles. (It should be noted that, in all 50 states and the District of Columbia, it is a crime to drive with a BAC of .08% or above.)

If you work a 10-hour shift, then attend court, then pick up your kids from school, drive home (hoping you do not fall asleep at the wheel), catch a couple hours of sleep, then get up and go back to work—and you do this for a week—you may be driving your patrol car while just as impaired as the last person you arrested for driving under the influence (DUI).

Bars and taverns are legally liable for serving too many drinks to people who then drive, have an accident, and kill someone. There is precedent for trucking companies and other employers being held responsible for drivers who cause accidents after working longer than permitted. It seems very likely that police departments eventually will be held responsible if an officer causes a death because he was too tired to drive home safely.

Sleep and fatigue are basic survival issues, just like patrol tactics, firearms safety, and pursuit driving. To reduce risks, stay alive, and keep healthy, officers and their managers have to work together to manage fatigue. Too-tired cops put themselves, their fellow officers, and the communities they serve at risk.

Accidental Deaths and Fatigue

The number of police officer deaths from both felonious assaults and accidents has decreased over the years. Contrary to what most people might think, however, more officers die as a result of accidents than criminal assaults. 91 percent of accidental deaths are caused by car crashes, being hit by vehicles while on foot, aircraft accidents, falls, or jumping.

It is known that the rate of these accidents increases with lack of sleep and time of day. Researchers have shown that the risk increases considerably after a person has been on duty 9 hours or more. After 10 hours on duty, the risk increases by approximately 90 percent; after 12 hours, 110 percent. The night shift has the greatest risk for accidents; they are almost 3 times more likely to happen during the night shift than the morning shift.

Countering Fatigue

Researchers who study officer stress, sleep, and performance have a number of techniques to counteract sleep deprivation and stress. They fall into two types:

- Things managers can do
- Things officers can do

The practices listed below have been well-received by departments that recognize that a tired cop is a danger both to her- or himself and to the public.

Things Managers Can Do

Review policies that affect overtime, moonlighting, and the number of consecutive hours a person can work. Make sure the policies keep shift rotation to a minimum and give officers adequate rest time. The Albuquerque (N.M.) Police Department, for example, prohibits officers from working more than 16 hours a day and limits overtime to 20 hours per week. This practice earned the Albuquerque team the Healthy Sleep Capital award from the National Sleep Foundation (NSF).

Give officers a voice in decisions related to their work hours and shift scheduling. People's work hours affect every aspect of their lives. Increasing the amount of control and predictability in one's life improves a host of psychological and physical characteristics, including job satisfaction.

Formally assess the level of fatigue officers experience, the quality of their sleep, and how tired they are while on the job, as well as their attitudes toward fatigue and work hours issues. Strategies include administering sleep quality tests, such as those available on the National Sleep Foundation's website (www.sleepfoundation.org), and training supervisors to be alert for signs that officers are overly tired (for example, falling asleep during a watch briefing) and on how to deal with those who are too fatigued to work safely.

Several Canadian police departments are including sleep screening in officers' annual assessments—something that every department should consider.

Create a culture in which officers receive adequate information about the importance of good sleep habits, the hazards associated with fatigue and shift work, and strategies for managing them. For example, the Seattle Police Department has scheduled an all-day fatigue countermeasures training course for every sergeant, lieutenant, and captain. In the Calgary Police Service, management and union leaders are conducting a long-term, research-based program to find the best shift and scheduling arrangements and to change cultural attitudes about sleep and fatigue.

Things Officers Can Do

- **Stay physically fit.** Get enough exercise, maintain a healthy body weight, eat several fruits and vegetables a day, and stop smoking.

- **Learn to use caffeine effectively by restricting routine intake** to the equivalent of one or two eight-ounce cups of coffee a day. When you need to combat drowsiness, drink only one cup every hour or two; stop doses well before bedtime.

- **Exercise proper sleep hygiene.** In other words, do everything possible to get seven or more hours of sleep every day. For example, go to sleep at the same time every day as much as possible; avoid alcohol just before bedtime; use room darkening curtains; make your bedroom a place for sleep, not for doing work or watching television. Do not just doze off in an easy chair or on the sofa with the television on.

If you have not been able to get enough sleep, try to take a nap before your shift. Done properly, a 20-minute catnap is proven to improve performance, elevate mood, and increase creativity.

If you are frequently fatigued, drowsy, snore, or have a large build, ask your doctor to check you for sleep apnea. Because many physicians have little training in sleep issues, it is a good idea to see someone who specializes in sleep medicine.

Section 11.4

Sleep Deprivation Affects Athletes

"Sleep Deprivation Affects Sports Performance,"
© 2017 Omnigraphics. Reviewed May 2019.

According to the National Institutes of Health (NIH), although there is still much that is not known about sleep, we do know that sleep is crucial to human physiology and cognition. Lack of sleep may cause autonomic nervous system imbalance, increase stress levels, and decrease glycogen and carbohydrate production. In athletes, reduced sleep can lead to a lack of energy, poor focus, fatigue, and slow recovery after a game.

Sports place a lot of demand on the muscles and tissues, depleting energy and fluids and breaking down muscle. Sleep helps the body recover quicker, repairs memory, and releases essential hormones. In sports, a split-second decision can make the difference between a win and a loss. And research indicates that poor sleep results in a decline in quick decision-making, while the proper amount of sleep shows an increase in this ability.

Effects of Sleep Deprivation

Reduced sleep can cause a decline in athletic performance, cognition, and immune function, and an increase in weight. The amount of sleep required for any given athlete depends on genetic factors, conditioning, and the level of physical activity demanded by the sport. Adolescence is a period of growth in which sleep is vital. However, it has become increasingly clear from research that most teens do not get the proper amount of sleep. Studies suggest that an average of ten hours of sleep per night can boost athletic performance. Athletes tend to focus on training and practice to achieve success; however, sleep has too often been an overlooked factor. Listed below are a few effects of lack of sleep:

- **Lower attention span.** Inability to stay focused on the game.

- **Decreased reaction time.** Overall reaction time is vital to athletic performance.

- **Longer recovery.** Some physical activities demand more energy; recovery and healing are slower when sleep is lost.

- **Higher cortisol levels.** High levels of the stress hormone cortisol can hinder tissue repair and growth. Over time, this may prevent an athlete from responding well to heavy training and may also lead to overtraining.

- **Lack of endurance.** Glycogen (stored glucose) is the main source of energy that is needed for endurance. Sleep deprivation causes slower storage of glycogen, preventing athletes from performing well in endurance events.

How Sleep Can Improve Sports Performance

Studies suggest that increased sleep enables better sports performance. Some benefits of proper sleep are noted below.

- In a study, basketball players who got an extra two hours of sleep per night tended to increase their speed by five percent and accuracy by nine percent.

- Athletes who sleep an average of eight to nine hours nightly are better able to perform high-intensity workouts, such as weight-lifting, running, or biking.

- Mental strain is a part of any sport. Sleep will help athletes improve their mood, memory, and alertness.

- Players have better reaction time and reflexes.

- Training and practice can cause physical exhaustion. The proper amount of sleep helps the body restore muscle and other tissue.

- Sleep promotes better coordination. While sleeping, the body recalls and consolidates memories linked to the motor skills that were practiced.

Sleep Tips for Athletes

Athletes have tight schedules when it comes to training and practice. However, experts say that as much as an athlete needs practice, so does she or he need sleep. Since the body is pushed on a regular basis, in order to recover, it needs rest and time. Below are a few tips that can help an athlete get better sleep.

- Establish a regular schedule for going to bed and waking up at the same time every day.

- Since traveling can upset sleep, it is best to get to the place of the competition two or three days early in order to allow the body adjust.

- Sleep medication should be avoided, unless prescribed by a doctor, since it can disturb the quality of sleep and hinder performance.

- It is best to avoid caffeine and alcohol, because they can disrupt healthful sleep patterns.

- Natural relaxation techniques, such as deep breathing or listening to soft music, can help promote sleep.

References

1. Fullagar, HH, S. Skorski, R. Duffield, D. Hammes, A.J. Coutts, and T. Meyer. "Sleep and Athletic Performance: The Effects of Sleep Loss on Exercise Performance, and Physiological and Cognitive Responses to Exercise," U.S. National Library of Medicine (NLM), February, 2015.

2. Griffin, R. Morgan. "Can Sleep Improve Your Athletic Performance?" WebMD, August 13, 2014.

3. "How Sleep Affects Athletes' Performance," Sleep.org, n.d.

4. Quinn, Elizabeth. "Sleep Deprivation and Athletes," Verywell. com, October 5, 2017.

5. Sherwood, Chris. "Does a Lack of Sleep Affect an Athlete's Performance?" Livestrong.com, August 14, 2017.

6. "Sleep and Athletes," Gatorade Sports Science Institute (GSSI), n.d.

7. "Sleep, Athletic Performance, and Recovery," National Sleep Foundation (NSF), n.d.

Chapter 12

Why Your Body and Brain Need Sleep

Chapter Contents

Section 12.1

Sleep for Good Health and Well-Being

This section includes text excerpted from "Sleep Deprivation and Deficiency," National Heart, Lung, and Blood Institute (NHLBI), April 22, 2019.

Sleep plays a vital role in good health and well-being throughout your life. Getting enough quality sleep at the right times can help protect your mental health, physical health, quality of life (QOL), and safety.

The way you feel while you are awake depends in part on what happens while you are sleeping. During sleep, your body is working to support healthy brain function and maintain your physical health. In children and teens, sleep also helps support growth and development.

The damage from sleep deficiency can occur in an instant (such as a car crash), or it can harm you over time. For example, ongoing sleep deficiency can raise your risk for some chronic health problems. It also can affect how well you think, react, work, learn, and get along with others.

Healthy Brain Function and Emotional Well-Being

Sleep helps your brain work properly. While you are sleeping, your brain is preparing for the next day. It is forming new pathways to help you learn and remember information.

Studies show that a good night's sleep improves learning. Whether you are learning math, how to play the piano, how to perfect your golf swing, or how to drive a car, sleep helps enhance your learning and problem-solving skills. Sleep also helps you pay attention, make decisions, and be creative.

Studies also show that sleep deficiency alters activity in some parts of the brain. If you are sleep deficient, you may have trouble making decisions, solving problems, controlling your emotions and behavior, and coping with change. Sleep deficiency also has been linked to depression, suicide, and risk-taking behavior.

Children and teens who are sleep deficient may have problems getting along with others. They may feel angry and impulsive, have mood swings, feel sad or depressed, or lack motivation. They also may have problems paying attention, and they may get lower grades and feel stressed.

Physical Health

Sleep plays an important role in your physical health. For example, sleep is involved in the healing and repairing of your heart and blood vessels. Ongoing sleep deficiency is linked to an increased risk of heart disease, kidney disease, high blood pressure, diabetes, and stroke.

Risk of obesity. Sleep deficiency also increases the risk of obesity. For example, one study of teenagers showed that with each hour of sleep lost, the odds of becoming obese went up. Sleep deficiency increases the risk of obesity in other age groups as well.

Sleep helps maintain a healthy balance of the hormones that make you feel hungry (ghrelin) or full (leptin). When you do not get enough sleep, your level of ghrelin goes up and your level of leptin goes down. This makes you feel hungrier than when you are well-rested.

Diabetes risk. Sleep also affects how your body reacts to insulin, the hormone that controls your blood glucose (sugar) level. Sleep deficiency results in a higher than normal blood sugar level, which may increase your risk for diabetes.

Growth and development. Sleep also supports healthy growth and development. Deep sleep triggers the body to release the hormone that promotes normal growth in children and teens. This hormone also boosts muscle mass and helps repair cells and tissues in children, teens, and adults. Sleep also plays a role in puberty and fertility.

Immunity. Your immune system relies on sleep to stay healthy. This system defends your body against foreign or harmful substances. Ongoing sleep deficiency can change the way in which your immune system responds. For example, if you are sleep deficient, you may have trouble fighting common infections.

Section 12.2

How Does Sleep Affect Your Heart Health?

This section includes text excerpted from "How Does
Sleep Affect Your Heart Health?" Centers for Disease
Control and Prevention (CDC), December 3, 2018.

Getting good sleep is not just important for your energy levels—it is
critical for your heart health too. Sleep is not a luxury. It is critical to
good health. Sleep helps your body repair itself. Getting enough good
sleep also helps you function normally during the day.

How Much Sleep Do You Need?

Most adults need at least seven hours of sleep each night. However,
more than one in three American adults say they do not get the recommended amount of sleep. While this may be fine for a day or two,
not getting enough sleep over time can lead to serious health problems
and make certain health problems worse.

What Health Conditions Are Linked to a Lack of Sleep?

Adults who sleep less than seven hours each night are more
likely to say they have had health problems, including heart attack,
asthma, and depression. Some of these health problems raise the risk
of heart disease, heart attack, and stroke. These health problems
include:

- **High blood pressure.** During normal sleep, your blood
  pressure goes down. Having sleep problems means your blood
  pressure stays higher for a longer amount of time. High blood
  pressure is one of the leading risks for heart disease and stroke.
  About 75 million Americans—1 in 3 adults—have high blood
  pressure.

- **Type 2 diabetes.** Diabetes is a disease that causes sugar to
  build up in your blood, a condition that can damage your blood
  vessels. Some studies show that getting enough good sleep may
  help people improve blood sugar control.

- **Obesity.** Lack of sleep can lead to unhealthy weight gain. This
  is especially true for children and adolescents, who need more

sleep than adults. Not getting enough sleep may affect a part of the brain that controls hunger.

What Sleep Conditions Can Hurt Your Heart Health?

Over time, sleep problems can hurt your heart health. Sleep apnea happens when your airway gets blocked repeatedly during sleep, causing you to stop breathing for short amounts of time. Sleep apnea can be caused by certain health problems, such as obesity and heart failure.

Sleep apnea affects how much oxygen your body gets while you sleep and increases the risk for many health problems, including high blood pressure, heart attack, and stroke. It is more common among Blacks, Hispanics, and Native Americans than among Whites.

Insomnia is trouble falling asleep, staying asleep, or both. As many as 1 in 2 adults experience short-term insomnia at some point, and 1 in 10 may have long-lasting insomnia. Insomnia is linked to high blood pressure and heart disease. Over time, poor sleep can also lead to unhealthy habits that can hurt your heart, including higher stress levels, less motivation to be physically active, and unhealthy food choices.

Section 12.3

Molecular Ties between Lack of Sleep and Weight Gain

This section includes text excerpted from "Molecular Ties between Lack of Sleep and Weight Gain," News and Events, National Institutes of Health (NIH), March 22, 2016.

A poor night's sleep can leave you feeling foggy and drowsy throughout the day. Sleep deprivation has also been associated with higher risks of weight gain and obesity in recent years.

A group led by Drs. Erin Hanlon and Eve Van Cauter at the University of Chicago wanted to better understand how sleep and weight gain interact biologically. They noticed that sleep deprivation has effects in the body similar to activation of the endocannabinoid (eCB) system, a key player in the brain's regulation of appetite and energy levels. Perhaps most well-known for being activated by chemicals found in marijuana, the eCB system affects the brain's motivation and reward circuits and can spark a desire for tasty foods.

The researchers enrolled 14 healthy, nonobese people—11 men and 3 women—who were between the ages of 18 and 30. The participants were placed on a fixed diet and allowed either a normal 8.5 hours of sleep or a restricted 4.5 hours of sleep for 4 consecutive days. All participants underwent both sleep conditions in a controlled clinical setting, with at least 4 weeks in between testing. For both conditions, the researchers collected blood samples from the participants beginning the afternoon following the second night.

When sleep deprived, participants had eCB levels in the afternoons that were both higher and lasted longer than when they had a full night's rest. This occurred around the same time that they reported increases in hunger and appetite.

After dinner on the fourth night, the participants fasted until the next afternoon. They were then allowed to choose their own meals and snacks for the rest of the day. All food was prepared and served in the clinical setting. Under both sleep conditions, people consumed about 90 percent of their daily calories at their first meal. But when sleep deprived, they consumed more and unhealthier snacks in between meals. This is when eCB levels were at their highest, suggesting that eCBs were driving hedonic, or pleasurable, eating.

Hanlon explains that if you see junk food and you have had enough sleep, you may be able to control some aspects of your natural response. "But if you are sleep deprived, your hedonic drive for certain foods gets stronger, and your ability to resist them may be impaired. So, you are more likely to eat it. Do that again and again, and you pack on the pounds."

The authors noted that though the results are based on a small sample size, they are consistent with evidence from other research. Additional studies are needed to look at how changes in eCB levels and timing are affected by other cues, such as the body's internal clock or meal schedules.

The study was supported in part by the National Institutes of Health's (NIH) National Center for Research Resources (NCRR) and National Heart, Lung, and Blood Institute (NHLBI). Results were published in the March 2016 issue of *Sleep*.

Section 12.4

How Sleep Clears the Brain

This section includes text excerpted from "How Sleep Clears the Brain," News and Events, National Institutes of Health (NIH), October 28, 2013. Reviewed May 2019.

A mouse study suggests that sleep helps restore the brain by flushing out toxins that build up during waking hours. The results point to a potential new role for sleep in health and disease.

Scientists and philosophers have long wondered why people sleep and how it affects the brain. Sleep is important for storing memories. It also has a restorative function. Lack of sleep impairs reasoning, problem-solving, and attention to detail, among other effects. However, the mechanisms behind these sleep benefits have been unknown.

Dr. Maiken Nedergaard and her colleagues at the University of Rochester Medical Center recently discovered a system that drains waste products from the brain. Cerebrospinal fluid, a clear liquid surrounding the brain and spinal cord, moves through the brain along a series of channels that surround blood vessels. The system is managed by the brain's glial cells, and so the researchers called it the "glymphatic system."

The scientists also reported that the glymphatic system can help remove a toxic protein called "beta-amyloid" from brain tissue. Beta-amyloid is renowned for accumulating in the brains of patients with Alzheimer disease (AD). Other research has shown that brain levels of beta-amyloid decrease during sleep. In their study, the team tested the idea that sleep might affect beta-amyloid clearance by regulating the glymphatic system. The work was funded by the National Institutes of Health's (NIH) National Institute of Neurological Disorders and Stroke (NINDS).

The researchers first injected dye into the cerebrospinal fluid of mice and monitored electrical brain activity as they tracked the dye flow through the animals' brains. As reported in the October 18, 2013 edition of *Science*, the dye barely flowed when the mice were awake. In contrast, when the mice were unconscious—asleep or anesthetized—it flowed rapidly.

Changes in the way fluid move through the brain between conscious and unconscious states may reflect differences in the space available for movement. To test the idea, the team used a method that measures the volume of the space outside brain cells. They found that this "extracellular" volume increased by 60 percent in the brain's cortex when the mice were asleep or anesthetized.

The researchers next injected mice with labeled beta-amyloid and measured how long it lasted in their brains when they were asleep and awake. Beta-amyloid disappeared twice as quickly in the brains of mice that were asleep.

Glial cells control flow through the glymphatic system by shrinking and swelling. The hormone noradrenaline, which increases alertness, is known to cause cells to swell. The researchers thus, tested whether the hormone might affect the glymphatic system. Treating mice with drugs that block noradrenaline induced a sleep-like state and increased brain fluid flow and extracellular brain volume. This result suggests a molecular connection between the sleep–wake cycle and the brain's cleaning system.

The study raises the possibility that certain neurological disorders might be prevented or treated by manipulating the glymphatic system. "These findings have significant implications for treating 'dirty brain' diseases like Alzheimer," Nedergaard says. "Understanding precisely how and when the brain activates the glymphatic system and clears waste is a critical first step in efforts to potentially modulate this system and make it work more efficiently."

Section 12.5

Making Up Sleep May Not Help

This section includes text excerpted from "Making Up Sleep May Not Help," *NIH News in Health*, National Institutes of Health (NIH), May 2019.

Catching up on sleep does not reverse damage to the body caused by sleep deprivation, according to a new study. In fact, so-called "recovery sleep" may make some things worse. About one of every three adults regularly gets less than seven hours of sleep a night. Over time, lack of sleep can lead to changes in metabolism. These increase the risk for obesity and diabetes.

Some people try to make up for a lack of sleep by sleeping more on their days off. A research team studied this strategy for 2 weeks in 36 men and women. After 3 nights of normal sleep, the participants were split into 3 groups. The first group slept up to 9 hours a night. The second group was allowed a maximum of 5 hours of sleep a night. The third group had a maximum of 5 hours a night for 5 days but were then allowed to sleep in for 2 days. They then had 2 more days of sleep deprivation.

Those who had only 5 hours of sleep a night gained about 3 pounds on average during the study. They also had a 13 percent decrease in a key measure of metabolism called "insulin sensitivity." Insulin sensitivity is the body's ability to use insulin properly and control blood sugar levels.

Those who had recovery sleep gained about 3 pounds but had a 27 percent decrease in insulin sensitivity. Their natural body rhythms were also disrupted. They were more likely to wake up during the nights following the period of recovery sleep. "Catch-up sleep does not appear to be an effective strategy to reverse sleep loss-induced disruptions of metabolism," says Dr. Kenneth Wright, Jr., who led the study at the University of Colorado.

Chapter 13

Sleep and Health of Middle- and High-School Students

Adequate sleep contributes to a student's overall health and well-being. Students should get the proper amount of sleep at night to help stay focused, improve concentration, and improve academic performance. Children and adolescents who do not get enough sleep have a higher risk for many health problems, including obesity, diabetes, poor mental health, and injuries. They are also more likely to have attention and behavior problems, which can contribute to poor academic performance in school.

How Much Sleep Do Students Need?

How much sleep someone needs depends on their age. The recommendations made by the American Academy of Sleep Medicine (AASM) for children and adolescents is shown in the following table.

This chapter includes text excerpted from "Sleep and Health," Centers for Disease Control and Prevention (CDC), September 18, 2018.

Table 13.1. Recommended Hours of Sleep Per Day for Children and Adolescents

Age Group	Recommended Hours of Sleep Per Day
6 to 12 years	9 to 12 hours per 24 hours
13 to 18 years	8 to 10 hours per 24 hours

Insufficient Sleep among Students

The data from the 2015 national and state Youth Risk Behavior Surveys, a Centers for Disease Control and Prevention (CDC) study, shows that a majority of middle-school and high-school students reported getting less than the recommended amount of sleep for their age.

Middle-school students (grades 6 to 8):

- Students in 9 states were included in the study.

- About 6 out of 10 students (57.8%) did not get enough sleep on school nights.

High-school students (grades 9 to 12):

- National sample

- About 7 out of 10 students (72.7%) did not get enough sleep on school nights.

What Schools Can Do
Provide Sleep Education

Schools can add sleep education to the K–12 curriculum to help children and adolescents learn why sleep is important to maintain a healthy lifestyle. Lessons in sleep patterns and sleep disorders, snoring, drowsy driving, and insomnia are among topics teachers can cover in the classroom to help students develop healthy sleep habits.

Sleep education programs in school may result in significantly longer weekday and weekend total sleep time and improved sleep hygiene (habits that support good sleep) after completion. However, more research is needed to determine how best to maintain these improvements long term. One possible strategy is to incorporate refresher sessions for students.

Review School Start Times

The combination of late bedtimes and early school start times results in most adolescents not getting enough sleep. In recent years, evidence has accumulated that later school start times for adolescents result in more students getting enough sleep.

School officials can learn more about the research connecting sleep and school start times. School districts can support adequate sleep among students by implementing delayed school start times as recommended by the American Academy of Pediatrics (AAP), the American Medical Association (AMA), and the AASM.

In 2014, the AAP recommended that middle schools and high schools start no earlier than 8:30 a.m. in order to allow adolescents to get the sleep they need. The AMA, the AASM, and other medical associations have since expressed support of delaying school start times for adolescents.

Good sleep hygiene in combination with later school times will enable adolescents to be healthier and better academic achievers.

What Parents Can Do

Model and encourage habits that help promote good sleep. Setting a regular bedtime and rise time, including on weekends, is recommended for everyone—children, adolescents, and adults alike. Adolescents with parent-set bedtimes usually get more sleep than those whose parents do not set bedtimes.

Dim lighting. Adolescents who are exposed to more light (such as room lighting or from electronics) in the evening are less likely to get enough sleep.

Implement a media curfew. Technology use (computers, video gaming, or mobile phones) may also contribute to late bedtimes. Parents should consider banning technology use after a certain time or removing these technologies from the bedroom.

What Healthcare Professionals Can Do

Healthcare professionals can educate adolescent patients and their parents about the importance of adequate sleep and factors that contribute to insufficient sleep among adolescents.

Chapter 14

Sleep Deprivation and Learning

The Learning Process and Sleep

Learning, sleep, and memory are interconnected processes that are not yet fully understood. The main function of sleep has generally been thought to be related to learning and memory, and research on humans and animals indicates that both the quality and quantity of sleep can impact those functions. Adequate sleep is required for the body and mind to repair and replenish energy. Sleep deprivation can, therefore, have a negative impact on the cognitive capacity of the brain. It can hinder spatial learning, along with other functions, such as memory, attention span, and reaction time. It can also take a toll on general health and the immune system, and in extreme cases may even result in hallucinations.

Learning and memory are characterized by three phases: acquisition, consolidation, and recall. During acquisition, the brain is fully alert and gathering new information. Consolidation occurs when a person is at rest, and the brain solidifies the freshly acquired information. The last phase, recall, is the process of retrieving stored information when the person is awake.

Though it is only during waking hours that acquisition and recall take place, research shows that memory consolidation, through the

"Sleep Deprivation and Learning," © 2016 Omnigraphics. Reviewed May 2019.

strengthening of neural connections, occurs during sleep. It is still not clear how this process takes place, but it is hypothesized by many researchers that certain characteristics of brainwaves at different sleep stages aid in the formation of memory.

Sleep researchers take two approaches when studying the effect of sleep on learning and memory. The first explores the various stages of sleep and changes in duration as they affect learning new tasks, and the second analyzes the impact of sleep deprivation on learning.

Sleep Stages and Types of Memory

Every learning situation provides different types of memories to be consolidated into the brain. Scientists, through various studies, are investigating the relationship between the consolidation of these types of memories and the stages of sleep. There is, however, speculation that it is most efficient for the brain to form strong neural connections and pathways during sleep, when there is little new information or external stimuli to process.

Lack of adequate sleep can impact attention and short-term (working) memory, thereby affecting retention of long-term (episodic) memories and also higher cognitive functions, such as reasoning and decision-making. Numerous studies have demonstrated how sleep promotes long-term memory processing, which includes both consolidation of short-term memory into long-term memory, and also reconsolidation of existing long-term memories.

Long-term memory can be classified into two main types: procedural memory (the unconscious storage of skills and the way we accomplish tasks) and declarative memory (the storage of facts and events). Studies show that rapid eye movement (REM) sleep, which usually occurs during the last two hours of sleep, benefits procedural memory, whereas deep slow-wave sleep (SWS), which occurs before REM sleep, benefits declarative memory. Other aspects that play an important role include motor learning, which seems to be dependent on lighter stages of non-REM sleep, and a few types of visual learning that seem to rely on timing and duration of both SWS and REM sleep. REM sleep has also been shown to aid in the retention of emotionally charged declarative memory.

Impact of Sleep Deprivation on Learning

Scientists are also examining the impact that sleep deprivation has on learning and the formation of new memories. Lack of adequate sleep can be partial (deprivation of either early or late sleep), total (no sleep at all), or selective (deprivation of specific stages of sleep).

Sleep deprivation can lead to poor focus, which makes it difficult to grasp information. It also causes the neurons to over-work, which in turn impairs the brain's ability to coordinate information. As a result, one's ability to recall previously stored information is affected. Furthermore, the interpretation of events and the capacity to make logical decisions may also be impeded.

Without proper rest, the body can feel tired to the extreme point of exhaustion. At such a stage, the muscles can weaken from lack of sleep, the body's organs are not synchronized, and neurons do not function optimally. Poor sleep can also have a negative impact on mood, which may affect the ability to acquire and retain new pieces of information. Although the effects of chronic sleep deprivation are not the same in each individual, it is evident that resting well has a profound impact on learning and memory.

References

1. "Sleep, Learning, and Memory," Division of Sleep Medicine, Harvard Medical School, December 18, 2007.

2. Mastin, Luke. "Why Do We Sleep? Memory Processing and Learning," howsleepworks.com, n.d.

3. Renee. "The Surprising Relationship between Sleep and Learning," Udemy.com, January 26, 2012.

Chapter 15

Drowsy Driving

Chapter Contents

Section 15.1

Drowsy Driving: An Overview

This section includes text excerpted from "Drowsy Driving," Centers for Disease Control and Prevention (CDC), March 21, 2017.

Drowsy driving is a major problem in the United States. The risk, danger, and sometimes tragic results of drowsy driving are alarming. Drowsy driving is the dangerous combination of driving and sleepiness or fatigue. This usually happens when a driver has not slept enough, but it can also happen due to untreated sleep disorders, medications, drinking alcohol, and shift work.

What Is Drowsy Driving?

Operating a motor vehicle while fatigued or sleepy is commonly referred to as "drowsy driving." Drowsy driving poses a serious risk not only for one's own health and safety, but also for the other people on the road. The National Highway Traffic Safety Administration (NHTSA) estimates that between 2005 and 2009 drowsy driving was responsible for an annual average of:

- 83,000 crashes
- 37,000 injury crashes
- 886 fatal crashes (846 fatalities in 2014)

These estimates are conservative, though, and up to 6,000 fatal crashes each year may be caused by drowsy drivers.

How Often Do Americans Fall Asleep While Driving?

Approximately 1 out of 25 adults 18 years of age and older surveyed reported that they had fallen asleep while driving in the past 30 days. Individuals who snored or slept 6 hours or less per day were more likely to fall asleep while driving.

How Does Sleepiness Affect Driving?

Falling asleep at the wheel is very dangerous, but being sleepy affects your ability to drive safely even if you do not fall asleep. Drowsiness:

- Makes drivers less attentive
- Slows reaction time
- Affects a driver's ability to make decisions

What Are the Warning Signs of Drowsy Driving?

The following are the warning signs of drowsy driving:

- Yawning or blinking frequently
- Difficulty remembering the past few miles driven
- Missing your exit
- Drifting from your lane
- Hitting a rumble strip

If you experience any of the warning signs of drowsy driving while driving, pull over to a safe place and take a nap for 15 to 20 minutes or change drivers. Simply turning up the radio or opening the window are not effective ways to keep you alert.

Who Is More Likely to Drive Drowsy?

Those who are more likely to be involved in drowsy driving include:

- Drivers who do not get enough sleep
- Commercial drivers who operate vehicles, such as tow trucks, tractor trailers, and buses
- Shift workers (work the night shift or long shifts)
- Drivers with untreated sleep disorders, such as one where breathing repeatedly stops and starts (sleep apnea)
- Drivers who use medications that make them sleepy

How to Prevent Drowsy Driving

There are four things you should do before taking the wheel to prevent driving while drowsy.

- **Get enough sleep.** Most adults need at least seven hours of sleep a day, while adolescents need at least eight hours.

- **Develop good sleeping habits**, such as sticking to a sleep schedule.

- **Seek treatment.** If you have a sleep disorder or have symptoms of a sleep disorder, such as snoring or feeling sleepy during the day, talk to your physician about treatment options.

- **Avoid drinking alcohol or taking medications that make you sleepy.** Be sure to check the label on any medications or talk to your pharmacist.

Drowsy Driving Is Similar to Drunk Driving

Your body needs adequate sleep on a daily basis. The more hours of sleep you miss, the harder it is for you to think and perform as well as you would like. Lack of sleep can make you less alert and affect your coordination, judgment, and reaction time while driving. This is known as "cognitive impairment."

Studies have shown that going too long without sleep can impair your ability to drive the same way as drinking too much alcohol.

- Being awake for at least 18 hours is the same as someone having a blood content (BAC) of 0.05 percent.

- Being awake for at least 24 hours is equal to having a blood alcohol content of 0.10 percent. This is higher than the legal limit (0.08% BAC) in all states.

Additionally, drowsiness increases the effect of even low amounts of alcohol.

Section 15.2

Some Sleep Drugs Can Impair Driving

This section includes text excerpted from "Some Sleep Drugs Can Impair Driving," U.S. Food and Drug Administration (FDA), January 10, 2013. Reviewed May 2019.

Many people take sedatives to help them sleep. The U.S. Food and Drug Administration (FDA) is reminding consumers that some drugs to treat insomnia could make them less able the next morning to perform activities for which they must be fully alert, including driving a car.

The U.S. Food and Drug Administration has informed manufacturers that the recommended dose should be lowered for sleep drugs approved for bedtime use that contain a medicine called "zolpidem." The FDA is also evaluating the risk of next-morning impairment in other insomnia medications.

People with insomnia have trouble falling or staying asleep. Zolpidem, which belongs to a class of medications called "sedative-hypnotics," is a common ingredient in widely prescribed sleep medications. Some sleep drugs contain an extended-release form of zolpidem that stays in the body longer than the regular form.

The U.S. Food and Drug Administration is particularly concerned about extended-release forms of zolpidem. They are sold as generic drugs and under the brand name "Ambien CR." Data show that the morning after use, many people who take products containing extended-release zolpidem have drug levels that are high enough to impair driving and other activities. The FDA says that women are especially vulnerable because zolpidem is cleared from the body more slowly in women than in men.

The U.S. Food and Drug Administration also found that some medicines containing the immediate-release form of zolpidem can impair driving and other activities the next morning. They are marketed as generic drugs and under the following brand names:

- Ambien (oral tablet)
- Edluar (tablet placed under the tongue)
- Zolpimist (oral spray)

The U.S. Food and Drug Administration has informed the manufacturers of products containing zolpidem that the recommended dose for women for both immediate- and extended-release products should be lowered. FDA is also suggesting a lower dose range for men.

Drowsiness is already listed as a side effect in the drug labels of insomnia drugs, along with warnings that patients may still feel drowsy the day after taking these products. However, people with high levels of zolpidem in their blood can be impaired even if they feel wide awake. "All insomnia drugs are potent medications, and they must be used carefully" says Russell Katz, M.D., Director of the FDA's Division of Neurology Products (DNP).

Recommended Doses

The U.S. Food and Drug Administration has informed manufacturers that changes to the dosage recommendations for the use of zolpidem products should be made:

- **For women,** the dose should be cut in half, from 10 mg to 5 mg for products containing the regular form of zolpidem (Ambien, Edluar, Zolpimist) and from 12.5 mg to 6.25 mg for zolpidem extended-release products (Ambien CR).

- **For men,** the lower dose of 5 mg for immediate-release zolpidem and 6.25 mg for extended-release should be considered.

Intermezzo, an approved drug containing zolpidem, is used when middle-of-the-night wakening is followed by difficulty returning to sleep and at least 4 hours remain available for sleep. The recommended dose for Intermezzo remains at 1.75 mg for women and 3.5 mg for men.

Most Widely Used Sleep Drug

Zolpidem—which has been on the market for nearly 20 years—is by far the most widely used active ingredient in prescription sleep medications, says Ronald Farkas, M.D., Ph.D., a medical team leader in the FDA's neurology products division. About 9 million patients received products containing zolpidem from retail pharmacies in 2011.

The U.S. Food and Drug Administration's Adverse Event Reporting System (AERS) has logged approximately 700 reports of zolpidem use and impaired driving ability and/or traffic accidents. However, the FDA cannot be certain that those incidents are conclusively linked to zolpidem. Many of those reports lacked important information, such as the dose of zolpidem and the time at which it was taken, the time of the accident, and whether alcohol or other drugs had also been used.

"We have had long-standing concern about sleep medications and driving. However, only recently have data from clinical trials and specialized driving simulation studies become available that enabled the FDA to better establish the risk of driving impairment and to make new recommendations about dosing," Farkas says.

An Individual Decision

The U.S. Food and Drug Administration is urging healthcare professionals to caution patients who use these products about the risks of next-morning impairment and its effect on activities, such as driving, that require alertness. The agency recommends that people who take sleep medications talk to their healthcare professional about ways to take the lowest effective dose. It should not be assumed that over-the-counter (OTC) sleep medicines are necessarily safer alternatives.

With zolpidem, Farkas notes that people must be aware of how this drug affects them personally. "Even with the new dosing recommendations, it's important to work with your healthcare professional to find the sleep medicine and dose that work best for you," he says.

Patients are asked to contact the FDA's MedWatch program if they suffer side effects from the use of zolpidem or another insomnia medication.

Part Three

Sleep Disorders

Chapter 16

Breathing Disorders of Sleep

Chapter Contents

Section 16.1

Sleep Apnea

This section includes text excerpted from "Struggling to Sleep?"
NIH News in Health, National Institutes of Health (NIH), July 2017.

Most people who have sleep apnea do not realize it. That is because this disorder only occurs during sleep. Sleep apnea is when you have pauses in breathing while you are asleep. These pauses can last from seconds to minutes. You may have difficulty breathing a few times or dozens of times an hour.

These breathing pauses can be dangerous if they cause the oxygen level in your body to drop or disturb your sleep. When oxygen drops, your brain does whatever it can to get you to resume breathing. And then you may snore, gasp, snort loudly, or make a choking sound. A family member or bed partner might be the first to notice these disruptions in your sleep.

Sleep apnea is a common disorder. Anyone can develop it. "Sleep apnea can occur in both genders, in all races and ethnicities, and in people of all sizes and shapes," says Dr. Michael Twery, a sleep expert at the National Institutes of Health (NIH).

The most common type of sleep apnea is obstructive sleep apnea. Any air that squeezes past a blocked airway can cause loud snoring. When you are awake, the muscles in your throat help keep your airway stiff and open. In adults, the throat muscles and tongue can relax during sleep, or fat tissue in the neck can narrow your airway to cause an obstruction. In children, the airway may become blocked if their tonsils are so large, they obstruct the airway opening.

The other type of sleep apnea is central sleep apnea. In central sleep apnea, the brain does not send the correct signals to your breathing muscles, so you stop breathing for brief periods.

So how can you tell whether you have this disorder? One of the most common symptoms is excessive daytime sleepiness. "Anyone who feels so tired on a regular basis that this is a drag on their daytime function—that even if they allow enough time to get enough sleep on a regular basis and they still feel this way—then they need to discuss it with their doctor," Twery says.

Another common symptom is loud, frequent snoring. But not everyone who snores has sleep apnea. Other symptoms of sleep apnea may include feeling irritable or depressed or having mood swings. You may have memory problems or trouble concentrating. Or, you may wake up with a headache or a dry mouth.

Your doctor can diagnose sleep apnea based on your symptoms, a physical exam, and a sleep study. For a sleep study, your doctor may send you to a sleep lab or provide a portable sleep monitor. Sleep studies record things such as heart rate and oxygen level while you sleep.

A sleep study can show whether the apnea is mild or severe. "The largest proportion of the population with sleep apnea has mild sleep apnea," Twery explains. "Mild may or may not be associated with any daytime symptoms." People who are so sleepy that they are at risk of a drowsy driving accident are probably in the moderate to severe range.

Doctors may prescribe breathing devices that pump air or mouthpieces that adjust the lower jaw or hold the tongue. Other treatments are available and may be considered with advice from a physician familiar with your health. Everyone deserves a good night's sleep. If you feel extremely sleepy during the day or your bed partner says that you stop breathing when you are asleep, go talk with your doctor.

Section 16.2

Obstructive Sleep Apnea

This section includes text excerpted from "Obstructive Sleep
Apnea," Genetics Home Reference (GHR), National
Institutes of Health (NIH), May 14, 2019.

Obstructive sleep apnea (OSA) is a condition in which individuals experience pauses in breathing (apnea) during sleep, which are associated with partial or complete closure of the throat (upper airway). Complete closure can lead to apnea while partial closure allows breathing but decreases the intake of oxygen (hypopnea).

Individuals with obstructive sleep apnea may experience interrupted sleep with frequent awakenings and loud snoring. Repeated pauses in breathing lead to episodes of lower-than-normal oxygen levels (hypoxemia) and a buildup of carbon dioxide (hypercapnia) in the bloodstream. Interrupted and poor-quality sleep can lead to daytime sleepiness and fatigue, impaired attention and memory, headaches, depression, and sexual dysfunction. Daytime sleepiness leads to a higher risk of motor vehicle accidents in individuals with obstructive sleep apnea. Obstructive sleep apnea is also associated with high blood pressure (hypertension), heart disease, stroke, and an increased risk of developing insulin resistance, which is an inability to regulate blood sugar levels effectively.

Causes of Obstructive Sleep Apnea

The causes of OSA are often complex. This condition results from a combination of genetic, health, and lifestyle factors, many of which have not been identified. Studies suggest that variations in multiple genes, each with a small effect, combine to increase the risk of developing the condition. However, it is unclear what contribution each of these genetic changes makes to disease risk. Most of the variations have been identified in single studies, and subsequent research has not verified them.

Genes thought to be associated with the development of OSA are involved in many bodily processes. These include communication between nerve cells, breathing regulation, control of inflammatory responses by the immune system, development of tissues in the head and face (craniofacial development), the sleep–wake cycle, and appetite control.

Obesity is a major risk factor for OSA, as 60 to 70 percent of individuals with this condition are obese. It is thought that excess fatty tissue in the head and neck constricts airways and abdominal fat may prevent the chest and lungs from fully expanding and relaxing. Other risk factors for OSA include alcohol use, frequent nasal congestion, and blockages of the airways, such as by enlarged tonsils.

Obstructive sleep apnea often occurs on its own, without signs and symptoms affecting other parts of the body. However, it can also occur as part of a syndrome, such as mucopolysaccharidosis type I or polycystic ovary syndrome (PCOS).

Obstructive Sleep Apnea: Frequency

Obstructive sleep apnea is a common condition. It is estimated to affect 2 to 4 percent of children and at least 10 percent of adults worldwide. Males are twice as likely as females to have OSA.

Section 16.3

Snoring

This section contains text excerpted from the following sources: Text
in this section begins with excerpts from "Snoring," MedlinePlus,
National Institutes of Health (NIH), August 4, 2016; Text under the
heading "Is Snoring a Problem?" is excerpted from "Your Guide to
Healthy Sleep," National Heart, Lung, and Blood Institute (NHLBI),
August 2011. Reviewed May 2019.

Snoring is the sound you make when your breathing is blocked while you are asleep. The sound is caused by tissues at the top of your airway that strike each other and vibrate. Snoring is common, especially among older people and people who are overweight.

When severe, snoring can cause frequent awakenings at night and daytime sleepiness. It can disrupt your bed partner's sleep. Snoring can also be a sign of a serious sleep disorder called "sleep apnea." You should see your healthcare provider if you are often tired during the day, do not feel that you sleep well, or wake up gasping.

To reduce snoring:

- Lose weight if you are overweight. It may help, but thin people can snore, too.

- Cut down or avoid alcohol and other sedatives at bedtime.

- Do not sleep flat on your back.

Is Snoring a Problem?

Long the material for jokes, snoring is generally accepted as common and annoying in adults but as nothing to worry about. However, snoring is no laughing matter. Frequent, loud snoring is often a sign of sleep apnea and may increase your risk of developing cardiovascular disease (CVD) and diabetes. Snoring also may lead to daytime sleepiness and impaired performance.

Snoring is caused by a narrowing or partial blockage of the airways at the back of your mouth, throat, or nose. This obstruction results in increased air turbulence when breathing in, causing the soft tissues in your upper airways to vibrate. The end result is a noisy snore that can disrupt the sleep of your bed partner. This narrowing of the airways is typically caused by the soft palate, tongue, and throat relaxing while you sleep, but allergies or sinus problems also can contribute to a narrowing of the airways, as can being overweight and having extra soft tissue around your upper airways.

The larger the tissues in your soft palate (the roof of your mouth in the back of your throat), the more likely you are to snore while sleeping. Alcohol or sedatives taken shortly before sleep also promote snoring. These drugs cause greater relaxation of the tissues in your throat and mouth. Surveys reveal that about one-half of all adults snore, and 50 percent of these adults do so loudly and frequently. African Americans, Asians, and Hispanics are more likely to snore loudly and frequently compared with Caucasians, and snoring problems increase with age.

Not everyone who snores has sleep apnea, but people who have sleep apnea typically do snore loudly and frequently. Sleep apnea is a serious sleep disorder, and its hallmark is loud, frequent snoring with pauses in breathing or shallow breaths while sleeping. Even if you do not experience these breathing pauses, snoring can still be a problem for you as well as for your bed partner. Snoring adds extra effort to your breathing, which can reduce the quality of your sleep and lead to many of the same health consequences as sleep apnea.

One study found that older adults who did not have sleep apnea, but who snored six to seven nights a week, were more than twice as likely to report being extremely sleepy during the day than those who never snored. The more people snored, the more daytime fatigue they reported. That sleepiness may help explain why snorers are more likely to be in car crashes than people who do not snore. Loud snoring also can disrupt the sleep of bed partners and strain marital relations, especially if snoring causes the spouses to sleep in separate bedrooms.

In addition, snoring increases the risk of developing diabetes and heart disease. One study found that women who snored regularly were twice as likely as those who did not snore to develop diabetes, even if they were not overweight (another risk factor for diabetes). Other studies suggest that regular snoring may raise the lifetime risk of developing high blood pressure, heart failure, and stroke.

About one-third of all pregnant women begin snoring for the first time during their second trimester. If you are snoring while pregnant, let your doctor know. Snoring in pregnancy can be associated with high blood pressure and can have a negative effect on your baby's growth and development. Your doctor will keep a close eye on your blood pressure throughout your pregnancy and can let you know if any additional evaluations for the snoring might be useful. In most cases, the snoring and any related high blood pressure will go away shortly after delivery. Snoring also can be a problem in children. As many as 10 to 15 percent of young children, who typically have enlarged adenoids and tonsils (both tissues in the throat), snore on a regular basis. Several studies show that children who snore (with or without sleep apnea) are more likely than those who do not snore to score lower on tests that measure intelligence, memory, and attention span. These children also have more problematic behavior, including hyperactivity. The end result is that children who snore do not perform as well in school as those who do not snore. Strikingly, snoring was linked to a greater drop in intelligence quotient (IQ) than that seen in children who had elevated levels of lead in their blood. Although the behavior of children improves after they stop snoring, studies suggest they may continue to get poorer grades in school, perhaps because of the lasting effects on the brain linked to the snoring. You should have your child evaluated by your doctor if the child snores loudly and frequently—three to four times a week—especially if you note brief pauses in breathing while asleep and if there are signs of hyperactivity or daytime sleepiness, inadequate school achievement, or slower than expected development.

Surgery to remove the adenoids and tonsils of children often can cure their snoring and any associated sleep apnea. Such surgery has been linked to a reduction in hyperactivity and improved ability to pay attention, even in children who showed no signs of sleep apnea before surgery.

Snoring in older children and adults may be relieved by less invasive measures, however. These measures include losing weight, refraining from the use of tobacco, sleeping on the side rather than on the back, or elevating the head while sleeping. Treating chronic congestion and refraining from alcohol or sedatives before sleeping also may decrease snoring. In some adults, snoring can be relieved by dental appliances that reposition the soft tissues in the mouth. Although numerous over-the-counter (OTC) nasal strips and sprays claim to relieve snoring, no scientific evidence supports those claims.

Chapter 17

Circadian Rhythm Disorders

What Are Circadian Rhythm Disorders?

Circadian rhythm sleep disorders are problems that occur when our internal sleep–wake timing does not match our outside environment.

We all have a master internal time clock in our brain. This internal time clock regulates a number of systems in of our body, including temperature and hormone levels. However, the primary job of this internal time clock is to control our sleep–wake times.

Typically, our brain will "set" our internal time clock with environmental cues. Light exposure is the most important way brains calibrate the internal time clock with the outside environment. There is even a direct pathway for light to travel from our eyes to the part of our brain with the internal time clock. Other cues include meals and exercise.

Examples of how our time clock can become mismatched with the environment include:

- Our internal time clock just wants to be a morning person or an evening person even with light exposure and environmental cues (advanced sleep–wake phase and delayed sleep–wake phase).

- We cannot time calibrate our internal time clock to light; for example, if we are blind and cannot see light or if we are working the night shift where there is less light (non-24-hour sleep–wake rhythm disorder and shift-work sleep disorder).

This chapter includes text excerpted from "Circadian Rhythm Disorders," U.S. Department of Veterans Affairs (VA), September 16, 2015. Reviewed May 2019.

- We travel to a different time zone and our internal time clock does not have time to adjust to the new environment (jet-lag disorder).

What Are the Types of Circadian Rhythm Sleep Disorders?

As hinted above, some common types of circadian rhythm sleep disorders are:

Advanced Sleep–Wake Phase Disorder

These are the "morning people" who wake up between 2 a.m. and 5 a.m. and want to go to sleep between 6 p.m. and 9 p.m. The person's time is "advanced," since they regularly go to sleep and wake up several hours earlier than most people in their environment. If allowed to go to bed at the preferred time on a regular basis, the person with the advanced sleep–wake disorder will have a very stable sleep pattern. Advanced sleep–wake phase disorder tends to increase with age.

Delayed Sleep-Wake Phase Disorder

These are the "evening people" who tend to stay awake until 1 a.m. or later and wake up in the late morning or afternoon. The person's time is "delayed," since they regularly go to sleep and wake up more than two hours later than most people. Again, if allowed to go to bed at the preferred late time on a regular basis, the sleep pattern for people with delayed sleep-wake phase disorder is stable. Delayed sleep–wake phase disorder tends to be more common in adolescents and young adults.

Non-24-Hour Sleep-Wake Disorder

Our brain's internal time clock actually runs slightly longer than 24 hours. On a daily basis, we synchronize our time clock to the 24-hour day primarily through light exposure. If the brain receives no light cues from the environment, the internal time clock will continue for more than 24 hours. Sleep–wake times will slightly shift later every day. Total blindness is the most important predisposition to a non-24-hour sleep-wake disorder (N24HSWD).

Shift-Work Disorder

Shift-work disorder occurs when scheduled work hours are during a person's normal sleep period. The internal time clock will expect to be asleep during the scheduled work time. Sleepiness during the work shift is common. It can be a struggle to stay awake during the shift. Once off work, the internal time clock will expect to be awake during the time allotted for sleep. Falling asleep then may be a struggle and a person may wake up frequently during the night.

Jet-Lag Disorder

Jet lag occurs when long travel by airplane quickly brings someone to another time zone. When the person arrives in the new time zone, their internal time clock sleep–wake times are misaligned with the environment. Jet lag tends to be worse with more time zones crossed. Eastward travel tends to be more difficult adjusting to than westward travel. Fortunately, jet lag is a temporary condition. As the brain takes in the new environmental cues, it can adjust the internal time clock to the new area.

What Can You Do for a Circadian Rhythm Sleep-Wake Disorder?

Treatment for the disorder depends on the type of circadian rhythm sleep disorder and how much it affects a person's quality of life (QOL).

Some lifestyle changes that can be tried at home include:

- Regular sleep–wake times

- Avoid naps

- Regular exercise

- Avoid caffeine or smoking prior to bedtime

- Avoid stimulating activities before bedtime

- For delayed sleep–wake phase disorder, avoiding light in the evening hours (including televisions and computer screens)

- For advanced sleep–wake phase disorder, increasing light in the evenings by keeping the lights on or spending more time outdoors

Chapter 18

Congenital Central Hypoventilation Syndrome

Congenital central hypoventilation syndrome (CCHS) is a disorder that affects breathing. People with this disorder take shallow breaths (hypoventilate), especially during sleep, resulting in a shortage of oxygen and a buildup of carbon dioxide in the blood. Ordinarily, the part of the nervous system that controls involuntary body processes (autonomic nervous system) would react to such an imbalance by stimulating the individual to breathe more deeply or wake up. This reaction is impaired in people with CCHS, and they must be supported with a machine to help them breathe (mechanical ventilation) or a device that stimulates a normal breathing pattern (diaphragm pacemaker). Some affected individuals need this support 24 hours a day, while others need it only at night.

Symptoms of Congenital Central Hypoventilation Syndrome

Symptoms of CCHS usually become apparent shortly after birth. Affected infants hypoventilate upon falling asleep and exhibit a bluish appearance of the skin or lips (cyanosis). Cyanosis is caused by

This chapter includes text excerpted from "Congenital Central Hypoventilation Syndrome," Genetics Home Reference (GHR), National Institutes of Health (NIH), April 30, 2019.

lack of oxygen in the blood. In some milder cases, CCHS may be diagnosed later in life. In addition to the breathing problem, people with this disorder may have difficulty regulating their heart rate and blood pressure, for example in response to exercise or changes in body position. They may have abnormalities in the nerves that control the digestive tract (Hirschsprung disease), resulting in severe constipation, intestinal blockage, and enlargement of the colon. They are also at an increased risk of developing certain tumors of the nervous system called "neuroblastomas," "ganglioneuromas," and "ganglioneuroblastomas."

Some affected individuals develop learning difficulties or other neurological problems, which may be worsened by oxygen deprivation if treatment to support their breathing is not completely effective.

Individuals with CCHS usually have eye abnormalities, including a decreased response of the pupils to light. They also have decreased perception of pain, low body temperature, and occasional episodes of profuse sweating.

People with CCHS, especially children, may have a characteristic appearance with a short, wide, somewhat flattened face often described as "box-shaped." Life expectancy and the extent of any cognitive disabilities depend on the severity of the disorder, timing of the diagnosis, and the success of treatment.

Causes of Congenital Central Hypoventilation Syndrome

Mutations in the *PHOX2B* gene cause congenital central hypoventilation syndrome. The *PHOX2B* gene provides instructions for making a protein that acts early in development to help promote the formation of nerve cells (neurons) and regulate the process by which the neurons mature to carry out specific functions (differentiation). The protein is active in the neural crest, which is a group of cells in the early embryo that gives rise to many tissues and organs. Neural crest cells migrate to form parts of the autonomic nervous system, many tissues in the face and skull, and other tissue and cell types.

Mutations are believed to interfere with the PHOX2B protein's role in promoting neuron formation and differentiation, especially in the autonomic nervous system, resulting in the problems regulating breathing and other body functions that occur in CCHS.

Frequency of Congenital Central Hypoventilation Syndrome

Congenital central hypoventilation syndrome is a relatively rare disorder. Approximately 1,000 individuals with this condition have been identified. Researchers believe that some cases of sudden infant death syndrome (SIDS) or sudden unexplained death in children may be caused by undiagnosed CCHS.

Chapter 19

Excessive Sleeping

Chapter Contents

Section 19.1

Hypersomnia

This section contains text excerpted from the following sources: Text in this section begins with excerpts from "Hypersomnia Information Page," National Institute of Neurological Disorders and Stroke (NINDS), March 27, 2019; Text under the heading "Support Groups" is excerpted from "Idiopathic Hypersomnia," Genetic and Rare Diseases Information Center (GARD), National Center for Advancing Translational Sciences (NCATS), May 1, 2019.

Hypersomnia is characterized by recurrent episodes of excessive daytime sleepiness or prolonged nighttime sleep. Unlike people who feel tired due to lack of or interrupted sleep at night, persons with hypersomnia are compelled to nap repeatedly during the day, and often at inappropriate times such as at work, during a meal, or in conversation. These daytime naps usually provide no relief from symptoms.

Symptoms of Hypersomnia

People with hypersomnia often have difficulty waking from a long sleep and may feel disoriented. Other symptoms may include:

- Anxiety
- Increased irritation
- Decreased energy
- Restlessness
- Slow thinking
- Slow speech
- Loss of appetite
- Hallucinations
- Memory difficulty

Some people with hypersomnia lose the ability to function in family, social, occupational, or other settings.

Causes of Hypersomnia

Hypersomnia may be caused by another sleep disorder (such as narcolepsy or sleep apnea), dysfunction of the autonomic nervous system, or drug or alcohol abuse. In some cases, it results from a physical problem, such as a tumor, head trauma, or injury to the central nervous system (CNS). Certain medications, or medicine withdrawal, may also cause hypersomnia. Medical conditions, including multiple sclerosis (MS), depression, encephalitis, epilepsy, or obesity may contribute to the disorder. Some people appear to have a genetic predisposition to hypersomnia; in others, there is no known cause. Typically, hypersomnia is first recognized in adolescence or young adulthood.

Treatment of Hypersomnia

Treatment is symptomatic in nature. Stimulants, such as amphetamine, methylphenidate, and modafinil, may be prescribed. Other drugs used to treat hypersomnia include clonidine, levodopa, bromocriptine, antidepressants, and monoamine oxidase inhibitors. Changes in behavior (for example, avoiding night work and social activities that delay bedtime) and diet may offer some relief. Patients should avoid alcohol and caffeine.

Prognosis for Hypersomnia

The prognosis for persons with hypersomnia depends on the cause of the disorder. While the disorder itself is not life-threatening, it can have serious consequences, such as automobile accidents caused by falling asleep while driving. The attacks usually continue indefinitely.

Support Groups

Support and advocacy groups can help you connect with other patients and families, and they can provide valuable services. Many develop patient-centered information and are the driving force behind research for better treatments and possible cures. They can direct you to research, resources, and services. Many organizations also have experts who serve as medical advisors or provide lists of doctors/clinics. Visit the group's website or contact them to learn about the services they offer.

Section 19.2

Kleine-Levin Syndrome

This section contains text excerpted from the following sources: Text in this section begins with excerpts from "Kleine-Levin Syndrome Information Page," National Institute of Neurological Disorders and Stroke (NINDS), March 27, 2019; Text under the heading "Find a Specialist" is excerpted from "Kleine Levin Syndrome," Genetic and Rare Diseases Information Center (GARD), National Center for Advancing Translational Sciences (NCATS), May 1, 2019.

Kleine-Levin syndrome (KLS) is a rare disorder that primarily affects adolescent males (approximately 70% of those with KLS are male). It is characterized by recurring but reversible periods of excessive sleep (up to 20 hours per day).

Symptoms of Kleine-Levin Syndrome

Symptoms occur as "episodes," typically lasting a few days to a few weeks. Episode onset is often abrupt and may be associated with flu-like symptoms. Excessive food intake, irritability, childishness, disorientation, hallucinations, and an abnormally uninhibited sex drive may be observed during episodes. The mood can be depressed as a consequence, but not a cause, of the disorder. Affected individuals are completely normal between episodes, although they may not be able to remember afterward everything that happened during the episode. It may be weeks or more before symptoms reappear. Symptoms may be related to malfunction of the hypothalamus and thalamus, parts of the brain that govern appetite and sleep.

Treatment of Kleine-Levin Syndrome

There is no definitive treatment for KLS and watchful waiting at home, rather than pharmacotherapy, is most often advised. Stimulant pills, including amphetamines, methylphenidate, and modafinil, are used to treat sleepiness but may increase irritability and will not improve cognitive abnormalities. Because of similarities between KLS and certain mood disorders, lithium and carbamazepine may be prescribed and, in some cases, have been shown to prevent further episodes. This disorder should be differentiated from cyclic re-occurrence of sleepiness during the premenstrual period in teenage girls, which may be controlled with birth control pills. It also should be differentiated from encephalopathy, recurrent depression, or psychosis.

Prognosis for Kleine-Levin Syndrome

Episodes eventually decrease in frequency and intensity over the course of 8 to 12 years.

Find a Specialist

If you need medical advice, you can look for doctors or other healthcare professionals who have experience with this disease. You may find these specialists through advocacy organizations, clinical trials, or articles published in medical journals. You may also want to contact a university or tertiary medical center in your area because these centers tend to see more complex cases and have the latest technology and treatments.

If you cannot find a specialist in your local area, try contacting national or international specialists. They may be able to refer you to someone they know through conferences or research efforts. Some specialists may be willing to consult with you or your local doctors over the phone or by email if you cannot travel to them for care.

Chapter 20

Fatal Familial Insomnia

Fatal familial insomnia (FFI) is an inherited prion disease that mainly affects the thalamus. The thalamus is the part of the brain that controls the sleep–wake cycle, but is also known as the "relay center" of the brain because it helps the different parts of the brain communicate with each other. Like all prion diseases, FFI is a progressive neurodegenerative disease, which means that over time there are fewer neurons (nerve cells). Loss of neurons in the thalamus, as well as other mechanisms not yet fully understood, cause the symptoms of fatal familial insomnia.

Almost all cases of FFI are caused by certain changes (mutations) in the *PRNP* gene and are inherited in an autosomal dominant manner. There are a very small number of reported sporadic cases of fatal familial insomnia. As of now there is no effective treatment for fatal familial insomnia, but research for a treatment and cure is ongoing. Death usually occurs within 12 to 18 months of the first symptoms.

Symptoms of Fatal Familial Insomnia

The first symptoms of FFI usually begin between the ages of 32 and 62 (mean average 51 years) but have been reported to begin as early as 18 and as late as 72. It is important to note that insomnia is not always the first symptom of fatal familial insomnia; sometimes

This chapter includes text excerpted from "Fatal Familial Insomnia," Genetic and Rare Diseases Information Center (GARD), National Center for Advancing Translational Sciences (NCATS), December 2, 2016.

the first symptom is progressive dementia. When insomnia begins, it usually comes on suddenly and steadily worsens over a period of a few months. Other symptoms may include panic attacks, phobias, weight loss, lack of appetite, and having a body temperature which is too low (hypothermia) or too high (hyperthermia). Autonomic disorders, such as high blood pressure, episodes of hyperventilation, excessive sweating and salivation, and/or erectile dysfunction, may occur.

As the disease progresses, most people with FFI develop abnormal, uncoordinated movements (ataxia), hallucinations, severe confusion (delirium), and muscle twitches and jerks (myoclonus). Although dementia may begin as forgetfulness and confusion, it leads eventually to the inability to walk and talk. Total inability to sleep is common toward the end of the course of the disease.

Causes of Fatal Familial Insomnia

Fatal familial insomnia is a very rare form of genetic prion disease. In almost every case it is caused by a very specific mutation in the *PRNP* gene. This mutation causes the prion protein (PrP) that is made from this gene to be a different shape (fold incorrectly). Since the protein has a different shape, it cannot work correctly.

The abnormally shaped PrP (prion protein) causes changes in the thalamus, including the progressive loss of neurons (nerve cells). The thalamus relays messages between different parts of the brain. It manages our sleep–wake cycle; the flow of visual, auditory, and motor information; our sense of balance; how we experience pain; aspects of learning, memory, speech and understanding language; and even emotional experiences, expression, and our personalities. Losing neurons in the thalamus causes many of the symptoms of FFI because the thalamus can no longer do all of its jobs well.

Although the main target of FFI is the thalamus, other parts of the brain are affected as well, including the inferior olives. The inferior olives are part of the medulla oblongata and are important for coordinating our movements (motor control). Losing neurons in the inferior olives can make it harder for a person to control their movements, as seen in later stages of FFI. Medical researchers are still working to understand how the abnormally folded PrP causes progressive changes in the thalamus and other affected brain areas.

In very rare cases of fatal familial insomnia, the cause is sporadic, meaning there is not a change in the *PRNP* gene. As of 2016, there have only been 24 reported cases of sporadic fatal familial insomnia. Sporadic FFI occurs when some of a person's normal PrP (prion protein) spontaneously changes into the abnormal shape that causes fatal familial insomnia, and then somehow changes the shape of PrP in other neurons in a chain reaction.

Inheritance of Fatal Familial Insomnia

In most cases, a person with fatal familial insomnia has inherited the genetic change from a parent with fatal familial insomnia. In order to have fatal familial insomnia, a person only needs one copy of their *PRNP* gene to carry the specific genetic change (mutation) that causes FFI. In other words, a person only needs to inherit the genetic change from one parent. In genetic terms, this is called "autosomal dominant inheritance." In rare cases, fatal familial insomnia may result from a *de novo* (new) change in the *PRNP* gene, however, it is not known how often a new mutation is the cause of fatal familial insomnia. New mutations can happen during the making of the egg or the sperm.

A person that has the genetic change that causes FFI has a 50-percent chance with each pregnancy of passing along the changed gene to offspring. In the rare sporadic cases of fatal familial insomnia, the disease is not inherited from either parent and cannot be passed down to their children.

Prognosis for Fatal Familial Insomnia

Presently, after symptoms of FFI begin, the disease usually causes death within 12 to 18 months, with a range of a few months to several years. As research continues, however, it is hoped that a treatment or even a cure will be developed that will dramatically change the outlook for people who have fatal familial insomnia.

Chapter 21

Insomnia

Insomnia is one of the most commonly reported sleep problems. One in four women has some insomnia symptoms, such as trouble falling asleep, trouble staying asleep, or both. About one in seven adults has chronic (long-term) insomnia. Chronic insomnia can affect your ability to do daily tasks, such as working, going to school, or caring for yourself. Insomnia is more common in women, especially older women, than in men.

What Is Insomnia?

Insomnia is a common sleep disorder. It is defined as an inability to go to sleep, waking up too early, or feeling unrested after sleep for at least three nights a week for at least three months. Most adult women need to get seven or more hours of sleep a night to feel rested.

Chronic or long-term insomnia makes it difficult to accomplish routine tasks, such as going to work or school and taking care of yourself. Insomnia can lead to or contribute to the development of other health problems, such as depression, heart disease, and stroke.

This chapter includes text excerpted from "Insomnia," Office on Women's Health (OWH), U.S. Department of Health and Human Services (HHS), November 21, 2018.

What Are the Different Types of Insomnia?

There are two types of insomnia:

- **Primary insomnia.** Primary insomnia is a disorder. It is not a symptom or a side effect of another medical condition. Your doctor may diagnose your sleeplessness as primary insomnia after ruling out other medical conditions as a cause.

- **Secondary insomnia.** Secondary insomnia is caused by or happens alongside other health conditions or as a side effect of prescribed medicines. It can be acute (short term) or chronic (long term). Most people with chronic insomnia have secondary insomnia.

What Causes Primary and Secondary Insomnia

The exact cause of primary insomnia is unknown. It may be lifelong, or it can happen because of changes in your routine during travel or stressful life events.

Conditions that may trigger, or happen at the same time as, secondary insomnia include:

- Mental-health conditions, such as depression, anxiety, or posttraumatic stress disorder (PTSD)

- Traumatic brain injury (TBI)

- Neurological (brain) disorders, such as Alzheimer disease (AD) or Parkinson disease (PD)

- Conditions that cause chronic pain, such as arthritis

- Conditions that make it hard to breathe, such as asthma and sleep apnea

- Trouble with hormones, including thyroid problems

- Gastrointestinal disorders, such as heartburn

- Stroke

- Other sleep disorders, such as restless legs syndrome (RLS)

- Menopause symptoms, such as hot flashes

- Cancer

- Side effects of medicines, such as those to treat cancer, asthma, heart disease, allergies, and colds

Talk to your doctor or nurse if you think another health problem could be causing insomnia.

Other things that can keep you from getting enough sleep include:

- **Caffeine, tobacco, and alcohol**. Caffeine and nicotine in tobacco products can disrupt sleep, especially if taken within several hours of going to bed. Alcohol may make it easier to fall asleep at first, but it can cause you to wake up too early and not be able to fall back asleep.

- **A traumatic event**. People who witness or experience a traumatic event, such as an accident, natural disaster, physical attack, or war, can have trouble falling and staying asleep. Getting treatment for symptoms of anxiety or PTSD as a result of the trauma can help insomnia get better.

- **A bad sleep environment**. Having a bed or place to sleep that is uncomfortable, unsafe, noisy, or too bright can make it difficult to fall asleep.

- **A partner with sleep problems**. If you sleep with a partner who snores or has sleep apnea, your sleep may be more restless and interrupted. Snoring and sleep apnea can be treated.

- **Pregnancy**. During pregnancy, especially in the third trimester, you may wake up more often than usual because of discomfort, leg cramps, or needing to use the bathroom.

- **Having a new baby.** Changing hormone levels after childbirth can disrupt your sleep. Very young babies do not usually sleep longer than a few hours at a time and need to be fed every few hours.

Who Gets Insomnia

Anyone can get insomnia, but it affects more women than men. More than one in four women in the United States experience insomnia, compared with fewer than one in five men. In one study, women of all ages reported worse sleep quality than men, including taking longer to fall asleep, sleeping for shorter periods of time, and feeling sleepier when awake.

Older women are at a higher risk of insomnia. Other people at risk for insomnia include those who:

- Have a lot of stress

- Have depression or other mental-health conditions

- Work nights or have an irregular sleep schedule, such as shift workers

- Travel long distances with time changes, such as air travelers

- Have certain medical conditions, such as sleep apnea, asthma, and fibromyalgia (FM)

Why Do More Women than Men Have Insomnia?

Women may be more likely to have insomnia than men because women experience unique hormonal changes that can cause insomnia symptoms. These include hormonal changes during:

- **The menstrual cycle**, especially in the days leading up to their period when many women report problems going to sleep and staying asleep. This is especially common in women who have premenstrual dysphoric disorder (PMDD), a more severe type of premenstrual syndrome (PMS).

- **Pregnancy**, especially in the third trimester, when women may wake up often because of discomfort, leg cramps, or needing to use the bathroom

- **Perimenopause and menopause**, when hot flashes and night sweats can disturb sleep

Also, some health problems that can cause secondary insomnia are more common in women than in men. These include:

- **Depression and anxiety**. People with insomnia are 10 times more likely to have depression and 17 times more likely to have anxiety. Researchers are not sure if mental-health conditions lead to insomnia or if insomnia leads to mental-health conditions, but not getting enough sleep may worsen mental-health conditions.

- **Fibromyalgia.** The pain experienced with fibromyalgia can make it difficult to fall asleep and stay asleep.

How Long Does Insomnia Last?

It depends. Insomnia can be acute (short term) or chronic (long term). While acute insomnia may last for only a few days or weeks, chronic insomnia can last for three months or more.

What Are the Symptoms of Insomnia?

The most common symptom of insomnia is difficulty sleeping—either going to sleep, staying asleep, or waking up too early. If you have insomnia, you may:

- Lie awake for a long time without going to sleep

- Wake up during the night and find it difficult to go back to sleep

- Not feel rested when you wake up

Lack of sleep may cause other symptoms during the daytime. For example, you may wake up feeling tired, and you may have low energy during the day. It can also cause you to feel anxious, depressed, or irritable, and you may have a hard time concentrating or remembering things.

How Does Insomnia Affect Women's Health?

Insomnia can cause you to feel tired, anxious, or irritable in the short term. Over time, lack of sleep may increase your risk for more serious problems, including:

- Accidents

- Health problems, including diabetes and high blood pressure

- Increased risk for falls, especially in older women

Women who have long-term insomnia may be more at risk than men with long-term insomnia for mood problems, heart disease and stroke, and obesity.

Chapter 22

Sleep-Related Movement Disorders

Chapter Contents

Section 22.1

Periodic Limb Movement Disorder

"Periodic Limb Movement Disorder,"
© 2016 Omnigraphics. Reviewed May 2019.

Periodic limb movement disorder (PLMD) is a type of sleep disorder in which patients experience repetitive, rhythmic jerking or twitching movements in the legs or other limbs during sleep. The movements typically occur in a regular pattern every 20 to 40 seconds. Episodes most commonly take place in the early part of the night and last for less than an hour. Although the person is usually not aware of them, the movements often disrupt sleep, resulting in such symptoms as daytime drowsiness and memory or attention problems.

Periodic limb movement disorder is often confused with restless legs syndrome (RLS). In this condition, patients experience uncomfortable sensations in their legs while awake that create an irresistible urge to move the affected limbs. Although approximately 80 percent of people with RLS also have periodic limb movement disorder, it is considered a separate condition and does not appear to increase the risk of restless legs syndrome.

Symptoms of Periodic Limb Movement Disorder

The main symptom of PLMD is tightening or flexing of muscles in the lower legs—including the big toe, foot, ankle, knee, or hip—during sleep. Although PLMD can also affect the arms or occur while awake, this is uncommon. The movements are usually concentrated during nonrapid eye movement (REM) sleep in the first half of the night. Each movement typically lasts around 2 seconds, and they tend to recur every 20 to 40 seconds, although the pattern can vary from night to night. The movements can range from slight twitches to strenuous kicks.

Most people with PLMD are unaware of the movements and only learn about them from another person who shares the same bed. For some patients, however, the repetitive movements can disrupt sleep and cause such symptoms as not feeling well rested after a good night's sleep, feeling tired or falling asleep during the day, having trouble remembering or paying attention, or becoming depressed.

Causes and Risk Factors of Periodic Limb Movement Disorder

Researchers have not uncovered the cause of primary periodic limb movement disorder, although some believe that it may be linked to abnormalities in the regulation of nerve impulses from the brain to the limbs. Periodic limb movement disorder affects males and females equally, and it can affect people of any age. The incidence of PLMD increases with age, however, and affects 34 percent of people over the age of 60.

Secondary PLMD is caused by underlying medical conditions, including the following:

- Diabetes

- Iron deficiency anemia

- Spinal cord injury (SCI)

- Restless legs syndrome (RLS)

- Sleep apnea

- Narcolepsy

- REM sleep behavior disorder

- Sleep-related eating disorder

- Multiple-system atrophy

Certain types of medications have also been found to increase the risk or worsen symptoms of periodic limb movement disorder, including antidepressants, such as amitriptyline (Elavil) and lithium; dopamine-receptor antagonists, such as Haldol; and withdrawal from sedatives, such as Valium.

Diagnosis of Periodic Limb Movement Disorder

Diagnosis of PLMD begins with a visit to a sleep specialist. Patients are typically asked to keep a sleep diary for several weeks (to evaluate their sleep using a rating system such as the Epworth Sleepiness Scale) and to provide a complete medical history, including any medications taken. In most cases, patients will then undergo an overnight sleep study, during which a polysomnogram keeps track of brain activity, heartbeat, breathing, and limb movement. In addition to diagnosing PLMD and other sleep disorders, the sleep specialist can help identify other potential causes of sleep problems, such as medical conditions, medications, substance abuse, or mental-health disorders.

Other medical tests can be used to detect underlying causes of periodic limb movement disorder, such as diabetes, anemia, or metabolic disorders. Doctors may take blood samples to check hormone levels, organ function, and blood chemistry. They may also look for infections or traces of drugs that can contribute to secondary periodic limb movement disorder. If no underlying cause can be found, the patient may be referred to a neurologist to rule out nervous system disorders and confirm the diagnosis of periodic limb movement disorder.

Treatment of Periodic Limb Movement Disorder

Many people with PLMD do not experience symptoms or require treatment. When sleep disruption makes treatment necessary, however, there are several medications available to help reduce the movements or help the person sleep through them. Some of the medications commonly prescribed to treat PLMD include:

- **Benzodiazepines,** such as clonazepam (Klonopin), which suppress muscle contractions

- **Anticonvulsant agents,** such as gabapentin (Neurontin), which also reduce muscle contractions

- **Dopaminergic agents,** such as levodopa/carbidopa (Sinemet) and pergolide (Permax), which increase the levels of the neurotransmitter dopamine in the brain and are also used to treat RLS and Parkinson disease (PD)

- **GABA agonists,** such as baclofen (Lioresal), which inhibit the release of neurotransmitters in the brain that stimulate muscle contractions.

References

1. "Periodic Limb Movement Disorder," WebMD, 2016.

2. "Sleep Education: Periodic Limb Movements," American Academy of Sleep Medicine (AASM), 2014.

Section 22.2

Restless Legs Syndrome

This section includes text excerpted from "Restless Legs Syndrome Fact Sheet," National Institute of Neurological Disorders and Stroke (NINDS), July 6, 2018.

What Is Restless Legs Syndrome?

Restless legs syndrome (RLS), also called "Willis-Ekbom disease" (WED), causes unpleasant or uncomfortable sensations in the legs and an irresistible urge to move them. Symptoms commonly occur in the late afternoon or evening hours and are often most severe at night when a person is resting, such as sitting or lying in bed. They also may occur when someone is inactive and sitting for extended periods (for example, when taking a trip by plane or watching a movie). Since symptoms can increase in severity during the night, it could become difficult to fall asleep or return to sleep after waking up. Moving the legs or walking typically relieves the discomfort but the sensations often recur once the movement stops. RLS is classified as a sleep disorder since the symptoms are triggered by resting and attempting to sleep, and as a movement disorder since people are forced to move their legs in order to relieve symptoms. It is, however, best characterized as a neurological sensory disorder with symptoms that are produced from within the brain itself.

Restless legs syndrome is one of several disorders that can cause exhaustion and daytime sleepiness, which can strongly affect mood, concentration, job and school performance, and personal relationships. Many people with RLS report they are often unable to concentrate, have impaired memory, or fail to accomplish daily tasks. Untreated moderate to severe RLS can lead to about a 20 percent decrease in work productivity and can contribute to depression and anxiety. It also can make traveling difficult.

It is estimated that up to 7 to 10 percent of the U.S. population may have restless legs syndrome. Restless legs syndrome occurs in both men and women, although women are more likely to have it than men. It may begin at any age. Many individuals who are severely affected are middle-aged or older, and the symptoms typically become more frequent and last longer with age.

More than 80 percent of people with RLS also experience periodic limb movement of sleep (PLMS). Periodic limb movement of sleep is characterized by involuntary leg (and sometimes arm) twitching or jerking movements during sleep that typically occur every 15 to 40 seconds, sometimes throughout the night. Although many individuals with RLS also develop periodic limb movement of sleep, most people with PLMS do not experience restless legs syndrome.

Fortunately, most cases of RLS can be treated with nondrug therapies and if necessary, medications.

What Are Common Signs and Symptoms of Restless Legs?

People with RLS feel the irresistible urge to move, which is accompanied by uncomfortable sensations in their lower limbs that are unlike normal sensations experienced by people without the disorder. The sensations in their legs are often difficult to define but may be described as aching throbbing, pulling, itching, crawling, or creeping. These sensations less commonly affect the arms, and rarely the chest or head. Although the sensations can occur on just one side of the body, they most often affect both sides. They can also alternate between sides. The sensations range in severity from uncomfortable to irritating to painful.

Because moving the legs (or other affected parts of the body) relieves the discomfort, people with RLS often keep their legs in motion to minimize or prevent the sensations. They may pace the floor, constantly move their legs while sitting, and toss and turn in bed.

A classic feature of RLS is that the symptoms are worse at night with a distinct symptom-free period in the early morning, allowing for more refreshing sleep at that time. Some people with RLS have difficulty falling asleep and staying asleep. They may also note a worsening of symptoms if their sleep is further reduced by events or activity.

Restless legs syndrome symptoms may vary from day to day, in severity and frequency, and from person to person. In moderately severe cases, symptoms occur only once or twice a week but often result in a significant delay of sleep onset, with some disruption of daytime function. In severe cases of restless legs syndrome, the symptoms occur more than twice a week and result in burdensome interruption of sleep and impairment of daytime function.

People with RLS can sometimes experience remissions—spontaneous improvement over a period of weeks or months before symptoms reappear—usually during the early stages of the disorder. In general, however, symptoms become more severe over time.

People who have both RLS and an associated medical condition tend to develop more severe symptoms rapidly. In contrast, those who have RLS that is not related to any other condition show a very slow progression of the disorder, particularly if they experience onset at an early age, and many years may pass before symptoms occur regularly.

What Causes Restless Legs Syndrome

In most cases, the cause of RLS is unknown (called "primary RLS"). However, RLS has a genetic component and can be found in families where the onset of symptoms is before age 40. Specific gene variants have been associated with restless legs syndrome. Evidence indicates that low levels of iron in the brain also may be responsible for restless legs syndrome.

Considerable evidence also suggests that RLS is related to a dysfunction in one of the sections of the brain that control movement (called the "basal ganglia") that use the brain chemical dopamine. Dopamine is needed to produce smooth, purposeful muscle activity and movement. Disruption of these pathways frequently results in involuntary movements. Individuals with Parkinson disease (PD), another disorder of the basal ganglia's dopamine pathway, have an increased chance of developing restless legs syndrome.

Restless legs syndrome also appears to be related to or accompany the following factors or underlying conditions:

- End-stage renal disease and hemodialysis

- Iron deficiency

- Certain medications that may aggravate RLS symptoms, such as antinausea drugs (e.g., prochlorperazine or metoclopramide), antipsychotic drugs (e.g., haloperidol or phenothiazine derivatives), antidepressants that increase serotonin (e.g., fluoxetine or sertraline), and some cold and allergy medications that contain older antihistamines (e.g., diphenhydramine)

- Use of alcohol, nicotine, and caffeine

- Pregnancy, especially in the last trimester; in most cases, symptoms usually disappear within four weeks after delivery

- Neuropathy (nerve damage)

Sleep deprivation and other sleep conditions, such as sleep apnea, also may aggravate or trigger symptoms in some people. Reducing or completely eliminating these factors may relieve symptoms.

How Is Restless Legs Syndrome Diagnosed?

Since there is no specific test for RLS, the condition is diagnosed by a doctor's evaluation. The five basic criteria for clinically diagnosing the disorder are:

- A strong and often overwhelming need or urge to move the legs that is often associated with abnormal, unpleasant, or uncomfortable sensations

- The urge to move the legs starts or get worse during rest or inactivity.

- The urge to move the legs is at least temporarily and partially or totally relieved by movements.

- The urge to move the legs starts or is aggravated in the evening or night.

- The above four features are not due to any other medical or behavioral condition.

A physician will focus largely on the individual's descriptions of symptoms, their triggers and relieving factors, as well as the presence or absence of symptoms throughout the day. A neurological and physical exam, plus information from the person's medical and family history and list of current medications, may be helpful. Individuals may be asked about frequency, duration, and intensity of symptoms; if movement helps to relieve symptoms; how much time it takes to fall asleep; any pain related to symptoms; and any tendency toward daytime sleep patterns and sleepiness, disturbance of sleep, or daytime function. Laboratory tests may rule out other conditions, such as kidney failure, iron deficiency anemia (which is a separate condition related to iron deficiency), or pregnancy that may be causing symptoms of RLS. Blood tests can identify iron deficiencies, as well as other medical disorders associated with RLS. In some cases, sleep studies such as polysomnography (a test that records the individual's brain waves, heartbeat, breathing, and leg movements during an entire night) may identify the presence of other causes of sleep disruption (e.g., sleep apnea), which may impact management of the disorder. Periodic limb movement of sleep during a sleep study can support the diagnosis of RLS but, again, is not exclusively seen in individuals with RLS.

Diagnosing RLS in children may be especially difficult since it may be hard for children to describe what they are experiencing, when and how often the symptoms occur, and how long symptoms last. Pediatric RLS can sometimes be misdiagnosed as "growing pains" or attention deficit disorder.

How Is Restless Legs Syndrome Treated?

Restless legs syndrome can be treated with care directed toward relieving symptoms. Moving the affected limb(s) may provide temporary relief. Sometimes, RLS symptoms can be controlled by finding and treating an associated medical condition, such as peripheral neuropathy, diabetes, or iron deficiency anemia.

Iron supplementation or medications are usually helpful, but no single medication effectively manages RLS for all individuals. Trials of different drugs may be necessary. In addition, medications taken regularly may lose their effect over time or even make the condition worse, making it necessary to change medications.

Treatment options for RLS include:

- **Lifestyle changes.** Certain lifestyle changes and activities may provide some relief in persons with mild to moderate symptoms of RLS. These steps include avoiding or decreasing the use of alcohol and tobacco; changing or maintaining a regular sleep pattern; a program of moderate exercise; and massaging the legs, taking a warm bath, or using a heating pad or ice pack. There are new medical devices that have been cleared by the U.S. Food and Drug Administration (FDA), including a foot wrap that puts pressure underneath the foot and another that is a pad that delivers vibration to the back of the legs. Aerobic and leg-stretching exercises of moderate intensity also may provide some relief from mild symptoms.

- **Iron.** For individuals with low or low-normal blood tests called "ferritin saturation" and "transferrin saturation," a trial of iron supplements is recommended as the first treatment. Iron supplements are available over-the-counter. A common side effect is upset stomach, which may improve with use of a different type of iron supplement. Because iron is not well-absorbed into the body by the gut, it may cause constipation that can be treated with a stool softeners, such as polyethylene glycol. In some people, iron supplementation does not improve a person's iron levels. Others may require iron given through an IV line in order to boost the iron levels and relieve symptoms.

- **Anti-seizure drugs.** Anti-seizure drugs are becoming the first-line prescription drugs for those with RLS. The FDA has approved gabapentin enacarbil for the treatment of moderate to severe RLS, This drug appears to be as effective as dopaminergic treatment (discussed below) and, at least to date, there have been no reports of problems with a progressive worsening of symptoms due to medication (called "augmentation"). Other medications may be prescribed "off-label" to relieve some of the symptoms of the disorder.

Other anti-seizure drugs, such as the standard form of gabapentin and pregabalin, can decrease such sensory disturbances as creeping and crawling as well as nerve pain. Dizziness, fatigue, and sleepiness are among the possible side effects. Recent studies have shown that pregabalin is as effective for RLS treatment as the dopaminergic drug pramipexole, suggesting this class of drug offers equivalent benefits.

- **Dopaminergic agents.** These drugs, which increase dopamine effect, are largely used to treat Parkinson disease. They have been shown to reduce symptoms of RLS when they are taken at nighttime. The FDA has approved ropinirole, pramipexole, and rotigotine to treat moderate to severe RLS. These drugs are generally well tolerated but can cause nausea, dizziness, or other short-term side effects. Levodopa plus carbidopa may be effective when used intermittently, but not daily.

Although dopamine-related medications are effective in managing RLS symptoms, long-term use can lead to worsening of the symptoms in many individuals. With chronic use, a person may begin to experience symptoms earlier in the evening or even earlier until the symptoms are present around the clock. Over time, the initial evening or bedtime dose can become less effective, the symptoms at night become more intense, and symptoms could begin to affect the arms or trunk. Fortunately, this apparent progression can be reversed by removing the person from all dopamine-related medications.

Another important adverse effect of dopamine medications that occurs in some people is the development of impulsive or obsessive behaviors such as obsessive gambling or shopping. Should they occur, these behaviors can be improved or reversed by stopping the medication.

- **Opioids.** Drugs such as methadone, codeine, hydrocodone, or oxycodone are sometimes prescribed to treat individuals with more severe symptoms of RLS who did not respond well to other medications. Side effects include constipation, dizziness, nausea, exacerbation of sleep apnea, and the risk of addiction; however, very low doses are often effective in controlling symptoms of RLS.

- **Benzodiazepines.** These drugs can help individuals obtain a more restful sleep. However, even if taken only at bedtime they can sometimes cause daytime sleepiness, reduce energy, and affect concentration. Benzodiazepines, such as clonazepam and lorazepam, are generally prescribed to treat anxiety, muscle spasms, and insomnia. Because these drugs also may induce or aggravate sleep apnea in some cases, they should not be used in people with this condition. These are last-line drugs due to their side effects.

What Is the Prognosis for People with Restless Legs Syndrome?

Restless legs syndrome is generally a lifelong condition for which there is no cure. However, current therapies can control the disorder, minimize symptoms, and increase periods of restful sleep. Symptoms may gradually worsen with age, although the decline may be some-what faster for individuals who also suffer from an associated medical condition. A diagnosis of RLS does not indicate the onset of another neurological disease, such as Parkinson disease. In addition, some individuals have remissions—periods in which symptoms decrease or disappear for days, weeks, months, or years—although symptoms often eventually reappear. If RLS symptoms are mild, do not produce significant daytime discomfort, or do not affect an individual's ability to fall asleep, the condition does not have to be treated.

Chapter 23

Narcolepsy

Chapter Contents

Section 23.1

Narcolepsy: An Overview

This section includes text excerpted from "Narcolepsy
Fact Sheet," National Institute of Neurological
Disorders and Stroke (NINDS), July 6, 2018.

What Is Narcolepsy?

Narcolepsy is a chronic neurological disorder that affects the brain's ability to control sleep–wake cycles. People with narcolepsy usually feel rested after waking but then feel very sleepy throughout much of the day. Many individuals with narcolepsy also experience uneven and interrupted sleep that can involve waking up frequently during the night.

Narcolepsy can greatly affect daily activities. People may unwillingly fall asleep even if they are in the middle of an activity, such as driving, eating, or talking. Other symptoms may include sudden muscle weakness while awake that makes a person go limp or be unable to move (cataplexy), vivid dreamlike images or hallucinations, and total paralysis just before falling asleep or just after waking up (sleep paralysis).

In a normal sleep cycle, a person enters rapid eye movement (REM) sleep after about 60 to 90 minutes. Dreams occur during REM sleep, and the brain keeps muscles limp during this sleep stage, which prevents people from acting out their dreams. People with narcolepsy frequently enter REM sleep rapidly, within 15 minutes of falling asleep. Also, the muscle weakness or dream activity of REM sleep can occur during wakefulness or be absent during sleep. This helps explain some symptoms of narcolepsy.

If left undiagnosed or untreated, narcolepsy can interfere with psychological, social, and cognitive function and development and can inhibit academic, work, and social activities.

Who Gets Narcolepsy

Narcolepsy affects both males and females equally. Symptoms often start in childhood, adolescence, or young adulthood (ages 7 to 25), but can occur at any time in life. It is estimated that anywhere from 135,000 to 200,000 people in the United States have narcolepsy. However, since this condition often goes undiagnosed, the number may be higher. Since people with narcolepsy are often misdiagnosed with other conditions, such as psychiatric disorders or emotional problems, it can take years for someone to get the proper diagnosis.

What Are the Symptoms of Narcolepsy?

Narcolepsy is a lifelong problem, but it does not usually worsen as the person ages. Symptoms can partially improve over time, but they will never disappear completely. The most typical symptoms are excessive daytime sleepiness, cataplexy, sleep paralysis, and hallucinations. Though all have excessive daytime sleepiness, only 10 to 25 percent of affected individuals will experience all of the other symptoms during the course of their illness.

- **Excessive daytime sleepiness (EDS).** All individuals with narcolepsy have EDS, and it is often the most obvious symptom. EDS is characterized by persistent sleepiness, regardless of how much sleep an individual gets at night. However, sleepiness in narcolepsy is more like a "sleep attack," where an overwhelming sense of sleepiness comes on quickly. In between sleep attacks, individuals have normal levels of alertness, particularly if doing activities that keep their attention.

- **Cataplexy.** This sudden loss of muscle tone while a person is awake leads to weakness and a loss of voluntary muscle control. It is often triggered by sudden, strong emotions such as laughter, fear, anger, stress, or excitement. The symptoms of cataplexy may appear weeks or even years after the onset of EDS. Some people may only have 1 or 2 attacks in a lifetime, while others may experience many attacks a day. In about 10 percent of cases of narcolepsy, cataplexy is the first symptom to appear and can be misdiagnosed as a seizure disorder. Attacks may be mild and involve only a momentary sense of minor weakness in a limited number of muscles, such as a slight drooping of the eyelids. The most severe attacks result in a total body collapse during which individuals are unable to move, speak, or keep their eyes open. But even during the most severe episodes, people remain fully conscious, a characteristic that distinguishes cataplexy from fainting or seizure disorders. The loss of muscle tone during cataplexy resembles paralysis of muscle activity that naturally occurs during REM sleep. Episodes last a few minutes at most and resolve almost instantly on their own. While scary, the episodes are not dangerous as long as the individual finds a safe place in which to collapse.

- **Sleep paralysis.** The temporary inability to move or speak while falling asleep or waking up usually lasts only a few seconds or minutes and is similar to REM-induced inhibitions of voluntary muscle activity. Sleep paralysis resembles cataplexy except it occurs at the edges of sleep. As with cataplexy, people remain fully conscious. Even when severe, cataplexy and sleep paralysis do not result in permanent dysfunction—after episodes end, people rapidly recover their full capacity to move and speak.

- **Hallucinations.** Very vivid and sometimes frightening images can accompany sleep paralysis and usually occur when people are falling asleep or waking up. Most often the content is primarily visual, but any of the other senses can be involved.

Additional symptoms of narcolepsy include:

- **Fragmented sleep and insomnia.** While individuals with narcolepsy are very sleepy during the day, they usually also experience difficulties staying asleep at night. Sleep may be disrupted by insomnia, vivid dreaming, sleep apnea, acting out while dreaming, and periodic leg movements.

- **Automatic behaviors.** Individuals with narcolepsy may experience temporary sleep episodes that can be very brief, lasting no more than seconds at a time. A person falls asleep during an activity (e.g., eating, talking) and automatically continues the activity for a few seconds or minutes without conscious awareness of what they are doing. This happens most often while people are engaged in habitual activities, such as typing or driving. They cannot recall their actions, and their performance is almost always impaired. Their handwriting may, for example, degenerate into an illegible scrawl, or they may store items in bizarre locations and then forget where they placed them. If an episode occurs while driving, individuals may get lost or have an accident. People tend to awaken from these episodes feeling refreshed, finding that their drowsiness and fatigue has temporarily subsided.

What Are the Types of Narcolepsy?

There are two major types of narcolepsy:

- **Type 1 narcolepsy** (previously termed "narcolepsy with cataplexy"). This diagnosis is based on the individual either having low levels of a brain hormone (hypocretin) or reporting cataplexy and having excessive daytime sleepiness on a special nap test.

- **Type 2 narcolepsy** (previously termed "narcolepsy without cataplexy"). People with this condition experience excessive daytime sleepiness but usually do not have muscle weakness triggered by emotions. They usually also have less severe symptoms and have normal levels of the brain hormone hypocretin.

A condition known as "secondary narcolepsy" can result from an injury to the hypothalamus, a region deep in the brain that helps regulate sleep. In addition to experiencing the typical symptoms of narcolepsy, individuals may also have severe neurological problems and sleep for long periods (more than 10 hours) each night.

What Causes Narcolepsy

Narcolepsy may have several causes. Nearly all people with narcolepsy who have cataplexy have extremely low levels of the naturally occurring chemical hypocretin, which promotes wakefulness and regulates REM sleep. Hypocretin levels are usually normal in people who have narcolepsy without cataplexy.

Although the cause of narcolepsy is not completely understood, current research suggests that narcolepsy may be the result of a combination of factors working together to cause a lack of hypocretin. These factors include:

- **Autoimmune disorders.** When cataplexy is present, the cause is most often the loss of brain cells that produce hypocretin. Although the reason for this cell loss is unknown, it appears to be linked to abnormalities in the immune system. Autoimmune disorders occur when the body's immune system turns against itself and mistakenly attacks healthy cells or tissue. Researchers believe that in individuals with narcolepsy, the body's immune system selectively attacks the hypocretin-containing brain cells because of a combination of genetic and environmental factors.

- **Family history.** Most cases of narcolepsy are sporadic, meaning the disorder occurs in individuals with no known family history. However, clusters in families sometimes occur—up to 10 percent of individuals diagnosed with narcolepsy with cataplexy report having a close relative with similar symptoms.

- **Brain injuries.** Rarely, narcolepsy results from traumatic injury to parts of the brain that regulate wakefulness and REM sleep or from tumors and other diseases in the same regions.

181

How Is Narcolepsy Diagnosed?

A **clinical examination and detailed medical history** are essential for diagnosis and treatment of narcolepsy. Individuals may be asked by their doctor to keep a sleep journal, noting the times of sleep and symptoms over a one- to two-week period. Although none of the major symptoms are exclusive to narcolepsy, cataplexy is the most specific symptom and occurs in almost no other diseases.

A **physical exam** can rule out or identify other neurological conditions that may be causing the symptoms. Two specialized tests, which can be performed in a sleep disorders clinic, are required to establish a diagnosis of narcolepsy:

- **Polysomnogram (PSG or sleep study).** The PSG is an overnight recording of brain and muscle activity, breathing, and eye movements. A PSG can help reveal whether REM sleep occurs early in the sleep cycle and if an individual's symptoms result from another condition, such as sleep apnea.

- **Multiple sleep latency test (MSLT).** The MSLT assesses daytime sleepiness by measuring how quickly a person falls asleep and whether they enter REM sleep. On the day after the PSG, an individual is asked to take 5 short naps separated by 2 hours over the course of a day. If an individual fall asleep in less than 8 minutes on average over the 5 naps, this indicates excessive daytime sleepiness. However, for individuals with narcolepsy, REM sleep starts abnormally quickly. If REM sleep happens within 15 minutes at least 2 times out of the 5 naps and the sleep study the night before, this is likely an abnormality caused by narcolepsy.

Occasionally, it may be helpful to measure the level of hypocretin in the fluid that surrounds the brain and spinal cord. To perform this test, a doctor will withdraw a sample of the cerebrospinal fluid (CBF) using a lumbar puncture (also called a "spinal tap") and measure the level of hypocretin-1. In the absence of other serious medical conditions, low hypocretin-1 levels almost certainly indicate type 1 narcolepsy.

What Treatments Are Available for Narcolepsy?

Although there is no cure for narcolepsy, some of the symptoms can be treated with medicines and lifestyle changes. When cataplexy is present, the loss of hypocretin is believed to be irreversible and lifelong.

Excessive daytime sleepiness and cataplexy can be controlled in most individuals with medications.

Medications

Modafinil. The initial line of treatment is usually a central nervous system stimulant, such as modafinil. Modafinil is usually prescribed first because it is less addictive and has fewer side effects than older stimulants. For most people, these drugs are generally effective at reducing daytime drowsiness and improving alertness.

Amphetamine-like stimulants. In cases where modafinil is not effective, doctors may prescribe amphetamine-like stimulants, such as methylphenidate, to alleviate EDS. However, these medications must be carefully monitored because they can have such side effects as irritability and nervousness, shakiness, disturbances in heart rhythm, and nighttime sleep disruption. In addition, healthcare professionals should be careful when prescribing these drugs and people should be careful using them because the potential for abuse is high with any amphetamine.

Antidepressants. Two classes of antidepressant drugs have proven effective in controlling cataplexy in many individuals: tricyclics (including imipramine, desipramine, clomipramine, and protriptyline) and selective serotonin and noradrenergic reuptake inhibitors (including venlafaxine, fluoxetine, and atomoxetine). In general, antidepressants produce fewer adverse effects than amphetamines. However, troublesome side effects still occur in some individuals, including impotence, high blood pressure, and heart rhythm irregularities.

Sodium oxybate. Sodium oxybate (also known as "gamma hydroxybutyrate" or "GHB") has been approved by the FDA to treat cataplexy and excessive daytime sleepiness in individuals with narcolepsy. It is a strong sedative that must be taken twice a night. Due to safety concerns associated with the use of this drug, the distribution of sodium oxybate is tightly restricted.

Lifestyle Changes

Not everyone with narcolepsy can consistently maintain a fully normal state of alertness using currently available medications. Drug therapy should accompany various lifestyle changes. The following strategies may be helpful:

- **Take short naps.** Many individuals take short, regularly scheduled naps at times when they tend to feel sleepiest.

- **Maintain a regular sleep schedule.** Going to bed and waking up at the same time every day, even on the weekends, can help people sleep better.

- **Avoid caffeine or alcohol before bed.** Individuals should avoid alcohol and caffeine for several hours before bedtime.

- **Avoid smoking,** especially at night.

- **Exercise daily.** Exercising for at least 20 minutes per day at least four or five hours before bedtime also improves sleep quality and can help people with narcolepsy avoid gaining excess weight.

- **Avoid large, heavy meals right before bedtime.** Eating very close to bedtime can make it harder to sleep.

- **Relax before bed.** Relaxing activities, such as a warm bath, before bedtime can help promote sleepiness. Also, make sure the sleep space is cool and comfortable.

- **Safety precautions,** particularly when driving, are important for everyone with narcolepsy. People with untreated symptoms are more likely to be involved in automobile although the risk is lower among individuals who are taking appropriate medication. EDS and cataplexy can lead to serious injury or death if left uncontrolled. Suddenly falling asleep or losing muscle control can transform actions that are ordinarily safe, such as walking down a long flight of stairs, into hazards.

The Americans with Disabilities Act (ADA) requires employers to provide reasonable accommodations for all employees with disabilities. Adults with narcolepsy can often negotiate with employers to modify their work schedules so they can take naps when necessary and perform their most demanding tasks when they are most alert. Similarly, children and adolescents with narcolepsy may be able to work with school administrators to accommodate special needs, such as taking medications during the school day, modifying class schedules to fit in a nap, and other strategies.

Additionally, support groups can be extremely beneficial for people with narcolepsy who want to develop better coping strategies or feel socially isolated due to embarrassment about their symptoms. Support groups also provide individuals with a network of social contacts who can offer practical help and emotional support.

Section 23.2

The Link between Narcolepsy and Autoimmunity

This section includes text excerpted from "Genetic Study Confirms the Immune System's Role in Narcolepsy," News and Events, National Institutes of Health (NIH), May 3, 2009. Reviewed May 2019.

Scientists funded by the National Institutes of Health (NIH) have identified a gene associated with narcolepsy, a disorder that causes disabling daytime sleepiness, sleep attacks, irresistible bouts of sleep that can strike at any time, and disturbed sleep at night. The gene has a known role in the immune system, which strongly suggests that autoimmunity, in which the immune system turns against the body's own tissues, plays an important role in the disorder.

"The link between narcolepsy and autoimmunity was proposed decades ago, but efforts to verify it have failed repeatedly. The findings leave little doubt that autoimmunity plays a role," says Merrill Mitler, Ph.D., a Program Director with the National Institute of Neurological Disorders and Stroke (NINDS). The study was funded principally by the NINDS, with additional support from the National Institute of Mental Health (NIMH), the National Heart, Lung and Blood Institute (NHLBI), and the National Institute of Allergy and Infectious Diseases (NIAID), all components of the NIH.

The study, which appeared in *Nature Genetics*, focused on narcolepsy with cataplexy—a sudden loss of muscle tone that can cause a person to collapse, with or without falling asleep. About 1 in 2,000 Americans have narcolepsy-cataplexy. The symptoms of narcolepsy-cataplexy have been shown to result from the death of a small group of brain cells that normally regulate the sleep–wake cycle by releasing chemicals called "hypocretins."

Genetic and environmental factors both clearly play a role in narcolepsy-cataplexy. Until now, the best evidence for autoimmunity as a cause of the disorder was the discovery that nearly everyone with the disorder has unique variants of a gene called "*HLA-DQB1*0602*." This is one of the genes that encodes human leukocyte antigen (HLA) proteins, which dot the surface of the body's cells and help the immune system identify foreign proteins. Some researchers theorize that the HLA variants found in people with narcolepsy-cataplexy predispose them to an autoimmune reaction that destroys their hypocretin-producing cells.

185

There are gaps in that theory, however, says Emmanuel Mignot, M.D., Ph.D., Director of the Center for Narcolepsy at Stanford University School of Medicine in Palo Alto, Calif., and a Howard Hughes Medical Institute investigator. Dr. Mignot discovered the link between narcolepsy and the hypocretins, and helped establish the link to the HLA system. HLA proteins are found in many tissues including the brain, where they may affect brain development, he says.

Human leukocyte antigen variations, however, do not fully account for narcolepsy-cataplexy. Dr. Mignot led a genome-wide association study to search for other genes associated with narcolepsy-cataplexy. These studies involve scanning the genome—the entire set of deoxyribonucleic acid (DNA)—for small differences between people who have a disorder and people who do not. Dr. Mignot's study included more than 4,000 individuals, all of whom had the HLA variants that predispose to narcolepsy-cataplexy but only about half of whom had the disorder. Participants were recruited so that many genetic groups were represented. Subjects were from the United States and eight countries in Europe and Asia; hundreds were African American, Korean, and Japanese, groups known to have a high incidence of the disorder.

The researchers discovered that in addition to unique HLA variants, people with narcolepsy-cataplexy are also more likely to have unique variants of the *TCRA* gene, which encodes a receptor protein on the surface of T cells. T cells are the mobile infantry of the immune system. In concert with the HLA proteins, the T cell receptor enables T cells to recognize and attack foreign invaders, such as bacteria and viruses. Changes to the T cell receptor could increase the likelihood that the cells will direct their attack against the body.

The findings of Dr. Mignot's group indicate that narcolepsy-cataplexy is linked to autoimmunity and involves T-cells. The research could lead to new approaches to prevention and treatment. One possibility may be preventing the disorder by stopping the effects of the autoimmune process. "If we can define the changes in the T cell receptor associated with narcolepsy-cataplexy, we might be able to develop drugs that block the protein's abnormal activity and prevent the onset of the disorder," says Dr. Mignot. Current treatments, such as stimulant drugs for combating daytime sleepiness and antidepressants for cataplexy, are only able to control symptoms and do not address the underlying loss of hypocretin cells.

It is important to note that this study, as with most genome-wide association studies, did not identify genetic variants that directly cause narcolepsy-cataplexy. Instead, it identifies groups that are more likely to show narcolepsy-cataplexy and groups that are less likely to show the disorder. In people with the HLA variants that predispose to narcolepsy-cataplexy, there is about a 20-fold higher frequency of the disorder if variants in the *TCRA* gene are present. It is yet to be known which people with the genetic variants will go on to develop narcolepsy-cataplexy.

Other risk factors for narcolepsy-cataplexy remain to be discovered, and Dr. Mignot's findings could provide clues to their identity. For example, further studies to characterize the T cells in people with narcolepsy-cataplexy could help reveal whether specific environmental factors—such as infections—contribute to the disorder. Dr. Mignot's findings also could lead to a better understanding of other autoimmune diseases where *HLA* genes are known to play a role, such as multiple sclerosis (MS) and type 1 diabetes.

Chapter 24

Parasomnias

What Are Parasomnias?

Parasomnias are "odd" actions that we do or unpleasant events that we experience while asleep or while partially asleep. Almost everyone has a nightmare. A nightmare is considered a parasomnia since it is an unpleasant event that occurs while we are asleep.

The term "parasomnia" is much broader than just nightmares, however. Other common parasomnia events include:

- Rapid eye movement (REM) behavior disorder (RBD)

- Sleep paralysis

- Sleepwalking

- Confusional arousals

What Are Common Parasomnias?

Parasomnias are typically classified by whether they occur during the REM sleep or the non-REM sleep. The REM sleep parasomnias tend to present as traits of wakefulness while in REM sleep, or as traits of REM sleep while awake. The non-REM sleep parasomnias tend to present as a middle ground where the patient is doing activities but is not fully awake.

This chapter includes text excerpted from "Parasomnia," U.S. Department of Veterans Affairs (VA), August 14, 2015. Reviewed May 2019.

Rapid Eye Movement Behavior Disorder

Most dreaming occurs in REM sleep. Normally in REM sleep, most of our body muscles are paralyzed to prevent us from acting out our dreams. In REM behavior disorder a person does not have this protective paralysis during REM sleep. A person, therefore, might "act out" their dream. Since dreams may involve violence and protecting oneself, a person acting out their dream may injure themselves or their bed partner. The person will usually recall the dream, but not realize that they were moving in real life.

Sleep Paralysis and Sleep Hallucinations

Rapid eye movement sleep is usually associated with dreams and the body paralyzing most of the muscles so dreams do not get acted out. Sometimes the REM-related paralysis or dream images can occur when falling asleep or when waking up from sleep. Sleep paralysis and sleep hallucinations can occur together or alone. The person is fully aware of what is happening. Events can be very scary. An event will usually last seconds to minutes and fortunately end on its own.

Sleepwalking

In sleepwalking, the person is just awake enough to be active but is still asleep and unaware of the activities. Sometimes, disorders such as sleepwalking are called "disorders of arousal" since the person is in a mixed state of awareness (not fully asleep or awake). Sleepwalking disorders can range from sitting up in bed to complex behaviors, such as driving a car. Sleepwalkers are unaware of their surroundings and can fall down or put themselves in danger. Despite the myths, it is not dangerous to awaken a sleepwalker. However, the person will not typically have recall of the sleepwalking event and may be confused or disoriented.

Confusional Arousals

We all have experienced that strange and confused feeling when we first wake up. Confusional arousal is a sleep disorder that causes a person to act that way for a prolonged period. Episodes usually start when someone is abruptly woken up. The person does not wake up completely and so remains in a foggy state of mind. The person with confusional arousal may have difficulty understanding situations around them, react slowly to commands or react aggressively as the first response to others.

What Can You Do for Parasomnias?

Many people with parasomnias see an improvement by improving their sleep habits. Some sleep healthy sleep tips include:

- Ensure you are getting enough sleep.
- Keep a regular schedule of going to bed and waking up.
- Avoid alcohol or other sedatives at night that might make it hard for you to completely wake up.
- Avoid caffeine or smoking.
- Keep the bedroom quiet to avoid getting disturbed.

Make sure that persons suffering from parasomnias remain safe. Some tips for bedroom safety with a parasomnia include:

- Avoid large objects that can fall by the bedside.
- Make sure there are no objects on the floor that can be tripped over.
- Close and lock bedroom doors and windows to ensure a person cannot go outside.
- Consider an alarm or bell on the door.
- Close shades over windows in case they are hit to protect a person from glass.
- Remove potentially dangerous objects and weapons in the bedroom.
- Avoid significant elevation. No bunk beds. Consider mattresses on the ground and ground-floor bedrooms.

Chapter 25

Nocturnal Sleep-Related Eating Disorder

About one to three percent of the general population appears to be affected by sleep-related eating disorder (SRED). Both men and women can have this disorder, but it is more common among women. Sleep eating is also known to run in the family. The onset of this disease is typically between the ages of 20 and 40. Sleep-related eating disorder can also be triggered by other sleep disorders or medical conditions.

What Is Nocturnal Sleep-Related Eating Disorder?

Sleep eating is a disorder in which the patient is hungry and eats at night. Patients diet during the day and are vulnerable to eating at night but have no memory of doing so. In most cases, people with SRED have a history of alcoholism, drug abuse, and other sleep disorders. They often eat different types of food at odd hours, and they may even eat inedible substances. They lose their appetite for food, which often results in anxiety, stress, or depression.

More than 50 percent of these individuals gain weight from consuming food during sleeping hours. They also feel drowsy and experience extreme emotions. Sometimes, low blood sugar (hypoglycemia) can also cause SRED. Dyssomnia is a conscious behavior, while parasomnia is an unconscious behavior. People with SRED usually:

"Nocturnal Sleep-Related Eating Disorder," © 2018 Omnigraphics. Reviewed May 2019.

- Become ill from inadequately cooked food or ingesting toxic substances

- Develop metabolic conditions (Type 2 diabetes or elevated cholesterol)

- Develop cavities or tooth decay from eating sugary foods

- Have unrefreshing sleep and feel sleepy or tired during the day

- Injure themselves preparing food (lacerations, burns)

- Gain weight

Sleep eating is an arousal disorder in which:

- The patient indulges in abnormal behavior during arousal from slow-wave sleep.

- The patient indulges in repetitive and automatic motor activity.

- The patient is unaware of the entire episode as it is occurring.

- The patient finds it difficult to wake up despite vigorous attempts.

Symptoms of Nocturnal Sleep-Related Eating Disorder

People with SREDs often eat toxic substances and often in strange combinations. Continuous episodes of binge eating only occur when the patients are partially awake. The following conditions are seen in people with sleep-related eating disorder:

- Do something dangerous while getting or cooking food

- Continuous episodes of binge eating and drinking during the time when they sleep

- Have eating episodes that disturb their sleep and cause insomnia, resulting in unrefreshing sleep

- Decline in health from eating foods that are high in calories

- Have a loss of appetite in the morning

If something else is causing the problem, it may be one of the following reasons:

- A mental-health disorder

- A medical condition
- Another sleep disorder
- Substance abuse
- Medication use

Risk Factors for Nocturnal Sleep-Related Eating Disorder

About 65 to 80 percent of SRED patients are females between the ages of 22 and 29. Sleep-related eating disorder can also occur from the use of certain medicines that are used to treat depression and other sleep problems. Sleep disorder is an ongoing problem, and most people with SRED were sleepwalkers as children. Sleep-related disorders include the following:

- Restless legs syndrome (RLS)
- Periodic limb movement disorder
- Obstructive sleep apnea (OSA)
- Irregular sleep–wake rhythm
- Sleep-related dissociative disorders

Sleep-related eating disorder symptoms typically include the following:

- Dieting during the day
- Daytime eating disorders
- Ending the abuse of alcohol or drugs
- Use of certain medications
- Quitting smoking

Sleep-related eating disorder may result in:

- Encephalitis (brain swelling)
- Hepatitis (liver infection)
- Narcolepsy
- Stress

Diagnosis of Sleep-Related Eating Disorder

It is important for patients to inform their doctor when this eating disorder begins. Keep your doctor informed about your complete medical history. Make sure to inform the doctor of any medication that you have been taking. Maintain a sleep diary to help the doctor understand your sleeping patterns. The doctor will do an overnight sleep study called a "polysomnogram." The polysomnogram will chart your brain waves, heartbeat, and breathing as you sleep. The unusual behaviors that occur during the night will be recorded on a video, which will help your doctor determine the patterns of your sleep-eating disorder.

Treatment of Sleep-Related Eating Disorder

Treatment for sleep-related disorders involves stress management classes, counseling, clinical interview, and a limited intake or avoidance of alcohol and caffeine. The physician may change some of your medicines to make it easier for you to treat SRED. Plenty of sleep is required on a daily basis. It is important to consult a sleep specialist to check for signs of sleep disorders.

Consulting a psychotherapist may help reduce stress and anxiety. The physician may recommend medicines, such as benzodiazepine, to treat your sleep-related disorder. Mirapex and Sinemet are effective dopaminergic agents for sleep eaters.

References

1. "Sleep-Related Eating Disorders," National Center for Biotechnology Information (NCBI), November 2006.

2. "Sleep-Related Eating Disorders," Cleveland Clinic, April 22, 2017.

3. "Sleep Eating Disorder—Overview and Facts," American Academy of Sleep Medicine (AASM), n.d.

Chapter 26

Myalgic Encephalomyelitis/ Chronic Fatigue Syndrome

Myalgic encephalomyelitis (ME)/chronic fatigue syndrome (CFS) is a disabling and complex illness.

People with ME/CFS are often not able to do their usual activities. At times, ME/CFS may confine them to bed. People with ME/CFS have overwhelming fatigue that is not improved by rest. ME/CFS may get worse after any activity, whether it is physical or mental. This symptom is known as "postexertional malaise" (PEM). Other symptoms can include problems with sleep, thinking and concentrating, pain, and dizziness. People with ME/CFS may not look ill. However:

- People with ME/CFS are not able to function the same way they did before they became ill.

- ME/CFS changes people's ability to do daily tasks, such as taking a shower or preparing a meal.

- ME/CFS often makes it hard to keep a job, go to school, and take part in family and social life.

- ME/CFS can last for years and sometimes leads to serious disability.

This chapter includes text excerpted from "What Is ME/CFS?" Centers for Disease Control and Prevention (CDC), July 12, 2018.

- At least one in four ME/CFS patients is bed- or house-bound for long periods during their illness.

Anyone can get ME/CFS. While most common in people between the ages of 40 and 60, the illness affects children, adolescents, and adults of all ages. Among adults, women are affected more often than men. Whites are diagnosed more than other races and ethnicities. But many people with ME/CFS have not been diagnosed, especially among minorities.

As noted in the Institute of Medicine (IOM) report:

- An estimated 836,000 to 2.5 million Americans suffer from ME/CFS.

- About 90 percent of people with ME/CFS have not been diagnosed.

- ME/CFS costs the U.S. economy about $17 to $24 billion annually in medical bills and lost incomes.

Some of the reasons that people with ME/CFS have not been diagnosed include limited access to healthcare and a lack of education about ME/CFS among healthcare providers.

- Most medical schools in the United States do not have ME/CFS as part of their physician training.

- The illness is often misunderstood and might not be taken seriously by some healthcare providers.

- More education for doctors and nurses is urgently needed so they are prepared to provide timely diagnosis and appropriate care for patients.

Researchers have not yet found what causes ME/CFS, and there are no specific laboratory tests to diagnose ME/CFS directly. Therefore, doctors need to consider the diagnosis of ME/CFS based on in-depth evaluation of a person's symptoms and medical history. It is also important that doctors diagnose and treat any other conditions that can cause similar symptoms. Even though there is no cure for ME/CFS, some symptoms can be treated or managed.

Possible Causes of Myalgic Encephalomyelitis/ Chronic Fatigue Syndrome

Scientists have not yet identified what causes ME/CFS. It is possible that ME/CFS has more than one cause, meaning that patients with ME/CFS could have illness resulting from different causes (see below). In addition, it is possible that two or more triggers might work together to cause the illness.

Some of the areas that are being studied as possible causes of ME/CFS are:

- Infections

- Immune system changes

- Stress affecting body chemistry

- Changes in energy production

- Possible genetic link

Symptoms of Myalgic Encephalomyelitis/Chronic Fatigue Syndrome
Primary Symptoms

Also called "core" symptoms, three primary symptoms are required for diagnosis:

- **Greatly lowered ability to do activities that were usual before the illness.** This drop in the activity level occurs along with fatigue and must last six months or longer.People with ME/CFS have fatigue that is very different from just being tired. The fatigue of ME/CFS:

  - Can be severe

  - Is not a result of unusually difficult activity

  - Is not relieved by sleep or rest

  - Was not a problem before becoming ill (not lifelong)

- **Worsening of ME/CFS symptoms after physical or mental activity that would not have caused a problem before illness.** This is known as "postexertional malaise" (PEM). People with ME/CFS often describe this experience as a "crash," "relapse," or "collapse." During PEM, any ME/CFS symptoms may get worse or first appear, including difficulty thinking, problems sleeping, sore throat, headaches, feeling dizzy, or severe tiredness. It may take days, weeks, or longer to recover from a crash. Sometimes patients may be house-bound or even completely bed-bound during crashes. People with ME/CFS may

199

not be able to predict what will cause a crash or how long it will last. As examples:

- Attending a child's school event may leave someone house-bound for a couple of days and not able to do needed tasks, such as laundry.

- Shopping at the grocery store may cause a physical crash that requires a nap in the car before driving home or a call for a ride home.

- Taking a shower may leave someone with ME/CFS bed-bound and unable to do anything for days.

- Keeping up with work may lead to spending evenings and weekends recovering from the effort.

- **Sleep problems.** People with ME/CFS may not feel better or less tired, even after a full night of sleep. Some people with ME/CFS may have problems falling asleep or staying asleep.

In addition to these core symptoms, one of the following two symptoms is required for diagnosis:

- **Problems with thinking and memory.** Most people with ME/CFS have trouble thinking quickly, remembering things, and paying attention to details. Patients often say they have "brain fog" to describe this problem because they feel "stuck in a fog" and not able to think clearly.

- **Worsening of symptoms while standing or sitting upright.** This is called "orthostatic intolerance." People with ME/CFS may be lightheaded, dizzy, weak, or faint while standing or sitting up. They may have vision changes, such as blurring or seeing spots.

Other Common Symptoms

Many but not all people with ME/CFS have other symptoms.

Pain is very common in people with ME/CFS. The type of pain, where it occurs, and how bad it is, varies a lot. The pain people with ME/CFS feel is not caused by an injury. The most common types of pain in ME/CFS are:

- Muscle pain and aches

- Joint pain without swelling or redness

- Headaches, either new or worsening

Some people with ME/CFS may also have:

- Tender lymph nodes in the neck or armpits
- A sore throat that happens often
- Digestive issues, such as irritable bowel syndrome (IBS)
- Chills and night sweats
- Allergies and sensitivities to foods, odors, chemicals, or noise

Part Four

Other Health Problems That Often Affect Sleep

Chapter 27

Attention Deficit Hyperactivity Disorder and Sleep

Attention deficit hyperactivity disorder (ADHD) is a problem of not being able to focus, being overactive, not being able control behavior, or a combination of these. For these problems to be diagnosed as ADHD, they must be out of the normal range for a person's age and development.

Causes of Attention Deficit Hyperactivity Disorder

Attention deficit hyperactivity disorder usually begins in childhood but may continue into the adult years. It is the most commonly diagnosed behavioral disorder in children. ADHD is diagnosed much more often in boys than in girls.

It is not clear what causes ADHD. A combination of genes and environmental factors likely plays a role in the development of the condition. Imaging studies suggest that the brains of children with

---

This chapter contains text excerpted from the following sources: Text in this chapter begins with excerpts from "Attention Deficit Hyperactivity Disorder (ADHD)," MentalHealth.gov, U.S. Department of Health and Human Services (HHS), August 22, 2017; Text under the heading "How Sleep Affects Attention Deficit Hyperactivity Disorder" is © 2017 Omnigraphics. Reviewed May 2019.

ADHD are different from those of children without attention deficit hyperactivity disorder.

Symptoms of Attention Deficit Hyperactivity Disorder

Symptoms of ADHD fall into three groups:

- Not being able to focus (inattentiveness)
- Being extremely active (hyperactivity)
- Not being able to control behavior (impulsivity)

Some people with ADHD have mainly inattentive symptoms. Some have mainly hyperactive and impulsive symptoms. Others have a combination of different symptom types. Those with mostly inattentive symptoms are sometimes said to have attention deficit disorder (ADD). They tend to be less disruptive and are more likely not to be diagnosed with attention deficit hyperactivity disorder.

Inattentive symptoms include:

- Fails to give close attention to details or makes careless mistakes in schoolwork
- Has difficulty keeping attention during tasks or play
- Does not seem to listen when spoken to directly
- Does not follow through on instructions and fails to finish schoolwork or chores and tasks
- Has problems organizing tasks and activities
- Avoids or dislikes tasks that require sustained mental effort (such as schoolwork)
- Often loses toys, assignments, pencils, books, or tools needed for tasks or activities
- Is easily distracted
- Is often forgetful in daily activities

Hyperactivity symptoms include:

- Fidgets with hands or feet or squirms in seat
- Leaves seat when remaining seated is expected
- Runs about or climbs in inappropriate situations

- Has problems playing or working quietly
- Is often "on the go," acts as if "driven by a motor"
- Talks excessively

Impulsivity symptoms include:

- Blurts out answers before questions have been completed
- Has difficulty awaiting turn
- Interrupts or intrudes on others (butts into conversations or games)

How Sleep Affects Attention Deficit Hyperactivity Disorder

Sleep deprivation among adolescents is a common problem in the United States, and researchers have found substantial links between ADHD and sleep issues. Adolescents who are diagnosed with ADHD tend to experience such problems as trouble falling asleep, staying asleep, and disrupted sleep. The National Sleep Foundation (NSF) studies have found that 50 percent of children and teens with ADHD suffer from sleep-disordered breathing and have more daytime sleepiness when compared to just 22 percent of other children and teens. Sleep issues can aggravate ADHD symptoms, and a few studies have even suggested that regular sleep patterns can help eliminate hyperactivity among some young people.

Interestingly, lack of sleep affects children and teens quite differently than it does adults. While adults who get very little sleep generally become lethargic, young people tend to get high-strung, inattentive, and often display disruptive behavior. As a result, sleep disorders in children and teens can lead to more serious issues in school, at home, and in social situations.

Here are some tips to help teens with ADHD get better sleep:

- Caffeine is a major stimulant; therefore, avoiding caffeinated beverages and foods can help ensure proper sleep.

- Consistent habits, such as specific bedtimes, waking times, and a healthy diet, can be helpful.

- A dark, quiet, and cozy room helps promote undisturbed sleep.

- Avoid sleep medication, which can result in daytime grogginess and lead to dependency.

- Daily exercise can help teens sleep better.
- Take a warm bath before bedtime to encourage relaxation.

References

1. "ADHD and Sleep," Sleep Foundation, n.d.

2. Bhandari, Smitha, MD. "ADHD and Sleep Disorders," WebMD, November 18, 2014.

3. "Diagnosing ADHD in Adolescence," CHADD The National Resource on ADHD, n.d.

4. Spruyt, Karen, Ph.D., and David Gozal, MD. "Sleep Disturbances in Children with Attention-Deficit/Hyperactivity Disorder," SleepMed, December 10, 2009.

Chapter 28

The Link between
Alzheimer Disease and Sleep

Alzheimer disease (AD) is an irreversible, progressive brain disorder that slowly destroys memory and thinking skills, and eventually the ability to carry out the simplest tasks. In most people with Alzheimer disease, symptoms first appear in their mid-60s. Estimates vary, but experts suggest that more than 5.5 million Americans may have AD. It is currently ranked as the sixth leading cause of death in the United States, but recent estimates indicate that the disorder may rank third, just behind heart disease and cancer, as a cause of death for older people.

Alzheimer disease is named after Dr. Alois Alzheimer. In 1906, Dr. Alzheimer noticed changes in the brain tissue of a woman who had died of an unusual mental illness. Her symptoms included memory loss, language problems, and unpredictable behavior. After she died, he examined her brain and found many abnormal clumps (now called "amyloid plaques") and tangled bundles of fibers (now called "neurofibrillary," or "tau," "tangles"). These plaques and tangles in the brain are still considered some of the main features of Alzheimer disease.

This chapter contains text excerpted from the following sources: Text in this chapter begins with excerpts from "Alzheimer Disease Fact Sheet," National Institute on Aging (NIA), National Institutes of Health (NIH), August 17, 2016; Text under the heading "What the Study Says about Alzheimer Disease and Sleep" is excerpted from "Does Poor Sleep Raise Risk for Alzheimer's Disease?" National Institute on Aging (NIA), National Institutes of Health (NIH), February 29, 2016.

What the Study Says about Alzheimer Disease and Sleep

Studies confirm what many people already know: sleep gets worse with age. Middle-aged and older adults often sleep less deeply, wake more frequently at night, or wake up too early in the morning. Could these problems be related to a risk of cognitive decline or AD?

Scientists are beginning to probe the complex relationship between the brain changes involved in poor sleep and those in very early-stage AD. It is an intriguing area of research, given that both the risk for disturbed sleep and AD increase with age.

"Nearly 60 percent of older adults have some kind of chronic sleep disturbance," said Phyllis Zee, Ph.D., a sleep expert at Northwestern University's Feinberg School of Medicine, Chicago.

It is long been known that people with AD often have sleep problems—getting their days and nights mixed up, for example. Now scientists are probing the link between sleep and AD earlier in the disease process and in cognitively normal adults. They wonder if improving sleep with existing treatments might help memory and other cognitive functions, and perhaps delay or prevent Alzheimer disease.

Which Comes First, Poor Sleep or Alzheimer Disease?

The chicken-and-egg question is whether AD-related brain changes lead to poor sleep, or whether poor sleep somehow contributes to Alzheimer disease. Scientists believe the answer may be both. Findings show that brain activity induced by poor sleep may influence AD-related brain changes, which begin years before memory loss and other disease symptoms appear.

National Institute on Aging (NIA)-funded scientists are studying the biological underpinnings of this relationship in animals and humans to better understand how these changes occur. Although evidence points to certain sleep problems as a risk factor for Alzheimer disease, "it is not known whether improving sleep will reduce the likelihood of developing Alzheimer," Dr. Mackiewicz said. He adds, "There is no scientific evidence that sleep medications or other sleep treatments will reduce risk for Alzheimer."

Effects of Good and Bad Sleep

At any age, getting a good night's sleep serves a number of important functions for our bodies and brains. Even though our bodies rest during sleep, our brains are active. The process is not totally understood, but researchers think that sleep might benefit the brain—and the whole body—by removing metabolic waste that accumulates in the brain during wakefulness. In addition, it has been shown that some memories are consolidated, moving from short-term to long-term storage, during periods of deep sleep. Other sleep stages may also influence memory and memory consolidation, research shows.

Disturbed sleep—whether due to illness, pain, anxiety, depression, or a sleep disorder—can lead to trouble concentrating, remembering, and learning. A return to normal sleep patterns usually eases these problems. But in older people, disturbed sleep may have more dire and long-lasting consequences.

Scientists long believed that the initial buildup of the beta-amyloid protein in the brain, an early biological sign of Alzheimer disease, causes disturbed sleep, Dr. Mackiewicz said. Though, evidence suggests the opposite may also occur—disturbed sleep in cognitively normal older adults contributes to the risk of cognitive decline and Alzheimer disease.

For example, in a study of older men free of dementia, poor sleep, including greater nighttime wakefulness, was associated with cognitive decline over a period of more than three years. Sleep was assessed through participants' reports and a device worn on the wrist that tracks movements during sleep.

Sleep disorders, such as sleep apnea, may pose an even greater risk of cognitive impairment. In a five-year study of older women, those with sleep-disordered breathing (SDB)—repeated arousals from sleep due to breathing disruptions, as with sleep apnea—had a nearly two-fold increase in risk for mild cognitive impairment (MCI) (a precursor to AD in some people) or dementia.

In addition, certain types of poor sleep seem to be associated with a risk of cognitive impairment, according to Kristine Yaffe, M.D., of the University of California, San Francisco. These include hypoxia (low oxygen levels that can be caused by sleep disorders) and difficulty in falling or staying asleep.

What Is the Connection between Sleep and Alzheimer Disease?

Evidence of a link between sleep and risk of AD has led to investigations to explain the brain activity that underlies this connection in humans. Some studies suggest that poor sleep contributes to abnormal levels of beta-amyloid protein in the brain, which leads to the amyloid plaques found in the AD brain. These plaques might then affect sleep-related brain regions, further disrupting sleep.

Studies in laboratory animals show a direct link between sleep and Alzheimer disease. One study in mice, led by researchers at Washington University, St. Louis, showed that beta-amyloid levels naturally rose during wakefulness and fell during sleep. Mice deprived of sleep for 21 days showed significantly greater beta-amyloid plaques than those that slept normally. Increasing sleep had the opposite effect—it reduced the amyloid load.

A subsequent study, also by Washington University researchers, showed that when mice with AD were treated with antibodies, beta-amyloid deposits decreased and sleep returned to normal. Mice that received a placebo saline solution continued to sleep poorly. The results suggest that sleep disruption could be a sign of AD beginning in the brain but not necessarily its cause.

Studies in humans have also addressed the relationship between sleep and biomarkers of Alzheimer disease. One study found that in cognitively normal older adults, poor sleep quality (more time awake at night and more daytime naps) was associated with lower beta-amyloid levels in cerebrospinal fluid (CSF), a preclinical sign of AD. Another study, by researchers at the NIA and Johns Hopkins University, Baltimore, found that healthy older adults who reported short sleep duration and poor sleep quality had more beta-amyloid in the brain than those without such sleep problems.

Emerging Insights

How exactly does poor sleep and Alzheimer disease influence each other? Research so far suggests a few possible mechanisms:

- **Orexin,** a molecule that regulates wakefulness and other functions, has been found to affect beta-amyloid levels in mice.

- **Chronic hypoxia,** insufficient oxygen in blood or tissue that is a feature of sleep apnea, increased the level of harmful beta-amyloid in brain tissue of mice.

- **Reduced slow-wave sleep** leads to increased neuronal activity.

Other factors may also be involved. For example, it has been shown in laboratory animals that the glymphatic system, the brain's waste removal system, removes beta-amyloid during sleep. A mouse study suggests that sleeping in different positions impacts waste removal from the brain. Sleeping on the side cleared beta-amyloid more efficiently than sleeping on the back or belly, researchers found. They pointed to the glymphatic system as a possible pathway for intervention.

Further biological and epidemiological studies and clinical trials should cast more light on the mechanisms behind the sleep-AD connection, and whether treating poor sleep might help delay or prevent cognitive decline in older adults.

"Sleep is something we can fix, and people with sleep problems should consult a doctor so that they can function at their best," Dr. Mackiewicz said. As for AD, for now, he said, improving sleep is "not the same as preventing Alzheimer disease. Researchers are committed to a achieving a better understanding of this complex dynamic in hopes of making a difference in the lives of older adults."

Studies to examine the value of a good night's sleep in delaying or preventing AD are underway.

Chapter 29

Brain Protein Affects Aging and Sleep

A study revealed how an aging-related protein in the brain affects sleep patterns. A better understanding of the connections between aging and sleep may lead to improved methods for treating or preventing certain diseases of aging.

Our sleep–wake cycle is governed by an internal circadian clock that is coordinated by a tiny brain region known as the "suprachiasmatic nucleus" (SCN). The circadian clock adjusts to several cues in your surroundings, especially light and darkness. Animal studies have shown that disrupting the circadian cycle may trigger health problems, such as obesity and diabetes. In contrast, a stable circadian cycle that includes healthy, consistent sleep is associated with longer lifespans in mice.

Many people develop sleeping problems as they age. Studies have linked circadian activity with SIRT1, a protein known to be involved in the aging process. Researchers have been searching for ways to raise SIRT1 activity in hope of warding off age-related diseases. Strategies include calorie restriction and the compound resveratrol, found in grapes and wine.

To further explore the links between SIRT1 and the circadian clock, a research team led by Dr. Leonard Guarente at the Massachusetts

This chapter includes text excerpted from "Brain Protein Affects Aging and Sleep," National Institutes of Health (NIH), July 15, 2013. Reviewed May 2019.

215

Institute of Technology altered SIRT1 levels in the brain tissue of mice. Their study, funded in part by the National Institutes of Health's (NIH) National Institute on Aging (NIA), appeared in the June 20, 2013 issue of *Cell*.

The team created genetically engineered mice that produce different amounts of SIRT1 in the brain. They studied groups of mice with normal levels of SIRT1, no SIRT1, and 2 groups with increased SIRT1—either 2 times or 10 times the normal amount. The researchers conducted "jet lag" experiments with the mice by shifting their light/dark cycles and observing their ability to adjust their sleep patterns.

Similar to previous findings, older mice with unaltered SIRT1 levels took much longer to adapt to shifting cycles than younger ones. Young mice lacking SIRT1 took twice as long to adapt as those with normal SIRT1 levels. Increasing SIRT1 levels, in contrast, had a protective effect. Old mice with 10 times the level of SIRT1 were able to adapt their sleep patterns much more quickly than normal SIRT1 mice of the same age.

A genetic analysis found that SIRT1 levels in the SCN affect the expression of genes involved in circadian control. All the circadian genes tested were expressed at significantly lower levels in mice lacking SIRT1. In contrast, the genes were expressed at higher levels in mice with more SIRT1. SIRT1 activated the two major circadian regulators, BMAL1 and CLOCK.

SIRT1 levels in the SCN declined with age in the mice—as did BMAL1 and other circadian regulatory proteins. These results suggest that SIRT1 plays a central role in the decline of circadian function as we age.

"What's now emerging is the idea that maintaining the circadian cycle is quite important in health maintenance," says Guarente, "and if it gets broken, there's a penalty to be paid in health and perhaps in aging." Further research will be needed to see whether dietary or other interventions that increase SIRT1 activity can help slow the onset and progression of sleep problems related to aging.

Chapter 30

Cancer Patients and Sleep Disorders

Sleep disorders keep you from having a good night's sleep. This may make it hard for you to stay alert and involved in activities during the day. Sleep disorders can cause problems for cancer patients. You may not be able to remember treatment instructions and may have trouble making decisions. Being well-rested can improve energy and help you cope better with side effects of cancer and treatment.

Sleep problems that go on for a long time may increase the risk of anxiety or depression. This chapter is about sleep disorders in adults who have cancer.

Sleep Disorders Are More Common in People with Cancer

While sleep disorders affect a small number of healthy people, as many as half of patients with cancer have problems sleeping. The sleep disorders most likely to affect patients with cancer are insomnia and an abnormal sleep–wake cycle.

There are many reasons a cancer patient may have trouble sleeping, including:

- Physical changes caused by the cancer or surgery

This chapter includes text excerpted from "Sleep Disorders (PDQ®)—Patient Version," National Cancer Institute (NCI), January 27, 2016.

- Side effects of drugs or other treatments
- Being in the hospital
- Stress about having cancer
- Health problems not related to the cancer

Tumors May Cause Sleep Problems

For patients with tumors, the tumor may cause the following problems that make it hard to sleep:

- Pressure from the tumor on nearby areas of the body
- Gastrointestinal (GI) problems (nausea, constipation, diarrhea, being unable to control the bowels)
- Bladder problems (irritation, being unable to control urine flow)
- Pain
- Fever
- Cough
- Trouble breathing
- Itching
- Feeling very tired

Certain Drugs or Treatments May Affect Sleep

Common cancer treatments and drugs can affect normal sleep patterns. How well a cancer patient sleeps may be affected by:

- Hormone therapy (HT)
- Corticosteroids
- Sedatives and tranquilizers
- Antidepressants
- Anticonvulsants

Long-term use of certain drugs may cause insomnia. Stopping or decreasing the use of certain drugs can also affect normal sleep. Other side effects of drugs and treatments that may affect the sleep–wake cycle include the following:

- Pain

- Anxiety

- Night sweats or hot flashes

- Gastrointestinal problems, such as nausea, constipation, diarrhea, and being unable to control the bowels

- Bladder problems, such as irritation or being unable to control urine

- Breathing problems

Being in the Hospital May Make It Harder to Sleep

Getting a normal night's sleep in the hospital is difficult. The following may affect how well a patient sleeps:

- **Hospital environment.** Patients may be bothered by an uncomfortable bed, pillow, or room temperature; noise; or sharing a room with a stranger.

- **Hospital routine.** Sleep may be interrupted when doctors and nurses come in to check on or administer drugs to the patient, other treatments, or exams.

Getting sleep during a hospital stay may also be affected by anxiety and the patient's age.

Stress Caused by Learning the Cancer Diagnosis Often Causes Sleeping Problems

Stress, anxiety, and depression are common reactions to initial learning of the cancer, receiving treatments, and being in the hospital. These are common causes of insomnia.

Other Health Problems Not Related to Cancer May Cause a Sleep Disorder

Cancer patients can have sleep disorders that are caused by other health problems. Conditions, such as snoring, headaches, and daytime seizures increase the chance of having a sleep disorder.

Chapter 31

Mental Health and Sleep

Chapter Contents

Section 31.1

Generalized Anxiety Disorder and Sleep

This section includes text excerpted from "Generalized Anxiety Disorder: When Worry Gets out of Control," National Institute of Mental Health (NIMH), October 5, 2016.

What Is Generalized Anxiety Disorder?

Occasional anxiety is a normal part of life. You might worry about things, such as health, money, or family problems. But, people with generalized anxiety disorder (GAD) feel extremely worried or feel nervous about these and other things—even when there is little or no reason to worry about them. People with GAD find it difficult to control their anxiety and stay focused on daily tasks.

The good news is that GAD is treatable. Call your doctor to talk about your symptoms so that you can feel better.

What Are the Signs and Symptoms of Generalized Anxiety Disorder?

Generalized anxiety disorder develops slowly. It often starts during the teen years or young adulthood. People with GAD may:

- Worry often about everyday things

- Have trouble controlling their worries or feelings of nervousness

- Know that they worry much more than they should

- Feel restless and have trouble relaxing

- Have a hard time concentrating

- Be easily startled

- Have trouble falling asleep or staying asleep

- Easily tire or feel tired all the time

- Have headaches, muscle aches, stomach aches, or unexplained pains

- Have a hard time swallowing

- Tremble or twitch

- Be irritable or feel "on edge"

- Sweat a lot, feel light-headed or out of breath
- Have to go to the bathroom a lot

Children and teens with GAD often worry excessively about:

- Their performance, such as in school or in sports
- Catastrophes, such as earthquakes or war

Adults with GAD are often highly nervous about everyday circumstances, such as:

- Job security or performance
- Health
- Finances
- The health and well-being of their children
- Being late
- Completing household chores and other responsibilities

Both children and adults with GAD may experience physical symptoms that make it hard to function and that interfere with daily life.

What Causes Generalized Anxiety Disorder

Generalized anxiety disorder sometimes runs in families, but no one knows for sure why some family members have it while others do not. Researchers have found that several parts of the brain, as well as biological processes, play a key role in fear and anxiety. By learning more about how the brain and body function in people with anxiety disorders, researchers may be able to create better treatments. Researchers are also looking for ways in which stress and environmental factors play a role.

What Is It like to Have Generalized Anxiety Disorder?

"I was worried all the time and felt nervous. My family told me that there were no signs of problems, but I still felt upset. I dreaded going to work because I could not keep my mind focused. I was having trouble falling asleep at night and was irritated at my family all the time.

I saw my doctor and explained my constant worries. My doctor sent me to someone who knows about GAD. Now I am working with a counselor to cope better with my anxiety. I had to work hard, but I feel better. I am glad I made that first call to my doctor."

Section 31.2

Depression and Sleep

This section includes text excerpted from "Depression," National Institute of Mental Health (NIMH), February 2018.

Depression (major depressive disorder or clinical depression) is a common but serious mood disorder. It causes severe symptoms that affect how you feel; think; and handle daily activities, such as sleeping, eating, or working. To be diagnosed with depression, the symptoms must be present for at least two weeks.

Some forms of depression are slightly different, or they may develop under unique circumstances, such as:

- **Persistent depressive disorder (PDD)** (also called "dysthymia") is a depressed mood that lasts for at least two years. A person diagnosed with persistent depressive disorder may have episodes of major depression along with periods of less severe symptoms, but symptoms must last for two years to be considered as persistent depressive disorder.

- **Postpartum depression** is much more serious than the "baby blues" (relatively mild depressive and anxiety symptoms that typically clear within two weeks after delivery) that many women experience after giving birth. Women with postpartum depression experience full-blown major depression during pregnancy or after delivery. The feelings of extreme sadness, anxiety, and exhaustion that accompany postpartum depression may make it difficult for new mothers to complete daily care activities for themselves and/or for their babies.

- **Psychotic depression** occurs when a person has severe depression plus some form of psychosis, such as having disturbing false fixed beliefs (delusions) or hearing or seeing upsetting things that others cannot hear or see (hallucinations). The psychotic symptoms typically have a depressive "theme," such as delusions of guilt, poverty, or illness.

- **Seasonal affective disorder (SAD)** is characterized by the onset of depression during the winter months when there is less natural sunlight. This depression generally lifts during spring and summer. Winter depression, typically accompanied by social withdrawal, increased sleep, and weight gain, predictably returns every year in seasonal affective disorder.

- **Bipolar disorder** is different from depression, but it is included in this list is because someone with bipolar disorder experiences episodes of extremely low moods that meet the criteria for major depression (called "bipolar depression"). But, a person with bipolar disorder also experiences extreme high—euphoric or irritable—moods called "mania" or a less severe form called "hypomania."

Examples of other types of depressive disorders newly added to the diagnostic classification of *Diagnostic and Statistical Manual of Mental Disorders, Fifth Edition* (DSM-5) include disruptive mood dysregulation disorder (DMDD) (diagnosed in children and adolescents) and premenstrual dysphoric disorder (PMDD).

Signs and Symptoms of Depression and Sleep

If you have been experiencing some of the following signs and symptoms most of the day, nearly every day, for at least two weeks, you may be suffering from depression:

- Persistent sad, anxious, or "empty" mood

- Feelings of hopelessness, or pessimism

- Irritability

- Feelings of guilt, worthlessness, or helplessness

- Loss of interest or pleasure in hobbies and activities

- Decreased energy or fatigue

- Moving or talking more slowly

- Feeling restless or having trouble sitting still

- Difficulty concentrating, remembering, or making decisions

- Difficulty sleeping, early-morning awakening, or oversleeping

- Appetite and/or weight changes

- Thoughts of death or suicide, or suicide attempts

- Aches or pains, headaches, cramps, or digestive problems without a clear physical cause and/or that do not ease even with treatment

Not everyone who is depressed experiences every symptom. Some people experience only a few symptoms, while others may experience many. Several persistent symptoms in addition to low mood are required for a diagnosis of major depression, but people with only a few—but distressing—symptoms may benefit from treatment of their "subsyndromal" depression. The severity and frequency of symptoms and how long they last will vary depending on the individual and her or his particular illness. Symptoms may also vary depending on the stage of the illness.

Risk Factors for Depression and Sleep

Depression is one of the most common mental disorders in the United States. Research suggests that depression is caused by a combination of genetic, biological, environmental, and psychological factors.

Depression can happen at any age, but it often begins in adulthood. Depression is now recognized as occurring in children and adolescents, although it sometimes presents with more prominent irritability than low mood. Many chronic mood and anxiety disorders in adults begin as high levels of anxiety in children.

Depression, especially in midlife or older adults, can co-occur with other serious medical illnesses, such as diabetes, cancer, heart disease, and Parkinson disease (PD). These conditions are often worse when depression is present. Sometimes, medications taken for these physical illnesses may cause side effects that contribute to depression. A doctor experienced in treating these complicated illnesses can help work out the best treatment strategy.

Risk factors include:

- Personal or family history of depression

- Major life changes, trauma, or stress

- Certain physical illnesses and medications

Section 31.3

Posttraumatic Stress Disorder and Sleep

This section includes text excerpted from "Sleep and PTSD,"
National Center for Posttraumatic Stress Disorder (NCPTSD),
U.S. Department of Veterans Affairs (VA), December 17, 2018.

Many people have trouble sleeping sometimes. This is even more likely, though, if you have posttraumatic stress disorder (PTSD). Trouble sleeping and nightmares are two symptoms of posttraumatic stress disorder.

Why Do People with Posttraumatic Stress Disorder Have Sleep Problems?

They may be "on alert." Many people with PTSD may feel as if they need to be on guard or "on the lookout," to protect herself or himself from danger. It is difficult to have restful sleep when you feel the need to be always alert. You might have trouble falling asleep, or you might wake up easily in the night if you hear any noise.

They may worry or have negative thoughts. Your thoughts can make it difficult to fall asleep. People with PTSD often worry about general problems or worry that they are in danger. If you often have trouble getting to sleep, you may start to worry that you will not be able to fall asleep. These thoughts can keep you awake.

They may use drugs or alcohol. Some people with PTSD use drugs or alcohol to help them cope with their symptoms. In fact, using too much alcohol can get in the way of restful sleep. Alcohol changes the quality of your sleep and makes it less refreshing. This is true of many drugs as well.

They may have bad dreams or nightmares. Nightmares are common for people with PTSD. Nightmares can wake you up in the middle of the night, making your sleep less restful. If you have frequent nightmares, you may find it difficult to fall asleep because you are afraid you might have a nightmare.

They may have medical problems. There are medical problems that are commonly found in people with PTSD, such as chronic pain, stomach problems, and pelvic-area problems in women. These physical problems can make going to sleep difficult.

What Can You Do If You Have Problems?

There are a number of things you can do to make it more likely that you will sleep well:

Change Your Sleeping Area

Too much noise, light, or activity in your bedroom can make sleeping harder. Creating a quiet, comfortable sleeping area can help. Here are some things you can do to sleep better:

- Use your bedroom only for sleeping and sex.

- Move the TV and radio out of your bedroom.

- Keep your bedroom quiet, dark, and cool. Use curtains or blinds to block out light. Consider using soothing music or a white noise machine to block out noise.

Keep a Bedtime Routine and Sleep Schedule

Having a bedtime routine and a set wake-up time will help your body get used to a sleeping schedule. You may want to ask others in your household to help you with your routine.

- Do not do stressful or energizing things within two hours of going to bed.

- Create a relaxing bedtime routine. You might want to take a warm shower or bath, listen to soothing music, or drink a cup of tea with no caffeine in it.

- Use a sleep mask and earplugs if light and noise bother you.

- Try to get up at the same time every morning, even if you feel tired. That will help to set your sleep schedule over time, and you will be more likely to fall asleep easily when bedtime comes. On weekends, do not to sleep more than an hour past your regular wake-up time.

Try to Relax If You Cannot Sleep

- Imagine yourself in a peaceful, pleasant scene. Focus on the details and feelings of being in a place that is relaxing.

- Get up and do a quiet activity, such as reading, until you feel sleepy.

Watch Your Activities during the Day

Your daytime habits and activities can affect how well you sleep. Here are some tips:

- Exercise during the day. Do not exercise within two hours of going to bed, though, because it may be harder to fall asleep.

- Get outside during daylight hours. Spending time in sunlight helps to reset your body's sleep and wake cycles.

- Cut out or limit what you drink or eat that has caffeine in it, such as coffee, tea, cola, and chocolate.

- Do not drink alcohol before bedtime. Alcohol can cause you to wake up more often during the night.

- Do not smoke or use tobacco, especially in the evening. Nicotine can keep you awake.

- Do not take naps during the day, especially close to bedtime.

- Do not drink any liquids after 6 p.m. if you wake up often because you have to go to the bathroom.

- Do not take medicine that may keep you awake or make you feel hyper or energized right before bed. Your doctor can tell you if your medicine may do this and if you can take it earlier in the day.

Talk to Your Doctor

If you cannot sleep because you are in pain or have an injury, you often feel anxious at night, or you often have bad dreams or nightmares, talk to your doctor.

There are a number of medications that are helpful for sleep problems associated with PTSD. Depending on your sleep symptoms and other factors, your doctor may prescribe some medication for you. There are also other skills you can learn to help improve your sleep.

Chapter 32

Multiple Sclerosis and Sleep Disorders

Multiple sclerosis (MS) is a nervous system disease that affects your brain and spinal cord. It damages the myelin sheath, the material that surrounds and protects your nerve cells. This damage slows down or blocks messages between your brain and your body, leading to the symptoms of MS. They can include:

- Visual disturbances

- Muscle weakness

- Trouble with coordination and balance

- Sensations such as numbness, prickling, or "pins and needles"

- Thinking and memory problems

No one knows what causes MS. It may be an autoimmune disease, which happens when your immune system attacks healthy cells in your body by mistake. Multiple sclerosis affects women more than men. It

This chapter contains text excerpted from the following sources: Text in this chapter begins with excerpts from "Multiple Sclerosis," MedlinePlus, National Institutes of Health (NIH), August 6, 2014. Reviewed May 2019; Text beginning with the heading "How Sleep Impacts People with Multiple Sclerosis" is excerpted from "VA Multiple Sclerosis Centers of Excellence—Where There's a Will, There's a Way," U.S. Department of Veterans Affairs (VA), 2015. Reviewed May 2019.

often begins between the ages of 20 and 40. Usually, the disease is mild, but some people lose the ability to write, speak, or walk.

There is no single test for MS. Doctors use a medical history, physical exam, neurological exam, magnetic resonance imaging (MRI), and other tests to diagnose it. There is no cure for MS, but medicines may slow it down and help control symptoms. Physical and occupational therapy may also help.

How Sleep Impacts People with Multiple Sclerosis

Sleep plays an important role in your physical health and well-being. Sleep supports healthy brain functioning, is involved in the healing and repair of your heart, and blood vessels, regulates mood, reduces stress, and even helps your immune system defend your body against foreign or harmful substances. The average adult needs seven to nine hours of sleep each night to function well. Yet, many people do not get adequate amounts of sleep.

People with multiple sclerosis (MS) often say they sleep poorly at night and are fatigued in the daytime. In the general population, the three most common sleep problems reported are insomnia, sleep apnea, and restless legs syndrome (RLS). Research suggests that people with MS have these problems even more often.

Insomnia

Insomnia is characterized by problems getting to sleep, staying asleep, or waking up too early. Insomnia can have multiple causes and is a significant problem at some point for almost half of people with MS. Insomnia can be caused by nighttime MS symptoms that disrupt sleep, such as pain, muscle spasms, and urinary frequency.

Medications, including some antidepressants (SSRIs), stimulants used to treat daytime fatigue, and corticosteroids used to treat MS exacerbations, can also contribute to insomnia. Depression, which is common with MS, is also associated with insomnia. Although occasional self-medication of insomnia with over-the-counter (OTC) sleep medications containing antihistamines can help, if you use them often, they will probably stop working and also make you sleepy or foggy during the day. Many approaches can be effective for treating insomnia, including adjusting your current medication regimen, addressing MS symptoms that are contributing to poor sleep, using nonmedication cognitive behavioral therapy (CBT) approaches, and, in resistant cases, using prescribed sleep-enhancing medications.

Sleep Apnea

Sleep apnea affects at least one in five Americans and probably an even greater proportion of people with multiple sclerosis. Sleep apnea is characterized by repeatedly stopping breathing during sleep. The frequent pauses in breathing can cause fragmented sleep, as well as low blood oxygen levels. Untreated sleep apnea is associated with poor daytime functioning; mood and memory problems; and, if severe, cardiovascular disorders (CVD), such as heart disease and stroke. Sleep apnea may also lead to worsened fatigue, poor energy, and daytime tiredness common in people with multiple sclerosis. Treatment of sleep apnea can reduce these symptoms which may have been attributed solely to multiple sclerosis.

Restless Legs Syndrome

Restless legs syndrome (RLS) is characterized by an uncomfortable urge to move your legs or, more rarely, other body areas. This urge is temporarily relieved by moving your legs. RLS symptoms are generally worst in the evening or at night. RLS is three times more common in people with MS than in the general population. RLS may affect up to one-third of individuals with MS and is more common in those who are older, have had MS for longer, have primary progressive MS, and have greater disability. The exact cause of RLS is not known, but RLS appears to be linked with iron metabolism in the brain. Checking for low iron levels with a blood test and replacing iron when low can improve symptoms. Decreasing the intake of caffeine, nicotine, and alcohol; massaging your legs; and taking warm baths before bedtime may decrease RLS symptoms. When these interventions fail, medications to treat RLS symptoms are available.

In summary, sleep problems, such as insomnia, sleep apnea, and RLS, are common in individuals with MS. These sleep problems may be troublesome on their own and may contribute to daytime fatigue, a poorer quality of life, and may be associated with greater disability. Fortunately, treatments are available for the most common sleep problems, so if you have poor quality, unrefreshing sleep, it is important that you discuss your symptoms with your healthcare provider. Good sleep practices, such as keeping a regular bedtime and wake time, protecting your sleep time from other activities, setting up your bedroom only for sleep, and limiting caffeinated beverages, can also help. While symptoms may not completely resolve with treatment, substantial improvements in daytime functioning and an improved sense of well-being are possible.

Chapter 33

Nocturia: When the Need to Urinate Interrupts Sleep

Nocturia, also known as "nocturnal polyuria" or "frequent nighttime urination," is a problem that affects an estimated 33 percent of adults. Normally, hormones signal the bladder to produce less urine at night, so most people can sleep for 6 to 8 hours without needing to get up to use the bathroom. Waking up once per night to empty the bladder is considered normal as well. People with nocturia, on the other hand, produce excessive amounts of urine and are regularly awakened several times per night by the need to urinate.

Waking up multiple times each night to use the bathroom can lead to chronic sleep deprivation. Since the incidence of nocturia increases with age, the majority of people affected are over the age of 60. Nocturia often appears as a symptom of underlying medical conditions, such as an enlarged prostate, diabetes, heart failure, or bladder problems. Nocturia should not be confused with enuresis—also known as "bed-wetting"—a condition in which urine is passed unintentionally during sleep. Nocturia also differs from urinary incontinence, in which patients experience a lack of voluntary control over urination in the daytime.

"Nocturia: When the Need to Urinate Interrupts Sleep," © 2016 Omnigraphics. Reviewed May 2019.

Causes of Nocturia

The main causes of nocturia are excessive urine production and reduced bladder capacity. Many different factors and conditions can contribute to nocturia, including the following:

- **Age.** Elderly people are more prone to nocturia because the bladder gradually loses elasticity over time. In addition, levels of the hormones that signal the bladder to reduce urine production at night tend to decline with age. Nocturia commonly affects older men who have an enlarged prostate, which can press on the urethra and prevent the bladder from emptying completely, but it affects older women as well.

- **Diabetes.** Poorly controlled diabetes leads to sugar in the urine, which stimulates the production of additional urine.

- **Congestive heart failure and other circulatory problems.** When the heart cannot adequately pump blood through the body, fluid tends to build up in the legs (edema). Lying down at night reduces the burden on the heart and improves circulation, causing the fluid to fill the bladder.

- **Pregnancy.** The growing fetus takes up space usually occupied by the bladder and restricts its capacity to hold fluids.

- **Lower urinary tract conditions.** Infections of the urinary tract or kidneys can cause nocturia by irritating the bladder and decreasing its capacity to hold urine. Conditions such as cystitis can result in an overactive bladder. Bladder obstructions can prevent the full elimination of urine, which may increase the frequency of urination at night.

- **Constipation.** Excessive waste in the bowels or intestines can put pressure on the bladder.

- **Medications.** Certain drugs, such as diuretics, increase the production of urine. Other examples include cardiac glycosides, demeclocycline, lithium, methoxyflurane, phenytoin, and propoxyphene. It is important to consult a doctor before stopping any prescribed medication, however, even if it causes nocturia as a side effect.

- **Diet.** Consuming excessive fluids before bedtime can contribute to nocturia. Alcohol and caffeinated beverages, in particular, act as diuretics to increase urine production.

- **Sleep disorders.** Obstructive sleep apnea (OSA) and other sleep disorders can disrupt the normal reduction in urine output at night.

- **Neurological disorders.** Conditions that affect the transmission of signals and hormones from the brain to the bladder—such as multiple sclerosis (MS), Parkinson disease (PD), or spinal cord injury (SCI)—can result in nocturia.

Symptoms and Diagnosis of Nocturia

Many experts consider nocturia to be a symptom rather than a health condition. As a result, doctors usually place an emphasis on diagnosing the underlying medical causes of frequent and excessive nighttime urination that disrupts sleep. To evaluate a patient with nocturia, medical practitioners generally collect detailed information about the problem, as well as the patient's overall health. The patient may be asked to keep a record of their bladder activity for several days, including the amount of fluid consumed, the frequency of urination during the day and at night, the amount of urine output, and any leaking of urine or wetting the bed. The patient will also be asked about any medications they take regularly, how much alcohol and caffeine they consume each day, and any discomfort they may experience during urination. The doctor may order a urinalysis to evaluate kidney function and check for a urinary tract infection (UTI).

Prevention and Treatment of Nocturia

Since nocturia is usually a symptom, most methods of treatment address the underlying medical conditions that contribute to frequent nighttime urination. Several of these conditions—such as an enlarged prostate or overactive bladder—can be managed with the help of medications. A number of lifestyle modifications can also help reduce urine production at night and prevent people from needing to get up to use the bathroom. Some of the recommended methods of prevention and treatment for nocturia include the following:

- Avoid consuming fluids in the evening (but be sure that total fluid intake is adequate during the day).

- Eliminate or reduce consumption of caffeinated beverages and alcohol.

- Take an afternoon nap to improve circulatory function and drain fluids from the extremities consistently throughout the day.

- Wear compression stockings or elevate the legs to reduce fluid accumulation.

- Perform Kegel exercises to strengthen the pelvic muscles and improve bladder control (these exercises are particularly helpful for pregnant women and for men with an enlarged prostate).

- Take diuretic medications in the late afternoon—six hours before bedtime—so that their therapeutic effects are completed before nighttime.

- Eliminate urinary tract infections with antibiotic medications.

- Treat an enlarged prostate with medications, such as tamsulosin (Flomax), finasteride, or dutasteride.

- Control an unstable or overactive bladder with anticholinergic medications, such as oxybutynin, tolterodine, or solifenacin.

- Reduce urine production at night with medications such as desmopressin (DDAVP).

References

1. Marchione, Victor. "Nocturia: Frequent Urination at Night," Doctors Health Press, 2016.

2. "Nocturia," Cleveland Clinic, 2016.

3. "Nocturia (Night-Time Urination)," NetDoctor, October 4, 2012.

Chapter 34

Pain Disorders That Impact Sleep

Chapter Contents

Section 34.1

Pain and Sleep: An Overview

"Pain and Sleep: An Overview,"
© 2016 Omnigraphics. Reviewed May 2019.

Pain is the leading cause of insomnia. People who experience chronic pain—which includes about 15 percent of the overall U.S. population and half of all elderly people—often have trouble falling asleep and staying asleep. In fact, about 65 percent of people with chronic pain report having disrupted sleep or nonrestorative sleep, resulting in an average deficit of 42 minutes between the amount of sleep they need and the amount they actually get. Shorter sleep duration and poorer sleep quality, in turn, exacerbate chronic pain and interfere with activities, work, mood, relationships, and other aspects of daily life.

How Pain Impacts Sleep

People who experience chronic pain often have trouble falling asleep. Most people prepare for sleep by eliminating distractions and trying to relax. This process may include preparing the covers and pillows, turning off the lights, quieting noises in the bedroom, and making themselves comfortable. For people with chronic pain, however, distractions may serve as a pain management tool. As long as they are able to focus on working, socializing, preparing meals, performing household tasks, reading, watching television, or engaging in recreational activities, their perception of pain tends to decrease. When they eliminate distractions and try to fall asleep, however, their brain tends to focus on the pain. Their level of stress and experience of pain may increase with the amount of time it takes them to fall asleep.

People dealing with pain also tend to have trouble sleeping through the night. Research has shown, for instance, that people with chronic back pain experience a number of microarousals—or changes from a deeper to a lighter stage of sleep—per hour each night. Such disruptions to the normal stages of sleep lead to frequent awakenings during the night and less restorative sleep. The poor quality of sleep means that people with chronic pain do not feel rested and refreshed in the morning. As a result, they often experience drowsiness, diminished energy, depressed mood, and increased pain throughout the day.

In some cases, people with pain also have other medical problems that disrupt sleep, such as restless legs syndrome or nocturnal leg cramps. People with restless legs syndrome experience an uncomfortable tingling or tickling sensation in their legs at night. This sensation creates an uncontrollable urge to move the legs, which can result in involuntary kicking or jerking motions during sleep. The symptoms of restless legs syndrome can contribute to problems falling asleep or staying asleep. They are sometimes relieved through massage, hot baths before bedtime, daily exercise, or eliminating caffeine or nicotine. They can also be treated with prescription medications.

Nocturnal leg cramps are sudden, painful muscle spasms that tend to occur during sleep or during the process of falling asleep. They may affect the feet, calves, or thighs and last between a few seconds and several minutes. Dehydration is the most common cause of muscle cramps, so staying well hydrated during the day can help prevent them from occurring. Overuse of the leg muscles is another factor that sometimes contributes to nocturnal cramping. Stretching before bedtime often helps with this problem. Deficiencies in calcium, magnesium, or potassium may also cause muscle cramps, so supplementing intake of these minerals in the diet may also prove helpful.

Improving Pain and Sleep

When pain impacts sleep, it is important to treat both problems together with a multidisciplinary approach. Since chronic pain and insomnia reinforce each other in a vicious cycle, treatments aimed at improving pain may also help improve sleep, while treatments aimed at improving sleep may also help improve pain. Many behavioral and psychological approaches are available to treat both pain and sleep issues.

Practices and habits that can lead to better quality sleep are known as "sleep hygiene." In many cases, people who experience chronic pain develop bad habits and poor sleep hygiene over time. Some of the practices that have proven safe and effective in improving sleep include the following:

- **Develop a regular routine to help the body get into a consistent, healthy sleep–wake cycle.** Try to go to bed at the same time every night, and wake up at the same time each morning. Chronic pain sufferers sometimes try to compensate for having trouble falling asleep by sleeping late the next morning, but this practice disrupts the sleep–wake pattern.

- **Avoid taking naps during the day,** which can make insomnia worse in the long run by disrupting the sleep–wake cycle.

- **Do not go to bed unless you are tired.** Instead, spend some time engaging in relaxing activities, such as listening to music, reading a book, or meditating.

- **Get out of bed if sleep does not come within 30 minutes.** Trying to fall asleep for hours on end only increases anxiety levels and turns the bedroom into a stressful place. Instead, get up and return to a relaxing activity until a feeling of drowsiness occurs.

- **Develop bedtime rituals to aid in relaxation and train the body to fall asleep.** Suggestions include taking a warm bath or shower, listening to music, reading a book, or having a light snack.

- **Avoid caffeine, nicotine, and alcohol before bedtime.** Research has shown that these substances can be disruptive to a good night's sleep.

- **Exercise at least four to six hours before bedtime.** Although regular exercise can help ease chronic pain and promote good sleep, vigorous exercise within a few hours of bedtime can disrupt sleep.

- **Create a comfortable, pleasant, relaxing sleep environment.** People with chronic pain tend to be highly sensitive to environmental factors, such as light, noise, temperature, mattresses, and bedding. As a result, choosing comfortable bedding, making sure the temperature is neither too hot nor too cold, and eliminating sources of distracting noise or light can make a big difference in helping them get a good night's sleep.

- **Try alternative techniques,** such as meditation, yoga, deep breathing, deep muscle relaxation, or hypnosis, to aid in chronic pain management and relaxation. These techniques can help people reduce stress, decrease the perception of pain, and improve sleep.

If these approaches are not effective in improving sleep, chronic pain sufferers should consult a doctor. A variety of medications are available to help address sleep problems. Before taking any sleep medication, however, patients must be sure to tell the doctor about any other medications they may be taking for chronic pain or other medical conditions.

References

1. "Chronic Pain and Insomnia: Breaking the Cycle," Drugs and Usage, December 23, 2015.

2. "Pain and Sleep," National Sleep Foundation (NSF), 2016.

3. Silberman, Stephanie. "What's Really Causing Your Sleepless Nights?" *Huffington Post*, July 21, 2011.

Section 34.2

Fibromyalgia and Sleep Problems

This section contains text excerpted from the following sources: Text in this section begins with excerpts from "Fibromyalgia," Centers for Disease Control and Prevention (CDC), October 11, 2017; Text beginning with the heading "Is There a Test for Fibromyalgia?" is excerpted from "Fibromyalgia—In Depth," National Institute of Arthritis and Musculoskeletal and Skin Diseases (NIAMS), July 30, 2014. Reviewed May 2019.

What Is Fibromyalgia?

Fibromyalgia (FM) is a condition that causes pain all over the body (also referred to as "widespread pain"), sleep problems, fatigue, and often emotional and mental distress. People with FM may be more sensitive to pain than people without fibromyalgia. This is called "abnormal pain perception processing." Fibromyalgia affects about four million U.S. adults, about two percent of the adult population. The cause of FM is not known, but it can be effectively treated and managed.

What Are the Signs and Symptoms of Fibromyalgia?

The most common symptoms of FM are:

- Pain and stiffness all over the body

- Fatigue and tiredness

- Depression and anxiety

- Sleep problems

- Problems with thinking, memory, and concentration

- Headaches, including migraines

Other symptoms may include:

- Tingling or numbness in hands and feet

- Pain in the face or jaw, including disorders of the jaw known as "temporomandibular joint syndrome" (also known as "TMJ").

- Digestive problems, such as abdominal pain, bloating, constipation, and even irritable bowel syndrome (also known as "IBS").

What Are the Risk Factors for Fibromyalgia?

Known risk factors include:

- **Age.** Fibromyalgia can affect people of all ages, including children. However, most people are diagnosed during middle age, and you are more likely to have FM as you get older.

- **Lupus or rheumatoid arthritis (RA).** If you have lupus or rheumatoid arthritis, you are more likely to develop fibromyalgia.

Some other factors have been weakly associated with the onset of fibromyalgia, but more research is needed to see if they are real. These possible risk factors include:

- **Sex.** Women are twice as likely to have FM as men.

- **Stressful or traumatic events,** such as car accidents, posttraumatic stress disorder (PTSD)

- **Repetitive injuries.** Injury from repetitive stress on a joint, such as frequent knee bending.

- Illness (such as viral infections)

- Family history

- Obesity

What Are the Complications of Fibromyalgia?

Fibromyalgia can cause pain, disability, and a lower quality of life. U.S. adults with FM may have complications such as:

- **More hospitalizations.** If you have fibromyalgia, you are twice as likely to be hospitalized as someone without fibromyalgia.

- **Lower quality of life (QOL).** Women with FM may experience a lower quality of life.

- **Higher rates of major depression.** Adults with FM are more than three times more likely to have major depression than adults without fibromyalgia. Screening and treatment for depression is extremely important.

- **Higher death rates from suicide and injuries.** Death rates from suicide and injuries are higher among FM patients, but overall mortality among adults with FM is similar to the general population.

- **Higher rates of other rheumatic conditions.** Fibromyalgia often co-occurs with other types of arthritis, such as osteoarthritis (OA), RA, systemic lupus erythematosus (SLE), and ankylosing spondylitis (AS).

Is There a Test for Fibromyalgia?

Currently there aren't any laboratory tests to diagnose fibromyalgia. You may see many doctors before receiving the diagnosis. This can happen because the main symptoms of fibromyalgia, pain and fatigue, are similar to many other conditions. Doctors often have to rule out other causes of these symptoms before making a diagnosis of fibromyalgia.

Doctors use guidelines to help diagnose fibromyalgia, which can include:

- A history of widespread pain lasting more than three months

- Physical symptoms including fatigue, waking unrefreshed, and cognitive (memory or thought) problems

- The number of areas throughout the body in which you had pain in the past week

Living with Fibromyalgia

In addition to taking medications to treat your fibromyalgia, there are many things you can do to minimize the impact of the disorder on your life.

Getting Enough Sleep

Getting enough sleep and getting the right kind of sleep can help you ease the pain and fatigue of fibromyalgia. However, many people with FM can experience symptoms that interfere with restful sleep, such as:

- Pain
- Restless legs syndrome (RLS)
- Brainwave irregularities

Try following these tips for good sleep:

- **Keep regular sleep habits.** You should try to get to bed at the same time and get up at the same time every day—even on weekends and vacations.

- **Avoid caffeine and alcohol in the late afternoon and evening.** If you consume caffeine found in coffee, tea, soft drinks, and chocolate, you may not get a good night's sleep. Even though it can make you feel sleepy, if you drink alcohol around bedtime it also can disturb your sleep.

- **Time your exercise.** Regular daytime exercise can improve your nighttime sleep. However, you should avoid exercising within three hours of bedtime because it can be stimulating, keeping you awake.

- **Avoid daytime naps.** Sleeping in the afternoon can interfere with your nighttime sleep. If you feel you cannot get by without a nap, set an alarm for one hour. When it goes off, get up and start moving.

- **Reserve your bed for sleeping.** Watching the late news, reading a suspenseful novel, or working on your laptop in bed can stimulate you, making it hard to sleep.

- **Keep your bedroom dark, quiet, and cool.**

- **Avoid liquids and spicy meals before bed.** Heartburn and late-night trips to the bathroom are not conducive to good sleep.

- **Wind down before going to bed.** Avoid working right up to bedtime. Instead, try some relaxing activities, such as listening to soft music or taking a warm bath, that get you ready to sleep. A warm bath also may soothe aching muscles.

It is important to discuss any sleep problems with your doctor, who can prescribe or recommend treatment for them.

Exercising

Pain and fatigue may make exercising and your daily activities difficult; however, it is important that you try to be as physically active as possible. Research has repeatedly shown that regular exercise is one of the most effective treatments for fibromyalgia. If you have too much pain or fatigue to do vigorous exercise, try starting with walking or other gentle exercise and build your endurance and intensity slowly.

Making Changes at Work

You can continue to work when you have fibromyalgia, but you may have to make some changes to do so. For example, you may need to:

- Lower the number of hours you work

- Switch to a less demanding job

- Make changes in your current job

If you face obstacles at work, such as an uncomfortable desk chair that leaves your back aching or difficulty lifting heavy boxes or files, your employer may make adaptations that will enable you to keep your job. An occupational therapist can help you design a more comfortable workstation or find more efficient and less painful ways to lift.

Eating Well

Although some people with FM report feeling better when they eat or avoid certain foods, no specific diet has been proven to influence fibromyalgia. Of course, it is important to have a healthy, balanced diet. Not only will proper nutrition give you more energy and make you generally feel better, it will also help you avoid other health problems.

Section 34.3

Headaches and Sleep

This section contains text excerpted from the following sources: Text in this section begins with excerpts from "Headaches and Sleep," National Institute of Neurological Disorders and Stroke (NINDS), July 6, 2018; Text under the heading "Genes and Migraines" is excerpted from "Sleep Gene Linked to Migraines," National Institutes of Health (NIH), May 21, 2013. Reviewed May 2019.

You are sitting at your desk, working on a difficult task, when it suddenly feels as if a belt or vice is being tightened around the top of your head. Or, you have periodic headaches that occur with nausea and increased sensitivity to light or sound. Maybe you are involved in a routine, nonstressful task when you are struck by head or neck pain.

Sound familiar? If so, you have suffered one of the many types of headache that can occur on its own or as part of another disease or health condition.

Anyone can experience a headache. Nearly 2 out of 3 children will have a headache by the age of 15. More than 9 in 10 adults will experience a headache sometime in their life. Headache is our most common form of pain and a major reason cited for days missed at work or school, as well as visits to the doctor. Without proper treatment, headaches can be severe and interfere with daily activities.

Certain types of headache run in families. Episodes of headache may ease or even disappear for a time and recur later in life. It is possible to have more than one type of headache at the same time.

Primary headaches occur independently and are not caused by another medical condition. It is uncertain what sets the process of a primary headache in motion. A cascade of events that affect blood vessels and nerves inside and outside the head causes pain signals to be sent to the brain. Brain chemicals called "neurotransmitters" are involved in creating head pain, as are changes in nerve cell activity (called "cortical spreading depression" (CSD)). Migraine, cluster, and tension-type headache are the more familiar types of primary headache.

Secondary headaches are symptoms of another health disorder that causes pain-sensitive nerve endings to be pressed on or pulled or pushed out of place. They may result from underlying conditions, including fever, infection, medication overuse, stress or emotional conflict, high blood pressure, psychiatric disorders, head injury or trauma, stroke, tumors, and nerve disorders (particularly trigeminal neuralgia (TN), a chronic pain condition that typically affects a major nerve on one side of the jaw or cheek).

Headaches can range in frequency and severity of pain. Some individuals may experience headaches once or twice a year, while others may experience headaches more than 15 days a month. Some headaches may recur or last for weeks at a time. Pain can range from mild to disabling and may be accompanied by symptoms such as nausea or increased sensitivity to noise or light, depending on the type of headache.

Why Headaches Hurt

Information about touch, pain, temperature, and vibration in the head and neck is sent to the brain by the trigeminal nerve, 1 of 12 pairs of cranial nerves (CNV) that start at the base of the brain.

The nerve has three branches that conduct sensations from the scalp; the blood vessels inside and outside of the skull; the lining around the brain (the meninges); and the face, mouth, neck, ears, eyes, and throat.

Brain tissue itself lacks pain-sensitive nerves and does not feel pain. Headaches occur when pain-sensitive nerve endings called "nociceptors" react to headache triggers (such as stress, certain foods or odors, or use of medicines) and send messages through the trigeminal nerve to the thalamus, the brain's "relay station" for pain sensation from all over the body. The thalamus controls the body's sensitivity to light and noise and sends messages to parts of the brain that manage awareness of pain and emotional response to it. Other parts of the brain may also be part of the process, causing nausea, vomiting, diarrhea, trouble concentrating, and other neurological symptoms.

Children and Headache

Headaches are common in children. Headaches that begin early in life can develop into migraines as the child grows older. Migraines in children or adolescents can develop into tension-type headaches at any time. In contrast to adults with migraine, young children often feel migraine pain on both sides of the head and have headaches that usually last less than two hours. Children may look pale and appear restless or irritable before and during an attack. Other children may become nauseous, lose their appetite, or feel pain elsewhere in the body during the headache.

Headaches in children can be caused by a number of triggers, including emotional problems, such as tension between family members, stress from school activities, weather changes, irregular eating and sleeping, dehydration, and certain foods and drinks. Of special concern among children are headaches that occur after head injury or those accompanied by rash, fever, or sleepiness.

It may be difficult to identify the type of headache because children often have problems describing where it hurts, how often the headaches occur, and how long they last. Asking a child with a headache to draw a picture of where the pain is and how it feels can make it easier for the doctor to determine the proper treatment.

Migraine in particular is often misdiagnosed in children. Parents and caretakers sometimes have to be detectives to help determine that a child has migraine. Clues to watch for include sensitivity to light and noise, which may be suspected when a child refuses to watch television or use the computer, or when the child stops playing to lie down in a dark room. Observe whether or not a child is able to eat during a headache. Very young children may seem cranky or irritable and complain of abdominal pain (abdominal migraine).

Headache treatment in children and teens usually includes rest, fluids, and over-the-counter (OTC) pain relief medicines. Always consult with a physician before giving headache medicines to a child. Most tension-type headaches in children can be treated with over-the-counter medicines that are marked for children with usage guidelines based on the child's age and weight. Headaches in some children may also be treated effectively using relaxation/behavioral therapy. Children with cluster headache may be treated with oxygen therapy early in the initial phase of the attacks.

Headache and Sleep Disorders

Headaches are often a secondary symptom of a sleep disorder. For example, tension-type headache is regularly seen in persons with insomnia or sleep–wake cycle disorders. Nearly three-fourths of individuals who suffer from narcolepsy complain of either migraine or cluster headache. Migraines and cluster headaches appear to be related to the number of and transition between rapid eye movement (REM) and other sleep periods an individual has during sleep. Hypnic headache (HH) awakens individuals mainly at night but may also interrupt daytime naps. Reduced oxygen levels in people with sleep apnea may trigger early morning headaches.

Getting the proper amount of sleep can ease headache pain. Generally, too little or too much sleep can worsen headaches, as can overuse of sleep medicines. Daytime naps often reduce deep sleep at night and can produce headaches in some adults. Some sleep disorders and secondary headache are treated using antidepressants. Check with a doctor before using OTC medicines to ease sleep-associated headaches.

Coping with Headache

Headache treatment is a partnership between you and your doctor, and honest communication is essential. Finding a quick fix to your headache may not be possible. It may take some time for your doctor or specialist to determine the best course of treatment. Avoid using OTC medicines more than twice a week, as they may actually worsen headache pain and the frequency of attacks. Visit a local headache support group meeting (if available) to learn how others with headache cope with their pain and discomfort. Relax whenever possible to ease stress and related symptoms, get enough sleep, regularly perform aerobic exercises, and eat a regularly scheduled and healthy diet that avoids food triggers. Gaining more control over your headache, stress, and emotions will make you feel better and let you embrace daily activities as much as possible.

Genes and Migraines

Migraines—pounding headaches sometimes preceded by a visual "aura," and often coupled with vomiting, nausea, distorted vision, and hypersensitivity to sound and touch—can be highly debilitating if recurrent and prolonged. A team of researchers funded by the National Institutes of Health (NIH), one of whom regularly suffered from migraines herself, found a gene that plays a part.

The clue that helped them to identify the rogue gene came from a family that suffers from both migraines and a rare sleep disorder, called "familial advanced sleep phase syndrome." The syndrome disrupts their sleep cycle, causing family members to fall asleep early, about 7 p.m., and rise around 4 a.m.

The researchers hunted for the cause of the sleep cycle disorder and discovered a mutation in the *casein kinase I delta (CKIδ)* gene. The gene produces an enzyme that is important for brain signaling and for regulating our circadian rhythms. The particular mutation in this family seemed to reduce the activity of the CKIδ enzyme and made the researchers wonder whether the mutation was also responsible for causing migraines. To test the hypothesis, they engineered mice that carried the same mutation.

As with the humans, the *CKIδ* mutant mice had disrupted sleep–wake cycles – but they were also more likely to suffer migraines compared to normal mice when given nitroglycerin. It is understood that you cannot exactly ask a mouse if it has a headache. But, because migraines cause a range of sensory issues, there are other physical signs the researchers could monitor in the mice. In this case, the *CKIδ* mutant mice became more sensitive to pain, temperature, and touch than normal mice. This mirrors the experience of many migraine sufferers.

The *CKIδ* mutant mice were also more vulnerable to a type of brain activity called "cortical spreading depression"—a wave of electrical silence that follows electrical stimulation. Brain cells called "astrocytes" from *CKIδ* mutants functioned differently from those from healthy mice, suggesting one possible mechanism through which the mutation wreaks havoc in the brain.

CKIδ affects several different proteins in the cell. The next step will be to tease apart which of these plays a role in triggering migraines. Once how migraines begin is identified, there is a better chance of identifying a new generation of drugs that can block that painful path.

Chapter 35

Parkinson Disease and Sleep

What Is Parkinson Disease?

Parkinson disease (PD) is a degenerative disorder of the central nervous system (CNS) that belongs to a group of conditions called "movement disorders." It is both chronic, meaning it persists over a long period of time, and progressive, meaning its symptoms grow worse over time. As nerve cells (neurons) in parts of the brain become impaired or die, people may begin to notice problems with movement, tremor, stiffness in the limbs or the trunk of the body, or impaired balance. As these symptoms become more pronounced, people may have difficulty walking, talking, or completing other simple tasks. Not everyone with one or more of these symptoms has PD, as the symptoms appear in other diseases as well.

The precise cause of PD is unknown, although some cases of PD are hereditary and can be traced to specific genetic mutations. Most cases are sporadic—that is, the disease does not typically run in families. It is thought that PD likely results from a combination of genetic susceptibility and exposure to one or more unknown environmental factors that trigger the disease.

This chapter includes text excerpted from "Parkinson's Disease: Hope through Research" National Institute of Neurological Disorders and Stroke (NINDS), October 11, 2018.

Parkinson disease is the most common form of parkinsonism, in which disorders of other causes produce features and symptoms that closely resemble Parkinson disease. While most forms of parkinsonism have no known cause, there are cases in which the cause is known or suspected, or where the symptoms result from another disorder.

No cure for PD exists nowadays, but research is ongoing and medications or surgery can often provide substantial improvement with motor symptoms.

What Causes Parkinson Disease

Parkinson disease occurs when nerve cells, or neurons, in the brain die or become impaired. Although many brain areas are affected, the most common symptoms result from the loss of neurons in an area near the base of the brain called the "substantia nigra (SN)." Normally, the neurons in this area produce an important brain chemical known as "dopamine." Dopamine is a chemical messenger responsible for transmitting signals between the substantia nigra and the next "relay station" of the brain—the corpus striatum—to produce smooth, purposeful movement. Loss of dopamine results in abnormal nerve firing patterns within the brain that cause impaired movement. Studies have shown that most people with Parkinson have lost 60 to 80 percent or more of the dopamine-producing cells in the substantia nigra by the time symptoms appear, and that people with PD also have loss of the nerve endings that produce the neurotransmitter norepinephrine. Norepinephrine, which is closely related to dopamine, is the main chemical messenger of the sympathetic nervous system, the part of the nervous system that controls many autonomic functions of the body, such as pulse and blood pressure. The loss of norepinephrine might explain several of the nonmotor features seen in PD, including fatigue and abnormalities of blood pressure regulation.

The affected brain cells of people with PD contain Lewy bodies— deposits of the protein alpha-synuclein. Researchers do not yet know why Lewy bodies form or what role they play in the disease. Some research suggests that the cell's protein disposal system may fail in people with PD, causing proteins to build up to harmful levels and trigger cell death. Studies have found evidence that clumps of protein that develop inside brain cells of people with PD may contribute to the death of neurons. Some researchers speculate that the protein buildup in Lewy bodies is part of an unsuccessful attempt to protect the cell from the toxicity of smaller aggregates, or collections, of synuclein.

Genetics. Scientists have identified several genetic mutations associated with Parkinson disease, including the alpha-synuclein gene, and many more genes have been tentatively linked to the disorder. Studying the genes responsible for inherited cases of PD can help researchers understand both inherited and sporadic cases. The same genes and proteins that are altered in inherited cases may also be altered in sporadic cases by environmental toxins or other factors. Researchers also hope that discovering genes will help identify new ways of treating PD.

Mitochondria. Several lines of research suggest that mitochondria may play a role in the development of PD. Mitochondria are the energy-producing components of the cell, and abnormalities in the mitochondria are major sources of free radicals—molecules that damage membranes, proteins, deoxyribonucleic acid (DNA), and other parts of the cell. This damage is often referred to as "oxidative stress." Oxidative stress-related changes, including free radical damage to DNA, proteins, and fats, have been detected in the brains of individuals with PD. Some mutations that affect mitochondrial function have been identified as causes of PD.

While mitochondrial dysfunction, oxidative stress, inflammation, toxins, and many other cellular processes may contribute to Parkinson disease, the actual cause of the cell loss death in PD is still undetermined.

Environmental Causes

Exposure to certain toxins has caused parkinsonian symptoms in rare circumstances (such as exposure to 1-methyl-4-phenyl-1,2,3,6-tetrahydropyridine (MPTP), an illicit drug, or in miners exposed to the metal manganese). Other still-unidentified environmental factors may also cause PD in genetically susceptible individuals.

Postencephalitic parkinsonism (PEP). Just after the First World War, the viral disease encephalitis lethargica (EL) affected almost five million people throughout the world, and then suddenly disappeared in the 1920s. Known as "sleeping sickness" in the United States, this disease killed one-third of its victims and led to postencephalitic parkinsonism in many others. This resulted in a movement disorder that appeared sometimes years after the initial illness. (In 1973, neurologist Oliver Sacks published Awakenings, an account of his work in the late 1960s with surviving postencephalitic patients in a New York hospital. Using the then-experimental drug levodopa, Dr. Sacks was able to temporarily "awaken" these individuals from their statue-like state). In rare cases, other viral infections, including western equine encephalomyelitis, eastern equine encephalomyelitis, and Japanese B encephalitis, have caused parkinsonian symptoms.

Drug-induced parkinsonism (DIP). A reversible form of parkinsonism sometimes results from the use of certain drugs, such as chlorpromazine and haloperidol, which are typically prescribed for patients with psychiatric disorders. Some drugs used for stomach disorders (metoclopramide); high blood pressure (reserpine); and others, such as valproate, can cause tremor and bradykinesia. Stopping the medication or lowering the dosage of these medications usually causes the symptoms to go away.

Toxin-induced parkinsonism. Some toxins can cause parkinsonism by various mechanisms. The chemical MPTP also causes a permanent form of parkinsonism that closely resembles Parkinson disease. Investigators discovered this reaction in the 1980s when heroin addicts in California who had taken an illicit street drug contaminated with MPTP began to develop severe parkinsonism. This discovery, which showed that a toxic substance could damage the brain and produce parkinsonian symptoms, led to a dramatic breakthrough in Parkinson research.

Parkinsonism-dementia complex (PDC) of Guam. This disease occurs among the Chamorro populations of Guam and the Mariana Islands and may be accompanied by a motor neuron disease resembling amyotrophic lateral sclerosis (ALS) (Lou Gehrig disease). The course of the disease is rapid, with death typically occurring within five years.

What Are the Symptoms of the Parkinson Disease?

The four primary symptoms of PD are:

- **Tremor.** The tremor associated with PD has a characteristic appearance. Typically, the tremor takes the form of a rhythmic back-and-forth motion at a rate of four to six beats per second. It may involve the thumb and forefinger, and appear as a "pill rolling" tremor. Tremor often begins in a hand; although, sometimes, a foot or the jaw is affected first. It is most obvious when the hand is at rest or when a person is under stress. Tremor usually disappears during sleep or improves with intentional movement. It is usually the first symptom that causes people to seek medical attention.

- **Rigidity.** Rigidity, or a resistance to movement, affects most people with PD. The muscles remain constantly tense and contracted so that the person aches or feels stiff. The rigidity becomes obvious when another person tries to move the individual's arm, which will move only in ratchet-like or short, jerky movements known as "cogwheel" rigidity.

- **Bradykinesia.** This slowing down of spontaneous and automatic movement is particularly frustrating because it may make simple tasks difficult. The person cannot rapidly perform routine movements. Activities once performed quickly and easily—such as washing or dressing—may take much longer. There is often a decrease in facial expressions.

- **Postural instability.** Postural instability, or impaired balance, causes affected individuals to fall easily.

Parkinson Disease and Sleep Problems

Sleep problems are common in PD and include difficulty staying asleep at night, restless sleep, nightmares, emotional dreams, and drowsiness or sudden sleep onset during the day. Another common problem is rapid eye movement (REM) behavior disorder (RBD), in which people act out their dreams, potentially resulting in injury to themselves or their bed partners. The medications used to treat PD may contribute to some of these sleep issues. Many of these problems respond to specific therapies.

Many people with PD often have fatigue, especially late in the day. Fatigue may be associated with depression or sleep disorders, but it may also result from muscle stress or from overdoing activities when the person feels well. Fatigue may also result from akinesia trouble initiating or carrying out movement. Exercise, good sleep habits, staying mentally active, and not forcing too many activities in a short time may help to alleviate fatigue.

257

How Is Parkinson Disease Diagnosed?

There are currently no blood or laboratory tests that diagnose sporadic PD. Therefore, the diagnosis is based on medical history and a neurological examination. In some cases, PD can be difficult to diagnose accurately early on in the course of the disease. Early signs and symptoms of PD may sometimes be dismissed as the effects of normal aging. Doctors may sometimes request brain scans or laboratory tests in order to rule out other disorders. However, computed tomography (CT) and magnetic resonance imaging (MRI) brain scans of people with PD usually appear normal. Since many other diseases have similar features but require different treatments, making a precise diagnosis is important so that people can receive the proper treatment.

What Is the Prognosis for Parkinson Disease?

The average life expectancy of a person with PD is generally the same as for people who do not have the disease. Fortunately, there are many treatment options available for people with PD. However, in the late stages, PD may no longer respond to medications and can become associated with serious complications, such as choking, pneumonia, and falls.

Parkinson disease is a slowly progressive disorder. It is not possible to predict what course the disease will take for an individual person. Hoehn and Yahr scale is a commonly used scale neurologists use for describing how the symptoms of PD have progressed in a patient.

Hoehn and Yahr Staging of Parkinson Disease

- Stage one—Symptoms on one side of the body only

- Stage two—Symptoms on both sides of the body. No impairment of balance.

- Stage three—Balance impairment. Mild to moderate disease. Physically independent.

- Stage four—Severe disability, but still able to walk or stand unassisted

- Stage five—Wheelchair-bound or bedridden unless assisted

Another commonly used scale is the Movement Disorders Society-Unified Parkinson Disease Rating Scale (MDS-UPDRS). This four-part scale measures motor movement in PD: non-motor experiences of daily living, motor experiences of daily living, motor examination, and motor complications. Both the Hoehn and Yahr scale and the MDS-UPDRS are used to describe how individuals are faring and to help assess treatment response.

Part Five

Preventing, Diagnosing, and Treating Sleep Disorders

Chapter 36

Sleep Hygiene: Tips for Better Sleep

As with eating well and being physically active, getting a good night's sleep is vital to your well-being. Here are tips to help you:

- **Stick to a sleep schedule.** Go to bed and wake up at the same time each day—even on the weekends.

- **Exercise is great, but not too late in the day.** Try to exercise at least 30 minutes on most days but not later than 2 to 3 hours before your bedtime.

- **Avoid caffeine and nicotine.** The stimulating effects of caffeine in coffee, colas, certain teas, and chocolate can take as long as eight hours to wear off fully. Nicotine is also a stimulant.

- **Avoid alcoholic drinks before bed.** A "nightcap" might help you get to sleep, but alcohol keeps you in the lighter stages of sleep. You also tend to wake up in the middle of the night when the sedating effects have worn off.

This chapter contains text excerpted from the following sources: Text in this chapter begins with excerpts from "In Brief: Your Guide to Healthy Sleep," National Heart, Lung, and Blood Institute (NHLBI), September 2011. Reviewed May 2019; Text under the heading "What Should You Do If You Cannot Sleep" is excerpted from "What Should I Do If I Can't Sleep," Centers for Disease Control and Prevention (CDC), March 9, 2017.

- **Avoid large meals and beverages late at night.** A large meal can cause indigestion that interferes with sleep. Drinking too many fluids at night can cause you to awaken frequently to urinate.

- **Avoid medicines that delay or disrupt your sleep, if possible.** Some commonly prescribed heart, blood pressure, or asthma medications, as well as some over-the-counter (OTC) and herbal remedies for coughs, colds, or allergies, can disrupt sleep patterns.

- **Do not take naps after 3 p.m.** Naps can boost your brain power, but late afternoon naps can make it harder to fall asleep at night. Also, keep naps to under an hour.

- **Relax before bed.** Take time to unwind. A relaxing activity, such as reading or listening to music, should be part of your bedtime ritual.

- **Take a hot bath before bed.** The drop in the body temperature after the bath may help you feel sleepy, and the bath can help you relax.

- **Have a good sleeping environment.** Get rid of anything in your bedroom that might distract you from sleep, such as noises, bright lights, an uncomfortable bed, or a TV or computer. Also, keeping the temperature in your bedroom on the cool side can help you sleep better.

- **Have the right sunlight exposure.** Daylight is key to regulating daily sleep patterns. Try to get outside in natural sunlight for at least 30 minutes each day.

- **Do not lie in bed awake.** If you find yourself still awake after staying in bed for more than 20 minutes, get up and do some relaxing activity until you feel sleepy. The anxiety of not being able to sleep can make it harder to fall asleep.

- **See a doctor if you continue to have trouble sleeping.** If you consistently find yourself feeling tired or not well-rested during the day despite spending enough time in bed at night, you may have a sleep disorder. Your family doctor or a sleep specialist should be able to help you.

What Should You Do If You Cannot Sleep

It is important to practice good sleep habits, but if your sleep problems continue or if they interfere with how you feel or function during the day, you should talk to your doctor. Before visiting your doctor, keep a diary of your sleep habits for about 10 days to discuss at the visit.

Include the following in your sleep diary, when you:

- Go to bed
- Go to sleep
- Wake up
- Get out of bed
- Take naps
- Exercise
- Drink alcohol
- Drink caffeinated beverages

Also, remember to mention if you are taking any medications (OTC or prescription) or supplements. They may make it harder for you to sleep.

Chapter 37

Identifying Common Sleep Disruptors

Chapter Contents

Section 37.1

Common Causes of Disturbed Sleep

This section includes text excerpted from "Your
Guide to Healthy Sleep," National Heart, Lung, and
Blood Institute (NHLBI), August 2011. Reviewed May 2019.

What Disrupts Sleep

Many factors can prevent a good night's sleep. These factors range
from well-known stimulants, such as coffee, to certain pain relievers,
decongestants, and other culprits. Many people depend on the caffeine
in coffee, cola, or tea to wake them up in the morning or to keep them
awake. Caffeine is thought to block the cell receptors that adenosine
(a substance in the brain) uses to trigger its sleep-inducing signals.
In this way, caffeine fools the body into thinking it is not tired. It can
take as long as six to eight hours for the effects of caffeine to wear off
completely. Thus, drinking a cup of coffee in the late afternoon may
prevent you from falling asleep at night.

Nicotine is another stimulant that can keep you awake. Nicotine
also leads to lighter than normal sleep, and heavy smokers tend to
wake up too early because of nicotine withdrawal. Although alcohol
is a sedative that makes it easier to fall asleep, it prevents deep sleep
and rapid eye movement (REM) sleep, allowing only the lighter stages
of sleep. People who drink alcohol also tend to wake up in the middle
of the night when the effects of an alcoholic "nightcap" wear off.

Certain commonly used prescription and over-the-counter (OTC)
medicines contain ingredients that can keep you awake. These ingredients include decongestants and steroids. Many medicines taken to
relieve headaches contain caffeine. Heart and blood pressure medications known as "beta-blockers" can make it difficult to fall asleep and
cause more awakenings during the night. People who have chronic
asthma or bronchitis also have more problems falling asleep and staying asleep than healthy people, either because of their breathing difficulties or because of the medicines they take. Other chronic painful or
uncomfortable conditions—such as arthritis, congestive heart failure,
and sickle cell anemia—can disrupt sleep too.

A number of psychological disorders—including schizophrenia,
bipolar disorder, and anxiety disorders—are well known for disrupting sleep. Depression often leads to insomnia, and insomnia can cause
depression. Some of these psychological disorders are more likely to

disrupt REM sleep. Psychological stress also takes its toll on sleep, making it more difficult to fall asleep or stay asleep. People who feel stressed also tend to spend less time in deep sleep and REM sleep. Many people report having difficulties sleeping if, for example, they have lost a loved one, are going through a divorce, or are under stress at work.

Menstrual cycle hormones can affect how well women sleep. Progesterone is known to induce sleep and circulates in greater concentrations in the second half of the menstrual cycle. For this reason, women may sleep better during this phase of their menstrual cycle. On the other hand, many women report trouble sleeping the night before their menstrual flow starts. This sleep disruption may be related to the abrupt drop in progesterone levels that occurs just before menstruation. Women in their late forties and early fifties, however, report more difficulties sleeping (insomnia) than younger women. These difficulties may be linked to menopause, when women have lower concentrations of progesterone. Hot flashes in women of this age also may cause sleep disruption and difficulties.

Certain lifestyle factors also may deprive a person of needed sleep. Large meals or vigorous exercise just before bedtime can make it harder to fall asleep. While vigorous exercise in the evening may delay sleep onset for various reasons, exercise in the daytime is associated with improved nighttime sleep.

If you are not getting enough sleep or are not falling asleep early enough, you may be over-scheduling activities that can prevent you from getting the quiet relaxation time you need to prepare for sleep. Most people report that it is easier to fall asleep if they have time to wind down into a less active state before sleeping. Relaxing in a hot bath or having a hot, caffeine-free beverage before bedtime may help. In addition, your body temperature drops after a hot bath in a way that mimics, in part, what happens as you fall asleep. Probably for both these reasons, many people report that they fall asleep more easily after a hot bath.

Your sleeping environment also can affect your sleep. Clear your bedroom of any potential sleep distractions, such as noises, bright lights, a TV, a cell phone, or computer. Having a comfortable mattress and pillow can help promote a good night's sleep. You also sleep better if the temperature in your bedroom is kept on the cool side.

Section 37.2

Alcohol and Its Effects on Sleep

This section includes text excerpted from "Alcohol Effects and Safer Drinking Habits," Mental Illness Research, Education and Clinical Centers (MIRECC), U.S. Department of Veterans Affairs (VA), June 2013. Reviewed May 2019.

Alcohol and the Body
Alcohol Entering the Body

After alcohol enters the stomach, it is absorbed quickly into the bloodstream through the stomach wall. The rest enters the bloodstream through the small intestine. How fast alcohol is absorbed into your bloodstream depends on several things. Higher concentrations of alcohol, such as shots, are absorbed faster than lower concentrations, such as a light beer. Absorption is faster for a person who weighs less. If you ate while you consumed the alcohol, the absorption of alcohol will be slower than if you drink on an empty stomach.

Alcohol Leaving the Body

Alcohol leaves your body in several ways. First, 90 percent of it is removed from the blood by the liver. Alcohol is then broken down into several chemicals, including carbon dioxide and water. The carbon dioxide and water come out in your urine. The final 10 percent is not removed by the liver and is expelled through sweat and breath. The reason why it is difficult to sober someone up is because the liver can only process about 1 drink per hour (this is slow considering the body absorbs alcohol through the stomach lining in about 10 minutes). There is not much that can influence how fast your liver processes alcohol. That is why cold showers, hot coffee, or vomiting do not help.

Tolerance

Over time, a person who drinks regularly has to drink more and more to feel the same effect as they did when they first began drinking. People develop a higher tolerance because they have adapted, both physically and psychologically, to having alcohol in their system. A low tolerance is similar to a built-in warning system to warn us when alcohol levels get too high in our body. A high tolerance may seem as if it is a good thing because it allows heavy drinkers to function when they have high levels of alcohol in their bodies, but it is not a good thing. People with a high alcohol tolerance short circuit this internal warning system. They do not experience negative reactions to the alcohol, and they continue drinking. Tolerant individuals are able to keep high levels of toxins in their bodies for long periods of time, which increases the stress on sensitive internal organs and the chances of developing long-term health problems. The good news about having a high tolerance is that you can decrease it (and the associated health risks) fairly easily. A high tolerance can be reversed gradually through either moderating the quantity and frequency of your drinking, or taking a break from the alcohol for a few weeks.

A standard drink of alcohol:

- One 12 oz beer
- One wine cooler
- One 5 oz glass of wine
- One shot of liquor
- One cocktail

Alcohol Intoxication and Performance
Sleep

The bottom line is that alcohol is bad for your sleep. Poor sleep can limit your ability to think, act quickly, and perform well. Alcohol intoxication shortens the time necessary to fall asleep, but sleep is usually disturbed and fragmented after just a few hours. Restful, restorative sleep decreases during the second half of the night. So, heavy drinking compromises your sleep throughout the night. Poor sleep decreases the body's ability to function optimally and your physical endurance. If you want peak performance (at work, sports, or other engagements), either plan to abstain from alcohol use altogether or drink in moderation.

Up and Down Response to Alcohol in Your Body

The up and down response refers to two different effects that alcohol produces. The up response is feeling stimulated or excited. This is followed by the down response of feeling depressed and tired. The initial up response is associated with low, but rising, blood alcohol levels (BALs). The BAL is the ratio of alcohol to blood in your bloodstream.

Table 37.1. Effects of Alcohol on the Body

Blood Alcohol Level	Effects of Alcohol on the Body
0.02%	Light to moderate drinkers begin to feel some effect
0.04%	Most people begin to feel relaxed
0.06%	Judgment is somewhat impaired; people are less able to make rational decisions about their capabilities (e.g., driving)
0.08%	Definite impairment of muscle coordination and driving skills. Increased risk of nausea and slurred speech. Legal intoxication.
0.10%	Clear deterioration of reaction time and control
0.15%	Balance and movement are impaired. Risk of blackouts and accidents.
0.30%	Many people lose consciousness. Risk of death.
0.45%	Breathing stops, death occurs

The down response is associated more with falling BALs. The up and down response is important because it allows you to test if "more" alcohol actually means "better." It also helps you understand how tolerance affects you physiologically when it comes to drinking alcohol.

Over time, as blood alcohol levels begin to fall, people experience the down effects of alcohol. This is the time when people begin to drink more in an attempt to get back their initial stimulated or excited state. However, the more alcohol that is consumed, the greater both the arousal and the depressant effects will be. At some point, the stimulating effects of a rising BAL will not amount to euphoria. The point at which an increase in BAL will not result in elevated mood or energy is known as the "point of diminishing returns." For most people, that point is a BAL of .05 percent.

Moderating Your Drinking

Decide what you want from drinking alcohol; think about the pros and cons (short- and long-term) for moderating your use versus maintaining your usual drinking behavior. Also, consider what you absolutely want to avoid when you drink.

Set Drinking Limits

- What is your upper limit on the number of drinks you consume per week?

- At what point do you decide you have had enough (consider a BAL limit)?

- What is the maximum number of days for drinking you will choose to give yourself?

- Use standard guidelines to determine what constitutes one drink: (1.25 oz of 80-proof liquor; 4 oz of wine; 10 oz of beer with 5 percent alcohol (microbrews and "ice" beer); 12 oz of beer with 4 percent alcohol (standard beer)

Count Your Drinks and Monitor Your Drinking Behavior

Most people are surprised by what they learn when they actually count how much they drink. Simply observe your behavior—this is similar to standing outside yourself and watching how you are acting when you are drinking. Some people put the bottle caps in their pockets while drinking to monitor how many beers they have had. You can also make tick marks with a pen on a napkin to monitor the number of drinks.

Alter How and What You Drink

- Switch to drinks that contain less alcohol (e.g., light beers).
- Slow down your pace of drinking.
- Space drinks further apart.
- Alternate drinking nonalcoholic beverages with alcoholic drinks.

Manage Your Drinking in the Moment

- Stay awake and on top of how you drink and what you are drinking when you are at a party
- Choose what is right for you, and ask a close friend to help you monitor your alcohol consumption.

Safe Drinking Guideline

- For women, no more than 3 drinks/day; no more than 9 drinks/week
- For men, no more than 4 drinks/day; no more than 14 drinks/week

Section 37.3

Caffeine, Nicotine, and Food and Their Impact upon Sleep

"Caffeine and Nicotine and Their Impact upon Sleep,"
© 2016 Omnigraphics. Reviewed May 2019.

Caffeine and Sleep

Caffeine has been called the most popular drug in the world. Millions of people consume it on a daily basis in the form of coffee, tea, soft drinks, energy drinks, chocolate, or certain medications. Many people depend on it to help them feel alert and energized throughout the day at work or at school. Some people become addicted to it and experience withdrawal symptoms, such as headaches, fatigue, anxiety, and irritability, if they do not get their daily dose. Yet, most people do not think of caffeine as a drug or realize that it can interfere with sleep.

Caffeine is typically absorbed into the bloodstream within 15 minutes after it is consumed, although it takes about an hour to reach peak levels. It acts as a stimulant to increase the heart rate and blood pressure and promote the production of adrenaline. As a result, caffeine temporarily increases alertness and reduces fatigue by suppressing sleep-inducing chemicals. These effects can last for 4 to 6 hours, although it takes a full 24 hours for the body to completely eliminate caffeine.

By stimulating the body to remain awake, caffeine can also weaken the body's ability to sleep. Consuming too much caffeine may cause insomnia. Most people can safely consume up to 250 milligrams per day, which is equivalent to 2 to 3 cups of coffee, without affecting their sleep. Consumption of 500 milligrams or more per day is considered excessive and can impair sleep.

Caffeine affects sleep in three ways: by making it harder to fall asleep, by reducing the quality of sleep, and by causing nocturia (frequent nighttime urination). These effects are particularly severe if the caffeine is consumed within four to six hours of bedtime. People with caffeine in their bloodstream are likely to feel jittery, anxious, or wired when they try to go to sleep. If they do manage to fall asleep, the stimulant effects of caffeine will make it difficult for their body to enter a deep, restorative phase of sleep. Finally, they are likely to wake up multiple times during the night to use the bathroom due to the diuretic effects of caffeine.

Nicotine and Sleep

Some people find smoking cigarettes relaxing and believe that smoking at bedtime or upon awakening in the middle of the night helps them sleep. But nicotine, the main addictive chemical in tobacco products, is actually a stimulant that can interfere with sleep. Smoking has countless other negative impacts on health, significantly increasing the risk of heart disease, lung disease, stroke, and cancer. In fact, smoking is the leading preventable cause of death in the United States. However, few people seem to recognize the impact of nicotine on sleep.

As with caffeine, nicotine is absorbed into the bloodstream quickly and acts as a stimulant, increasing the heart rate and breathing rate and releasing stress hormones in the body. The stimulant effects of nicotine persist for several hours, affecting brain waves, body temperature, and other systems. These effects make it more difficult to fall asleep and stay asleep. As a result, smokers tend to sleep lightly and spend less time in deep, restorative sleep than nonsmokers.

In addition to sleep disruptions from the stimulant effects of nicotine, which tend to occur in the early part of the night, smokers may also experience withdrawal symptoms closer to morning that interfere with sleep. These symptoms may include headaches, nausea, diarrhea or constipation, irritability, anxiety, fatigue, and depression. Although quitting smoking is the best way to avoid the negative effects of nicotine on sleep, the effects can be reduced by avoiding nicotine for at least two hours before bedtime.

Food and Sleep

Food also has the capacity to enhance or disrupt sleep. Eating a healthy, balanced diet has been shown to improve overall well-being, providing people with increased energy during the day and enabling them to sleep better at night. But, eating large meals or spicy foods close to bedtime can have a negative impact on sleep. Experts recommend allowing two to three hours between the last large meal of the day and bedtime. Since going to bed hungry can also impair sleep, they also suggest eating a small, light snack or drinking a glass of milk as needed to assuage late-night hunger.

References

1. "Caffeine, Food, Alcohol, Smoking, and Sleep," Sleep Health Foundation, May 21, 2013.

2. Stewart, Kristin. "The Chemistry of Caffeine, Nicotine, and Sleep," Everyday Health, January 7, 2013.

Section 37.4

Opioid Misuse and Poor Sleep

This section includes text excerpted from "HEAL Initiative: Science Taking on Pain, Opioid Misuse—And Poor Sleep," National Heart, Lung, and Blood Institute (NHLBI), April 22, 2019.

The story of the U.S. opioid crisis is often told through numbers. And for many, that makes sense because the numbers are staggering; more than 2 million Americans suffer from opioid-use disorder (OUD), a serious but treatable chronic illness that claims the lives of more than 130 people every day. Many with OUD carry another burden, however: they are among the more than 50 million adults affected by chronic, often debilitating pain, and their addiction, often the fallout of their quest for relief.

Opioids accounted for nearly 68 percent of the more than 70,000 deaths from U.S. drug overdoses in 2017. And those deaths are no longer confined mainly to White communities. While the epidemic still kills more White Americans, the number of deaths is increasing faster among African Americans and Latinos, according to a report by the Centers for Disease Control and Prevention (CDC).

Why Focus on Opioid Use and Sleep

Sleep deficiency, such as insufficient sleep duration, irregular sleep schedules, and poor-sleep quality, are prevalent comorbidities in individuals with OUD. There is a need to determine if sleep deficiency contributes to the overuse of opioids, to addiction, and to how individuals respond to medication treatments to overcome addiction. That way, new therapeutic targets for the prevention and treatment of opioid addiction can be identified and investigated.

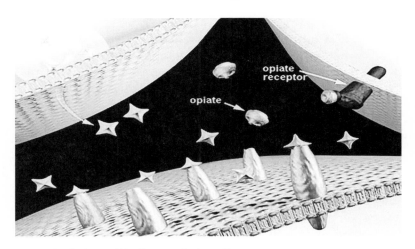

Figure 37.1. *Opiates Binding to Opiate Receptors*

Opiates binding to opiate receptors in the nucleus accumbens: increased dopamine release.

Are People Who Misuse Opioids More Susceptible to Sleep Disorders? Conversely, Are People with Sleep Disorders More Prone to Opioid Misuse?

The relationship between sleep and OUD is likely a two-way street. People with OUD often complain of sleep disturbance and insomnia, particularly during withdrawal and periods of abstinence following medication treatment.

Are Racial and Ethnic Minorities Particularly Affected by Opioid-Related Sleep Disorders?

American Indian/Alaska Natives and Whites have higher rates of nonmedical opioid use and overdose deaths when compared to African Americans and Latinos. These disparities make it difficult to fight the national epidemic. Studies suggest that sleep deficiency and untreated sleep disorders may be more common among minorities and women. However, the direct contribution of racial and ethnic differences in sleep to opioid overuse, addiction, and medication treatment outcomes are not yet well understood and require further study.

Are There Common Pathways or Biological Mechanisms That Could Provide Answers about This Relationship?

Sleep deprivation, irregular sleep schedules, and poor-quality sleep weaken the network of circadian gene regulation in brain cells and affect how well the brain can adapt to stress. Impaired emotional regulation, increased risk-taking behavior, and greater sensitivity to pain increase susceptibility to substance use.

There is a need to identify the mechanisms that directly connect sleep to the biological causes of opioid-use disorder. Once that is done, we can explore these mechanisms as potential therapeutic targets in the prevention and treatment of opioid addiction.

Research has already started to make important connections. Studies have demonstrated that sleep deprivation alters regions of the brain involved in reward (pleasure-seeking) mechanisms. There are indications that behavioral and molecular mechanisms that trigger OUDs may be directly influenced by the circadian clock. Lastly, opioid withdrawal and sleep are regulated by some of the same brain regions and neurochemical systems.

Chapter 38

Stress and Sleep

Stress is a complex biological response that is designed to help people focus their attention, energy, and physical resources to deal with a problem or threat. Everyone faces sources of stress in their daily lives, such as traffic jams, work deadlines, relationship issues, or hectic schedules. In fact, surveys show that 70 percent of American adults experience stress, anxiety, or worry on a daily basis. Most people report that stress interferes with their lives, particularly by reducing the quantity and quality of their sleep.

People under stress often have trouble falling asleep because their minds race with thoughts rather than shut down. Sleep usually gives the brain a chance to rest by switching functions over from the active sympathetic nervous system to the calmer parasympathetic nervous system. Excessive worry prevents this switch from happening, so the brain remains on high alert. Stress also reduces the quantity of sleep by causing people to awaken frequently or toss and turn restlessly during the night. Among American adults, 43 percent report lying awake at night due to stress, with over half experiencing this problem more than once per week.

Stress also impacts the quality of sleep. Around 42 percent of American adults report feeling less satisfied with the quality of their sleep when they are under stress. In addition, people who experience ongoing stress have an increased risk of developing sleep disorders and insomnia. In fact, each additional source of stress in a person's

---

life has been shown to increase their risk of insomnia by 19 percent. As a result, people with high levels of stress report sleeping only 6.2 hours per night on average, with only 33 percent feeling that they get enough sleep. People with lower levels of stress, on the other hand, sleep an average of 7.1 hours per night, and 79 percent feel that they get enough sleep.

Compounding the problem, research indicates that sleep deprivation leads to even higher levels of stress. Among people whose sleep is affected by stress or anxiety, 75 percent report that the lack of sleep increases their levels of stress and anxiety. People with high stress are also more likely to feel the physical and emotional effects of getting too little sleep, such as fatigue, sluggishness, daytime drowsiness, trouble concentrating, irritability, lack of patience, and depression. When stress causes sleep problems, and then sleep problems increase stress levels, people become locked in a vicious cycle that can be hard to break.

Managing Stress and Improving Sleep

There are a number of stress-management tools and techniques available to help people cope with anxiety and thus improve the quantity and quality of their sleep. Some helpful approaches for dealing with stress-related sleep issues include the following:

- **Identify sources of stress**. The first step in managing stress involves figuring out its main causes, which will vary by individual. Common sources of stress include one's job, health, and finances, and experiencing trauma or going through a divorce.

- **Reduce exposure to stressors**. Once the main sources of stress have been identified, the next step is to find ways to handle them better. With job-related stress, for instance, it may be possible to delegate some responsibilities in order to reduce workload.

- **Adjust thought processes and expectations**. Often, the way of looking at a problem or situation can determine whether or not it is stressful. It is possible to change negative thought patterns and lower expectations in order to reduce stress. It is particularly important to avoid generalizing concerns and blowing small things out of proportion. Many self-help books and websites offer tips and exercises for managing negative thoughts. For instance, one approach might be to write down worries and concerns, and then throw away the paper in order to symbolically clear the mind.

- **Build a social support system**. Spending time relaxing with family and friends is a valuable way to reduce stress. Talking with supportive loved ones can also make problems seem more manageable or lead to positive new approaches and solutions.

- **Exercise**. Getting regular exercise is a proven way to relieve stress and improve mood. It can also lead to improvements in sleep; although, vigorous exercise should be undertaken at least two hours before bedtime to allow body temperature to return to normal.

- **Eat a healthy diet**. A healthy diet with plenty of fruits, vegetables, whole grains, and lean proteins promotes overall health, increases energy, and helps reduce stress. On the other hand, consuming refined sugars, caffeine, and alcohol can negatively impact sleep and leave people feeling sluggish.

- **Try relaxation techniques**. Deep-breathing exercises can activate the parasympathetic nervous system and help calm nerves. Yoga, meditation, progressive muscle relaxation, and other techniques can also help quiet the mind and promote sleep.

- **Practice good sleep hygiene**. Since sleep problems increase stress levels, getting a good night's sleep is vital to effective stress management. Sleep hygiene methods that can improve the quality of sleep include making sleep a priority, blocking out eight full hours for sleep, establishing a regular sleep schedule and a relaxing bedtime routine, avoiding naps during the day, and creating a comfortable and inviting sleep environment.

If these steps are ineffective in reducing stress and improving sleep, it may be helpful to consult with a doctor. Therapists can help patients identify sources of stress and find productive ways of dealing with them. Sleep specialists can assess patients for sleep disorders and recommend approaches or medications to address the problem. Since stress and sleep often go hand in hand, both kinds of professional help may be needed to enable people to manage stress successfully and sleep soundly through the night.

References

1. Holmes, Lindsay. "Five Ways Stress Wrecks Your Sleep (And What to Do about It)," *Huffington Post*, September 17, 2014.

2. "Stress and Anxiety Interfere with Sleep," Anxiety and Depression Association of America (ADAA), 2016.

3. "Tips to Reduce Stress and Sleep Better," WebMD, 2016.

Chapter 39

Shift Work and Sleep

In the current competitive economy, an increasing number of U.S. businesses operate to meet customers' demand for 24/7 services. These around-the-clock operations are required in order to maintain a place in the global market where transactions with clients, suppliers, and colleagues can span multiple time zones. Consequently, for many men and women, the workday no longer fits the traditional 9-to-5 model. They may clock in at midnight and clock out at eight in the morning, or they may follow a rotating shift work schedule, consisting of periodic day shifts, evening shifts, and night shifts.

Since our body clocks are typically set for a routine of daytime activity and nighttime sleep, working irregular shifts or night hours can be associated with disrupted or insufficient sleep. In turn, drowsiness, fatigue, and circadian rhythm disruption from too little sleep or interrupted sleep are associated with risks for immune system dysfunction, diabetes, cardiovascular disease (CVD), and other chronic health problems. As nontraditional schedules become more common, it becomes increasingly important to understand who may be at risk of unintended job-related outcomes and why. From that knowledge, employers, workers, and practitioners can better craft practical, effective interventions.

This chapter contains text excerpted from the following sources: Text in this chapter begins with excerpts from "Shift Work and Sleep," Centers for Disease Control and Prevention (CDC), October 5, 2016; Text under the heading "Steps You Can Take to Improve Your Sleep" is excerpted from "Wake Up and Get Some Sleep," National Highway Traffic Safety Administration (NHTSA), February 2002, Reviewed May 2019.

Scientists know little about the prevalence of sleep disorders in the United States workforce because, to date, most studies have been limited to selected occupational groups, geographic areas, and types of sleep disorders. A study was published online on October 5, 2016 in the peer-reviewed journal Occupational and Environmental Medicine. Data were used from the National Health and Nutrition Examination Survey (NHANES), conducted by the National Center for Health Statistics (NCHS), one of the partner centers of the U.S. Centers for Disease Control and Prevention (CDC).

The National Health and Nutrition Examination Survey was the first-ever study to use a nationally representative sample of the U.S. working population to examine the role of shift work in sleep quality, sleep-related activities of daily living, and insomnia.

The nationally representative sample included 6,338 adults, all 18 years of age and older. They were asked to complete a survey questionnaire that covered sleep duration, sleep disorders, sleep quality, impairment of sleep-related activities of daily living (ADL), and insomnia. To determine the shift schedule worked by each individual, they were asked which choice best described the hours they usually worked: regular daytime (any hours between 6 a.m. and 6 p.m.), regular evening shift (any hours between 4 p.m. and midnight), regular night shift (any hours between 7 p.m. and 8 a.m.), rotating shift, or another schedule. Based on a recommendation by the National Sleep Foundation that adults should sleep 7 to 9 hours per night, the NCHS created 2 categories of sleep duration for the study: either less than 7 hours, referred to as "short sleep duration," or seven or more hours.

From a study of this large, nationally representative sample, the NCHS concluded that sleep-related problems were common among workers, especially among night-shift workers who had the highest risks for sleep problems. Moreover, these risks among night-shift workers persisted even after the NCHS adjusted for potentially confounding factors, such as long working hours, sociodemographic characteristics, and health/lifestyle/work factors. Findings included these:

- 37.6 percent of the respondents reported experiencing short sleep duration, representing 54.1 million U.S. workers. Short sleep duration was more prevalent among night-shift workers (61.8% of those who reported short duration) than among daytime workers (35.9%).

- Daytime workers had the lowest prevalence (31%) of "prolonged sleep-onset latency," which is when at bedtime, 30 or more minutes are required to go from full wakefulness to sleep—compared with the night shift (46.2%), evening shift (43%) and rotating shift (42.1%).

- Poor sleep quality was reported by 30.7 percent of night-shift workers, and moderate sleep quality by 34.1 percent of workers on another schedule. Night- and evening-shift workers more frequently had difficulty falling asleep (21.7% and 21.2%, respectively, versus 12.7% of daytime workers). Night-shift workers had a higher prevalence of feeling excessively or overly sleepy during the day (22.3% versus 16.2%).

- Insomnia, which is defined as having both poor sleep quality and impaired sleep-related ADL, was reported by 18.5 percent of night-shift workers compared to 8.4 percent of daytime workers.

- Workers 60 years of age or older had a lower prevalence of short sleep duration, impaired sleep-related activities of daily living (ADL), and insomnia than those between the ages of 30 and 59.

- Female workers had a lower prevalence of short sleep duration but a higher prevalence of the other three sleep outcomes (poor sleep quality, impaired sleep-related ADL, and insomnia) than male workers.

- Obese workers had a higher prevalence of short sleep duration and poor sleep quality than those who were normal weight/ underweight.

- Current smokers had a higher prevalence of short sleep duration, poor sleep quality, and insomnia (but not impaired sleep-related ADL) than nonsmokers.

- Workers who worked 48 hours or more per week had a higher prevalence of short sleep duration, poor sleep quality, and insomnia than those who worked less than 48 hours per week.

- Workers who frequently used sleeping pills had a higher prevalence of poor sleep quality, impaired sleep-related ADL, and insomnia (but not short sleep duration) than those who did not.

- A higher prevalence of all four sleep outcomes (short sleep duration, poor sleep quality, insomnia, and impaired sleep-related ADL) was observed among workers who were widowed, divorced or separated; workers who reported fair or poor health;

285

workers with symptomatic depression; and workers who had a physician-diagnosed sleep disorder-than among workers who did not have those characteristics.

Although the study was not subject to limitations of earlier investigations with smaller sample sizes, it was subject to other limitations inherent in the kind of investigation we conducted. As the NCHS notes, the limitations of their study are mitigated to some degree by the consistency of their methods and findings with those of other well-designed studies in the literature.

Particularly in light of the likely continuing increase in nontraditional working schedules, work-based prevention strategies and policies should be adopted to improve the quantity and quality of sleep among workers. Unfortunately, there is no single ideal strategy to successfully address the sleep risks of every demanding shift work situation. Instead, interventions often need to be customized to the specific employer and worker. These include designing new shift schedules with frequent rest breaks, avoiding night shifts that exceed eight hours, improving one's sleep environment, taking a long nap before a night shift begins, accelerating the modulation of circadian rhythms using bright lights, improving physical fitness, engaging in stress reduction activities, and strengthening family and social support.

Steps You Can Take to Improve Your Sleep

Make your room dark—the darker, the better. As a shift worker, you are waking and sleeping against the natural rhythms of lightness and darkness—the most powerful regulators of our internal clocks. Your body wants to be active when it is light, and it craves rest when it is dark. Try using special room-darkening shades, lined drapes, or a sleep mask to simulate nighttime. Sleep without a night light, block the light that comes from your doorway, and if your alarm clock is illuminated, cover it up.

Block outside sounds. Sleep can be easily interrupted by sudden, unexpected sounds—the screech of a passing siren, a plane flying overhead, construction work or a barking dog, to name a few. Use earplugs, a fan, or turn the FM radio or TV to in between stations so the "shhhh" blocks out other noises and lulls you to sleep. (Just be sure to turn off the brightness on your TV or cover the screen.) You might even want to consider a white noise machine, which plays a steady stream of lulling sounds, such as ocean waves.

Adjust your thermostat before going to bed. A room that is too hot or too cold can disturb your sleep. Some research shows that 60 to 65 °F or 16 to 18 °C is ideal.

Keep a regular schedule. Go to bed and get up at the same time every day. The best way to ensure a good night's sleep is to stick to a regular schedule, even on your days off, holidays, or when traveling.

Maintain or improve your overall health. Eat well and establish a regular exercise routine. It can be as simple as a 20- to 30-minute walk, jog, swim, or bicycle ride 3 times a week. Exercising too close to bedtime may actually keep you awake because your body has not had a chance to unwind. Allow at least 3 hours between working out and going to bed.

Avoid caffeine several hours before bedtime. Its stimulating effects will peak two to four hours later and may linger for several hours more. The result is diminished deep sleep and increased awakenings.

Avoid alcohol before going to sleep. It may initially make you fall asleep faster, but it can make it much harder to stay asleep. As the immediate effects of the alcohol wear off, it deprives your body of deep rest and you end up sleeping in fragments and waking often.

Know the side effects of medications. Some medications can increase sleepiness and make it dangerous to drive. Other medications can cause sleeping difficulties as a side effect.

Change the time you go to sleep. After driving home from work, do not go right to bed. Take a few hours to unwind and relax.

Develop a relaxing sleep ritual. Before going to sleep, try taking a warm bath, listening to soothing music or reading until you feel sleepy—but do not read anything exciting or stimulating.

Do not make bedtime the time to solve the day's problems. Try to clear your mind. Make a list of things you are concerned about or need to do the next day so you do not worry about them when you are trying to sleep.

Set house rules. Speak with your family about your sleep schedule and why your sleep time is so important. Establish guidelines for everyone in your household to help maintain a peaceful sleeping environment, such as wearing headphones to listen to music or watch TV and avoiding vacuuming, dishwashing, and noisy games.

Keep a sleep schedule. Let family and friends know your sleep schedule and ask them to call or visit at times that are convenient for you. Plan ahead for activities together.

Switch off the phone. Be sure unimportant calls do not wake you up. Switch off the phone and, if necessary, get a beeper so your family can reach you in an emergency.

Hang a "do not disturb" sign on your door. Make sure your family understands the conditions under which they should wake you. Make a deal with them. If they let you sleep, you will be less grumpy. And make sure delivery people and solicitors understand your sleeping rules by hanging a "do not disturb" sign on your front door too.

By following as many tips as possible, you should start to experience improvements in the quality of your sleep. It will not happen right away, but if you stick with it for a week or two, you will begin to notice positive changes. Staying alert on the job will be much easier. Drowsy driving will no longer be a problem. And you will be able to enjoy more quality time with your family, and they will enjoy you.

Chapter 40

Daylight Saving: Helping Workers to Prevent Sleep Deprivation

Spring forward, fall back.

We all know the saying to help us remember to adjust our clocks for the daylight-saving time changes, but what can we do to help workers adjust to the effects of the time change? A few studies have examined these issues, but many questions remain, including the best strategies to cope with the time changes.

By moving the clocks ahead one hour in the Spring, we lose one hour, which shifts work times and other scheduled events one hour earlier. This pushes most people to go to bed and wake up one hour earlier than normal. In the Fall, time moves back one hour. We gain one hour, which shifts work times and other scheduled events one hour later, thereby pushing most people to go to bed and wake up one hour later than normal.

It can take about one week for the body to adjust to the new times for sleeping, eating, and activity. Until they have adjusted, people can have trouble falling asleep, staying asleep, and waking up at the right time. This can lead to sleep deprivation and a reduction in

This chapter includes text excerpted from "Daylight Saving: Suggestions to Help Workers Adapt to the Time Change," Centers for Disease Control and Prevention (CDC), August 15, 2016.

performance, increasing the risk for mistakes. Workers can experience somewhat higher risks to both their health and safety after the time changes. A study by Kirchberger and colleagues* reported that persons with heart disease may be at higher risk for a heart attack during the week after the time changes in the Spring and Fall.

* Kirchberger I, Wolf K, Heier M, Kuch B, von Scheidt W, Peters A, Meisinger C [2015]. Are daylight saving time transitions associated with changes in myocardial infarction incidence? Results from the German MONICA/KORA Myocardial Infarction Registry. BMC Public Health. 14;15(1):778.

The reason for these problems is thought to be disruption to circadian rhythms and sleep. Circadian rhythms are daily cycles of numerous hormones and other body functions that prepare us for the expected times for sleeping, eating, and activity. Circadian rhythms have difficulty adjusting to an abrupt one-hour time change.

Other hazards for workers related to the time change in the Fall include a sudden change in the driving conditions in the late-afternoon rush hour—from driving home from work during daylight hours to driving home in darkness. People may not have changed their driving habits to nighttime driving and might be at somewhat higher risk for a vehicle crash. Additionally, the Spring time change leads to more daylight in the evening, which may disturb some people's sleep.

To help reduce risks about one and a half weeks before the time changes in the Fall and Spring, employers can relay these points to help their workers.

- Remind workers that several days after the time changes are associated with somewhat higher health and safety risks due to disturbances to circadian rhythms and sleep.

- It can take one week for the body to adjust sleep times and circadian rhythms to the time change, so consider reducing demanding physical and mental tasks as much as possible that week to allow oneself time to adjust.

- Remind workers to be especially vigilant while driving, at work, and at home to protect themselves as others around them may be sleepier and at risk for making an error that can cause a vehicle crash or other accident.

- Research found that people with existing heart disease may be at risk for a heart attack after the time change.

- Workers can improve their adaptation to the time change by using these suggestions. Circadian rhythms and sleep are strongly influenced by several factors including timing of exposure to light and darkness, times of eating and exercise, and time of work. One way to help the body adjust is to gradually change the times for sleep, eating, and activity.

- For the Spring time change, starting about 3 days before, one can gradually move up the timing of going to bed and waking up, meals, exercise, and exposure to light earlier by 15 to 20 minutes each day until these are in line with the new time. About 1 hour before bedtime, keep the lights dim and avoid electronic lit screens on computers, tablets, etc. to help the body adjust its internal clock in regards to bedtime and waking up.

- For the Fall time change, starting about 3 days before, one can gradually move the timing of going to bed and waking up, meals, exercise, and exposure to light later by 15 to 20 minutes each day until these are in line with the new time. About 1 hour after waking up in the morning, keep the lights dim and avoid the electronic screens on computers, tablets, etc. to help the body adjust its internal clock in regards to bedtime and waking up.

- Being sleep deprived before the time change will increase the health and safety risks, so make it a priority to get enough sleep and be well rested several days before the time change.

Does the Time Change Affect Everyone Equally?

In short, no. People who sleep seven or less hours per day tend to have more problems with the time changes. Additionally, a person's natural tendency to get up early and go to bed early or get up late and go to bed late may also influence their ability to adjust to the one-hour time changes in the Spring and Fall. Those prone to naturally follow an "early to bed and early to rise" pattern (morningness) will tend to have more difficulties adjusting to the Fall time change because this goes against their natural tenancies. Conversely, those who naturally follow a "late to bed and late to rise" routine (eveningness) will tend to have more trouble with the Spring time change.

Morningness/eveningness tends to change as people age. Teenagers and young adults tend to be "evening" types, and researchers theorize this may be due to brain and body development at those ages. Younger workers, therefore, may have more difficulty adjusting to the Spring time change. Morningness increases as people age, so older adults tend to be "morning" types. As a result, older workers may have more trouble adjusting to the Fall time change. Finally, people who are on the extreme end of the eveningness or the morningness trait may tend to have more trouble adjusting their sleep to the time changes.

Chapter 41

Bedding and Sleep Environment

Although sleep is vital to emotional and physical health, millions of people do not get the recommended eight hours of sleep per night. Some have chronic, long-term sleep disorders, while others experience occasional trouble sleeping. Sleep deprivation can lead to daytime drowsiness, poor concentration, stress, irritability, and a weakened immune system. Among the many factors that can impact the amount and quality of sleep, bedding and the sleep environment are perhaps the easiest to control or change. Choosing a high-quality mattress; selecting the right pillow; and creating a comfortable, inviting sleep sanctuary can help people improve their sleep as well as their overall quality of life.

Environmental factors—such as light, noise, temperature, color, accessories, and bedding—play an important role in the sleep experience. Choosing comfortable bedding, making sure the bedroom temperature is neither too hot nor too cold, and eliminating sources of distracting noise or light can make a big difference in helping people get a good night's sleep. The goal is to turn the bedroom into a soothing, relaxing, indulgent escape from the everyday pressures and hassles of life. Inviting colors and attractive accessories are available from many sources to fit any space or budget.

"Bedding and Sleep Environment," © 2016 Omnigraphics. Reviewed May 2019.

Choosing a Mattress

The centerpiece of any bedroom, and the most important aspect of ensuring a comfortable, high-quality night's sleep, is the mattress. Mattresses generally have a lifespan of 5 to 7 years, depending on usage, before the comfort and support they offer begins to decline. At this point, experts recommend evaluating the mattress and comparing it to newer models. A mattress is likely to need replacing if it shows signs of wear, such as sagging, lumps, or exposed springs. A new mattress may also be warranted if users tend to sleep better elsewhere or frequently wake up with numbness, stiffness, or pain. Research has shown that 70 percent of people report significant improvements in sleep comfort, 62 percent report improvements in sleep quality, and more than 50 percent report reductions in back pain and spine stiffness when sleeping on a new mattress rather than one that is 5 years old.

The search for a new mattress begins at a reputable mattress store with educated salespeople who can explain the various options and guide customers through the purchasing process. Since quality mattresses are major expenditures, it is important for customers to test different types and models to find the one that best meets their personal needs. Testing a mattress involves lying down for several minutes in various sleep positions while concentrating on the feel of each surface.

The main qualities to look for in a new mattress include comfort, support, durability, and size. Many types of cushioning materials are available to create a soft, plush feel. Beneath the surface, the mattress and foundation should provide gentle support that keeps the spine in alignment. The quality of materials and construction determine the durability of the mattress. The main mattress sizes, from smallest to largest, are:

- Twin (38" x 75")

- Full or double (53" x 75")

- Queen (60" x 80")

- California king (72" x 84")

- King (76" x 80")

Since twin- and full-sized mattresses are only 75" long, they may be too short to accommodate taller adults. If 2 people will be sharing a bed, experts recommend buying a queen-sized or larger mattress. King-sized mattresses provide maximum sleeping space. Since an average person shifts position between 40 and 60 times per night, many people feel that a larger mattress provides them with greater freedom to move around comfortably.

There are many different types of mattresses to choose from, including:

- **Innerspring**, which features tempered steel coils for support beneath layers of insulation and cushioning for comfort

- **Foam**, which can be made of solid foam or layers of different kinds of foam, including visco-elastic "memory" foam that molds to individual sleepers

- **Airbeds**, which feature an air-filled core rather than springs for support and are usually adjustable to fit sleepers' preferences

- **Waterbeds**, which feature a water-filled core for support beneath layers of upholstery for comfort and insulation

- **Adjustable beds**, which feature an electric motor to allow sleepers to change the position of the head and foot of the bed to increase comfort

- **Futons**, which offer a space-saving alternative by converting into a sofa during the day

Caring for a Mattress

After purchasing a new mattress, proper care is key to getting the most out of the investment. The first step is to ensure that the mattress and foundation are properly installed. If they have a slight "new-product" odor, proper ventilation should solve the problem within a few hours. Although it is not illegal to remove the tag, it is best to leave it attached to the mattress in case it is required for a warranty claim.

Sleep sets retain their comfort and support longer if they are placed on a sturdy, high-quality bed frame. Boards should never be placed beneath the mattress to increase support. Instead, the mattress should be replaced when it reaches that stage. To keep the mattress fresh and prevent stains, it is important to use a washable mattress pad. If the mattress should require cleaning, the recommended methods are vacuuming or spot cleaning with mild soap and cold water. Mattresses should never be dry cleaned, which can damage the material or become soaked with water.

Basic mattress care involves not allowing children to jump on the bed, which can damage its interior construction. In addition, periodically rotating the mattress from top to bottom and end to end will help extend its useful life. For other issues, it is best to follow the manufacturer's guidelines.

Choosing a Pillow

Pillows, as with mattresses, need to be replaced periodically to ensure that they provide adequate support and comfort. The useful life of a pillow depends on its quality and the amount of use it receives. Most pillows should be replaced on an annual basis. A pillow generally must be replaced when it becomes lumpy or shows signs of dirt, stains, or wear and tear. An easy test to see whether a pillow has lost its capacity to support the head involves folding it in half and squeezing the air out. If it springs back to its original shape quickly, it still retains its support. If not, it may be time to buy a new pillow.

Ideally, a pillow should support the head in the same position as if the person were standing with an upright posture. Different amounts of cushioning are available for different sleeping positions. People who sleep on their side may want a firm pillow, while people who sleep on their back may want a somewhat softer pillow. A wide variety of pillows are available to fit any budget. Some of the different types of pillows include feather, down, memory foam, microbead, neck, lumbar, body, and wedge. Special pillows are also available for people who are pregnant or have sleep apnea.

References

1. "The Better Sleep Guide," Better Sleep Council (BSC), n.d.

2. "Pillows," Better Sleep Council (BSC), n.d.

Chapter 42

Exercise and Sleep

Exercise is an essential aspect of a healthy lifestyle. It not only promotes physical fitness, cardiovascular health, and weight management, but it can also help people sleep better. Regular exercise has been shown to reduce stress and anxiety, which often contribute to sleep problems. It can also improve physical health conditions that contribute to sleep disorders. For instance, exercise can help people lose weight, which can reduce the symptoms of sleep apnea. Improvements in sleep duration and quality, in turn, lead to greater energy, vitality, and mood—all of which can increase people's motivation to exercise, as well as improve their athletic performance.

The link between exercise and sleep is particularly important for people who are middle-aged or older. Around half of the adults in this age group experience symptoms of chronic insomnia. Regular aerobic exercise can help this population combat insomnia without medication and improve their sleep and overall health. A 2010 study followed a group of sedentary women 60 years of age and older who had been diagnosed with chronic insomnia. Half of the group remained inactive, while the other half engaged in a moderate exercise program over a 4-month period. By the end of the study, the women who exercised 30 minutes per day were sleeping 45 to 60 minutes longer each night than the women who did not exercise. They also reported sleeping more soundly, waking up fewer times during the night, and feeling more refreshed in the morning.

"Exercise and Sleep," © 2016 Omnigraphics. Reviewed May 2019.

Enhancing the Effects of Exercise on Sleep

Although exercise has the potential to positively impact sleep, getting the full effect depends on the timing and intensity of the workout, as well as the length of time that an exercise program is sustained. The following tips can help people with sleep difficulties maximize the benefits of exercise:

- **Time workouts at least five to six hours before bedtime**, if possible. Body temperature tends to rise during exercise and slowly drop back to normal afterward. This process can take several hours. Since cooler body temperatures coincide with feelings of drowsiness, exercising too close to bedtime can interfere with sleep. On the other hand, exercising in the late afternoon or early evening can help people fall asleep faster at night.

- **Exercise at a moderate intensity.** It is not necessary to exercise at peak intensity or to the point of exhaustion to see improvements in sleep. In fact, moderate aerobic activities, such as brisk walking or bicycling, seem to provide the maximum benefits. Although any increase in physical activity can lead to improvements in insomnia, studies have shown that the more people exercise, the better they tend to sleep.

- **Stick with the program for at least three months.** For people with insomnia or other sleep issues, research has shown that it takes time for an exercise regimen to show results. At first, they may not sleep any better than they did before starting to exercise. Researchers theorize that people with existing sleep problems have highly aroused stress systems, and that it may take several months for the effects of regular exercise to overcome this stress response. Eventually, however, people with insomnia can see improvements in sleep duration and quality that are better than those offered by other treatments or medications.

Finally, it is important to note that the connection between exercise and sleep works both ways. Just as exercise can help people sleep better, getting a good night's sleep can help people feel motivated to exercise and remain active. Studies have shown that people with insomnia often shorten or skip their workouts following nights when they have trouble sleeping. Sleep deprivation makes exercise feel harder and more tiring, and it can also detract from athletic performance. On the flip side, getting a good night's sleep can help athletes reach their potential. One study showed that college basketball players ran faster and made a higher percentage of shots when they got extra sleep the night before.

References

1. Andrews, Linda Wasmer. "How Exercise Helps You Get a Good Night's Sleep," Health Grades, November 10, 2014.

2. Hendrick, Bill. "Exercise Helps You Sleep," WebMD, September 17, 2010.

3. Reynolds, Gretchen. "How Exercise Can Help Us Sleep Better." New York Times, August 21, 2013.

Chapter 43

How to Discuss Sleep with Your Doctor

Doctors may not detect sleep problems during routine office visits because patients are awake. Thus, you should let your doctor know if you think you might have a sleep problem. For example, talk with your doctor if you often feel sleepy during the day, do not wake up feeling refreshed and alert, or are having trouble adapting to shift work.

Be Prepared

To get a better sense of your sleep problem, your doctor will ask you about your sleep habits. Before you see the doctor, think about how to describe your problems, including:

- How often you have trouble sleeping and how long you have had the problem

- When you go to bed and get up on workdays and days off

- How long it takes you to fall asleep, how often you wake up at night, and how long it takes you to fall back asleep

- Whether you snore loudly and often or wake up gasping or feeling out of breath

---

This chapter includes text excerpted from "Sleep Deprivation and Deficiency," National Heart, Lung, and Blood Institute (NHLBI), April 22, 2019.

301

- How refreshed you feel when you wake up, and how tired you feel during the day

- How often you doze off or have trouble staying awake during routine tasks, especially driving

Your doctor also may ask questions about your personal routine and habits. For example, she or he may ask about your work and exercise routines. Your doctor also may ask whether you use caffeine, tobacco, alcohol, or any medicines (including over-the-counter (OTC) medicines).

Keep a Sleep Diary

To help your doctor, consider keeping a sleep diary for a couple of weeks. Write down when you go to sleep, wake up, and take naps. (For example, you might note: Went to bed at 10 p.m.; woke up at 3 a.m. and could not fall back asleep; napped after work for 2 hours.)

Also, write down how much you sleep each night, how alert and rested you feel in the morning, as well as how sleepy you feel at various times during the day. Share the information in your sleep diary with your doctor.

Diagnostic Procedures That Doctors May Consider

Doctors can diagnose some sleep disorders by asking questions about sleep schedules and habits, and by getting information from sleep partners or parents. To diagnose other sleep disorders, doctors also use the results from sleep studies and other medical tests. Sleep studies allow your doctor to measure how much and how well you sleep. They also help show whether you have sleep problems and how severe they are.

Your doctor will do a physical exam to rule out other medical problems that might interfere with sleep. You may need blood tests to check for thyroid problems or other conditions that can cause sleep problems.

Chapter 44

What You Need to Know about Sleep Studies

The more common sleep studies monitor and record data about your body during a full night of sleep. Other types of sleep studies include multiple sleep latency and daytime maintenance of wakefulness tests. Multiple sleep latency tests measure how quickly you fall asleep during a series of daytime naps and use sensors to record your brain activity and eye movements. A daytime maintenance of wakefulness test measures your ability to stay awake and alert.

Sleep studies can help your doctor diagnose sleep-related breathing disorders, such as sleep apnea; sleep-related seizure disorders; sleep-related movement disorders; and sleep disorders that cause extreme daytime tiredness, such as narcolepsy. Doctors also may use sleep studies to help diagnose or rule out restless legs syndrome (RLS).

Your doctor will determine whether you must have your sleep study at a sleep center or if you can do it at home with a portable diagnostic device. If your sleep study will be done at a sleep center, you will sleep in a bed at the sleep center for the duration of the study. Removable sensors will be placed on your scalp, face, eyelids, chest, limbs, and finger. These sensors record your brain waves, heart rate, breathing

This chapter contains text excerpted from the following sources: Text in this chapter begins with excerpts from "Sleep Studies," National Heart, Lung, and Blood Institute (NHLBI), October 12, 2018; Text beginning with the heading "Types of Sleep Studies" is excerpted from "Your Guide to Healthy Sleep," National Heart, Lung, and Blood Institute (NHLBI), August 2011. Reviewed May 2019.

effort and rate, oxygen levels, and muscle movements before, during, and after sleep. There is a small risk of irritation from the sensors, but this will go away after they are removed.

Your doctor will review your sleep study test results and develop a treatment plan for any diagnosed sleep disorder. Untreated sleep disorders can raise your risk for heart failure, high blood pressure, stroke, diabetes, and depression. Sleep disorders also have been linked to an increased risk for injury and car accidents.

Types of Sleep Studies

Depending on your symptoms, your doctor will gather information and consider several possible tests when trying to diagnose a sleep disorder:

Sleep History and Sleep Log

Your doctor will ask you how many hours you sleep each night, how often you awaken during the night and for how long, how long it takes you to fall asleep, how well rested you feel upon awakening, and how sleepy you feel during the day. Your doctor may ask you to keep a sleep diary for a few weeks. Your doctor also may ask you whether you have any symptoms of sleep apnea or restless legs syndrome, such as loud snoring, snorting or gasping, morning headaches, tingling or unpleasant sensations in the limbs that are relieved by moving them, and jerking of the limbs during sleep. Your sleeping partner may be asked whether you have some of these symptoms, as you may not be aware of them yourself.

Polysomnogram

A sleep recording or polysomnogram (PSG) is usually done while you stay overnight at a sleep center or sleep laboratory. Electrodes and other monitors are placed on your scalp, face, chest, limbs, and finger. While you sleep, these devices measure your brain activity, eye movements, muscle activity, heart rate and rhythm, blood pressure, and how much air moves in and out of your lungs. This test also checks the amount of oxygen in your blood. A PSG test is painless. In certain circumstances, the PSG can be done at home. A home monitor can be used to record heart rate, how air moves in and out of your lungs, the amount of oxygen in your blood, and your breathing effort.

Multiple Sleep Latency Test

This daytime sleep study measures how sleepy you are and is particularly useful for diagnosing narcolepsy. The multiple sleep latency test (MSLT) is conducted in a sleep laboratory and typically done after an overnight sleep recording (PSG). In this test, sleep-stage monitoring devices are placed on your scalp and face. You are asked to nap 4 or 5 times for 20 minutes every 2 hours during the day. Technicians note how quickly you fall asleep and how long it takes you to reach various stages of sleep, especially rapid eye movement (REM) sleep, during your naps. Normal individuals either do not fall asleep during these short-designated nap times or take a long time to fall asleep. People who fall asleep in less than 5 minutes are likely to require treatment for a sleep disorder, as are those who quickly reach REM sleep during their naps. It is important to have a sleep specialist interpret the results of your PSG or MSLT.

How to Find a Sleep Center and Sleep Specialist

If your doctor refers you to a sleep center or sleep specialist, make sure that center or specialist is qualified to diagnose and treat your sleep problem. To find sleep centers accredited by the American Academy of Sleep Medicine (AASM), go to www.aasmnet.org and click on "Find a Sleep Center" (under the patients and public menu), or call 708-492-0930. To find sleep specialists certified by the American Board of Sleep Medicine (ABSM), go to www.absm.org and click on "verification of diplomates of the American Board of Sleep Medicine."

Chapter 45

Treatment for Insomnia

If your insomnia is caused by a short-term change in your sleep–wake schedule, such as with jet lag, your sleep schedule will probably return to normal on its own. Chronic or long-term insomnia can be treated with steps you can try at home to sleep better, cognitive behavioral therapy (CBT), and prescription medicines.

If insomnia is a symptom or side effect of another health problem, your doctor may recommend treating the other health problem at the same time. When the other health problem is treated, secondary insomnia often goes away on its own. For example, if menopause symptoms, such as hot flashes, are keeping you awake, your doctor might try treating your hot flashes first. Research suggests that older women who use hormone replacement therapy (HRT), eat healthy foods based on a Mediterranean diet, and limit how much caffeine and alcohol they drink may have fewer sleep problems than women who do not do these things.

Talk to your doctor or nurse if you have symptoms of insomnia, and ask about the best ways to treat insomnia.

How Does Cognitive Behavioral Therapy Help Treat Insomnia?

Research shows that CBT works as well as prescription medicine for many people who have chronic or long-term insomnia. Cognitive

This chapter includes text excerpted from "Insomnia," Office on Women's Health (OWH), U.S. Department of Health and Human Services (HHS), November 21, 2018.

behavioral therapy helps you change thoughts and actions that may get in the way of sleep. This type of therapy is also used to treat conditions, such as depression, anxiety disorders, and eating disorders. For success with CBT, you may need to see a therapist weekly for two months or more. Cognitive behavioral therapy may involve:

- Keeping a diary to track your sleep

- Replacing negative thoughts about sleep with positive thinking. This includes linking being in bed to being asleep and not to the problems you have falling asleep.

- Talking with a therapist alone or in group sessions. This can help you identify and change any unhelpful thoughts and behaviors about sleep.

- Learning habits that can help you sleep better

What Prescription Medicines Treat Insomnia?

Prescription medicines can help treat short-term or long-term insomnia. But, your doctor or nurse may have you try cognitive behavioral therapy first rather than medicine to treat insomnia.

The types of prescription medicines used to treat insomnia include sedatives and certain kinds of antidepressants. Prescription sleep medicines can have serious side effects, including sleepiness during the daytime and increased risk of falls for older adults. They can also affect women differently than men. In 2013, the U.S. Food and Drug Administration (FDA) required drug companies to lower the recommended dose for women of certain prescription sleep medicines with zolpidem because women's bodies do not break down the medicine as quickly as men's bodies do.

If you decide to use a prescription sleep medicine:

- Ask your doctor, nurse, or pharmacist about any warnings and potential side effects of the medicine.

- Take the medicine at the time of day your doctor tells you to.

- Do not drive or do other activities that require you to be alert and sober.

- Take only the amount of medicine prescribed by your doctor.

- Tell your doctor, nurse, or pharmacist about all other medicines you take, both over-the-counter (OTC) and prescription.

- Call your doctor or nurse right away if you have any problems while using the medicine.

- Do not drink alcohol.

- Do not take medicines that your doctor has not prescribed to you.

- Talk to your doctor or nurse if you want to stop using the sleep medicine. You need to stop taking some sleep medicines gradually (a little at a time).

When taking sleep medicine, make sure to give yourself enough time to get a full night of sleep. A full night of sleep is usually at least seven hours. Ask your doctor or pharmacist to tell you about any side effects of taking sleep medicine, such as grogginess that may make it difficult to drive. Talk to your doctor or nurse if your insomnia symptoms continue longer than four weeks.

Can You Take an Over-the-Counter Medicine for Insomnia?

Over-the-counter medicines, or sleep aids, may help some people with insomnia symptoms, but they are not meant for regular or long-term use. Many OTC sleep medicines contain antihistamines that are usually used to treat allergies.

If you decide to use OTC sleep medicine:

- Ask your doctor, nurse, or pharmacist about any warnings and potential side effects of the medicine.

- Take the medicine at the time of day your doctor tells you to.

- Do not drive or do other activities that require you to be alert and sober.

- Take only the amount of medicine suggested by your doctor.

- Tell your doctor, nurse, or pharmacist about all other medicines you take, both OTC and prescription.

- Call your doctor or nurse right away if you have any problems while using the medicine.

- Do not drink alcohol.

- Do not use drugs that your doctor has not prescribed to you.

Chapter 46

Treatment for Myalgic Encephalomyelitis/Chronic Fatigue Syndrome

There is no cure or approved treatment for myalgic encephalomyelitis (ME)/chronic fatigue syndrome (CFS). However, some symptoms can be treated or managed. Treating these symptoms might provide relief for some patients with ME/CFS but not others. Other strategies, such as learning new ways to manage activity, can also be helpful.

Patients, their families, and healthcare providers need to work together to decide which symptom causes the most problems. This should be treated first. Patients, families, and healthcare providers should discuss the possible benefits and harms of any treatment plans, including medicines and other therapies.

Healthcare providers need to support their patients' families as they come to understand how to live with this illness. Providers and families should remember that this process might be hard on people with ME/CFS.

This chapter includes text excerpted from "Treatment of ME/CFS," Centers for Disease Control and Prevention (CDC), July 12, 2018.

Symptoms of Myalgic Encephalomyelitis/Chronic Fatigue Syndrome That Healthcare Providers Might Try to Address

Symptoms that healthcare providers might try to address are discussed below.

Sleep Problems

Patients with ME/CFS often feel less refreshed and restored after sleep than they did before they became ill. Common sleep complaints include difficulty falling or staying asleep, extreme sleepiness, intense and vivid dreaming, restless legs, and nighttime muscle spasms.

Good sleep habits are important for all people, including those with ME/CFS. When people try these tips but are still unable to sleep, their doctor might recommend taking medicine to help with sleep. First, people should try over-the-counter sleep products. If this does not help, doctors can offer a prescription sleep medicine, starting at the smallest dose and using for the shortest possible time.

People might continue to feel unrefreshed even after the medications help them to get a full night of sleep. If so, they should consider seeing a sleep specialist. Most people with sleep disorders, such as sleep apnea (symptoms include brief pausing in breathing during sleep) and narcolepsy (symptoms include excessive daytime sleepiness), respond to therapy. However, for people with ME/CFS, not all symptoms may go away.

Postexertional Malaise

Postexertional malaise (PEM) is the worsening of symptoms after even minor physical, mental or emotional exertion. The symptoms typically get worse 12 to 48 hours after the activity and can last for days or even weeks.

PEM can be addressed by activity management, also called "pacing." The goal of pacing is to learn to balance rest and activity to avoid PEM flare-ups, which can be caused by exertion that patients with ME/CFS cannot tolerate. To do this, patients need to find their individual limits for mental and physical activity. Then they need to plan activity and rest to stay within these limits. Some patients and doctors refer to staying within these limits as staying within the "energy envelope." The limits may be different for each patient. Keeping activity and symptom diaries may help patients find their personal limits, especially early on in the illness.

For some patients with ME/CFS, even daily chores and activities such as cleaning, preparing a meal, or taking a shower can be difficult and may need to be broken down into shorter, less strenuous pieces. Rehabilitation specialists or exercise physiologists who know ME/CFS may help patients with adjusting to life with ME/CFS. Patients who have learned to listen to their bodies might benefit from carefully increasing exercise to improve fitness and avoid deconditioning. However, exercise is not a cure for ME/CFS.

Patients with ME/CFS need to avoid "push-and-crash" cycles through carefully managing activity. Push-and-crash cycles are when someone with ME/CFS is having a good day and tries to push to do more than they would normally attempt (do too much, crash, rest, start to feel a little better, do too much once again). This can then lead to a "crash" (worsening of ME/CFS symptoms). Finding ways to make activities easier may be helpful, such as sitting while doing the laundry or showering, taking frequent breaks, and dividing large tasks into smaller steps.

Any activity or exercise plan for people with ME/CFS needs to be carefully designed with input from each patient. While vigorous aerobic exercise can be beneficial for many chronic illnesses, patients with ME/CFS do not tolerate such exercise routines. Standard exercise recommendations for healthy people can be harmful for patients with ME/CFS. However, it is important that patients with ME/CFS undertake activities that they can tolerate, as described above.

Pain

People with ME/CFS often have deep pain in their muscles and joints. They might also have headaches (typically pressure-like) and soreness of their skin when touched.

Patients should always talk to their healthcare provider before trying any medication. Doctors may first recommend trying over-the-counter (OTC) pain-relievers, such as acetaminophen, aspirin, or ibuprofen. If these do not provide enough pain relief, patients may need to see a pain specialist. People with chronic pain, including those with ME/CFS, can benefit from counseling to learn new ways to deal with pain.

Other pain management methods include stretching and movement therapies, gentle massage, heat, toning exercises, and water therapy for healing. Acupuncture, when done by a licensed practitioner, might help with pain for some patients.

Depression, Stress, and Anxiety

Adjusting to a chronic, debilitating illness sometimes leads to other problems, including depression, stress, and anxiety. Many patients with ME/CFS develop depression during their illness. When present, depression or anxiety should be treated. Although treating depression or anxiety can be helpful, it is not a cure for ME/CFS.

Some people with ME/CFS might benefit from antidepressants and antianxiety medications. However, doctors should use caution in prescribing these medications. Some drugs used to treat depression have other effects that might worsen other ME/CFS symptoms and cause side effects. When healthcare providers are concerned about patient's psychological condition, they may recommend seeing a mental-health professional.

Some people with ME/CFS might benefit from trying techniques, such as deep breathing and muscle relaxation, massage, and movement therapies (stretching, yoga, and tai chi). These can reduce stress and anxiety, and promote a sense of well-being.

Dizziness and Light-Headedness or Orthostatic Intolerance

Some people with ME/CFS might also have symptoms of orthostatic intolerance that are triggered when-or made worse by-standing or sitting upright. These symptoms can include:

- Frequent dizziness and light-headedness
- Changes in vision (blurred vision, seeing white or black spots)
- Weakness
- Feeling, such as your heart is beating too fast or too hard, fluttering, or skipping a beat

For patients with these symptoms, their doctor will check their heart rate and blood pressure, and may recommend they see a specialist, such as a cardiologist or neurologist.

For people with ME/CFS who do not have heart or blood vessel disease, doctor might suggest patients increase daily fluid and salt intake and use support stockings. If symptoms do not improve, prescription medication can be considered.

Memory and Concentration Problems

Memory aids, such as organizers and calendars, can help with memory problems. For people with ME/CFS who have concentration problems, some doctors have prescribed stimulant medications, such as those typically used to treat attention deficit hyperactivity disorder (ADHD). While stimulants might help improve concentration for some patients with ME/CFS, they might lead to the push-and-crash cycle and worsen symptoms. Push-and-crash cycles are when someone with ME/CFS is having a good day and tries to push to do more than they would normally attempt (do too much, crash, rest, start to feel a little better, do too much once again).

Living with Myalgic Encephalomyelitis/Chronic Fatigue Syndrome

Strategies that do not involve use of medications and might be helpful to some patients are:

- **Professional counseling.** Talking with a therapist to help find strategies to cope with the illness and its impact on daily life and relationships.

- **Balanced diet.** A balanced diet is important for everyone's good health and would benefit a person with or without any chronic illness.

- **Nutritional supplements.** Doctors might run tests to see if patients lack any important nutrients and might suggest supplements to try. Doctors and patients should talk about any risks and benefits of supplements, and consider any possible interactions that may occur with prescription medications. Follow-up tests to see if nutrient levels improve can help with treatment planning.

- **Complementary therapies.** Therapies, such as meditation, gentle massage, deep breathing, or relaxation therapy, might be helpful.

Patients should talk with their doctors about all potential therapies because many treatments that are promoted as cures for ME/CFS are unproven, often costly, and could be dangerous.

Chapter 47

Sleep Medication

Chapter Contents

Section 47.1

Prescription Sleep Aid Use among Adults

This section includes text excerpted from "Prescription
Sleep Aid Use among Adults: United States, 2005–2010,"
Centers for Disease Control and Prevention (CDC),
November 6, 2015. Reviewed May 2019.

Sedative and hypnotic medications, often referred to as "sleep aids," are used to induce or maintain sleep by suppressing activities in the central nervous system (CNS). In the past two decades, both popular media and pharmaceutical companies have reported an increased number of prescriptions filled for sleep aids in the United States. In fact, a market research firm has reported a tripling in sleep aid prescriptions from 1998 to 2006 for young adults between the ages of 18 and 24. This section presents person-based nationally representative estimates on prescription sleep aid use in the past 30 days, describes sociodemographic differences in use, and examines sleep aid use by self-reported sleep duration and insomnia.

Data from the National Health and Nutrition Examination Survey (NHANES), 2005 to 2010 shows that:

- About 4 percent of U.S. adults 20 years of age and older used prescription sleep aids in the past month.

- The percentage of adults using a prescription sleep aid increased with age and education. More adult women (5.0%) used prescription sleep aids than adult men (3.1%).

- Non-Hispanic White adults were more likely to use sleep aids (4.7%) than non-Hispanic Black (2.5%) and Mexican-American (2.0%) adults.

- Prescription sleep aid use varied by sleep duration and was highest among adults who sleep less than 5 hours (6.0%) or sleep 9 or more hours (5.3%).

- One in six adults with a diagnosed sleep disorder, and one in eight adults with trouble sleeping reported using sleep aids.

Prescription Sleep Aid Use in the past 30 Days Increased with Age

During 2005 to 2010, about 4 percent of U.S. adults 20 years of age and older reported that they took prescription sleep aids in the past 30 days. Prevalence of use was lowest among the youngest age group (those between the ages of 20 and 39) at about 2 percent, increased to 6 percent among those between the ages of 50 and 59, and reached 7 percent among those 80 years of age and older.

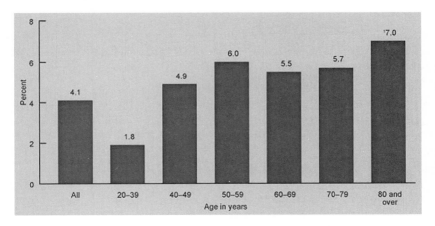

Figure 47.1. *Percentage of Adults Aged 20 and over Who Used Prescription Sleep Aids in the Past 30 Days, by Age: United States, 2005 to 2010* (Source: Centers for Disease Control and Prevention (CDC)/National Center for Health (NCHS), National Health and Nutrition Examination Survey (NHANES).)

[1] *Significant increasing linear trend by age (p < 0.05).*
Note: *Sleep aids include all hypnotic drugs and four antidepressant or sedative medications commonly prescribed for insomnia or depression.*

Prescription Sleep Aid Use in the past 30 Days Varied by Sex and Race and Ethnicity

Reported prescription sleep aid use in the past 30 days was higher among women (5.0%) than men (3.1%). Non-Hispanic White adults reported higher use of sleep aids (4.7%) than non-Hispanic Black (2.5%) and Mexican American (2.0%) adults. No difference was shown between non-Hispanic Black adults and Mexican American adults in use of prescription sleep aids.

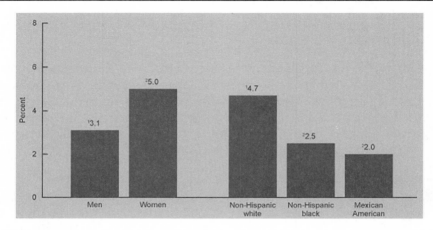

Figure 47.2. *Age-Adjusted Percentage of Adults 20 Years of Age and Older Who Used Prescription Sleep Aids in the Past 30 Days, By Sex and Race and Ethnicity: United States, 2005 to 2010* (Source: Centers for Disease Control and Prevention (CDC)/National Center for Health (NCHS), National Health and Nutrition Examination Survey (NHANES).)

[1] *Reference group.*
[2] *Significantly different from reference group (p < 0.05).*
Note: *Data are age-adjusted to the 2000 projected U.S. standard population using the age groups 20 to 39, 40 to 59, and 60 and over. Sleep aids include all hypnotic drugs and four antidepressant or sedative medications commonly prescribed for insomnia or depression.*

Prescription Sleep Aid Use in the past 30 Days Increased with Higher Education

3 percent of adults with less than a high-school education reported using sleep aids in the past 30 days, compared with 3.9 percent with a high-school diploma and 4.4 percent of adults with greater than a high-school education.

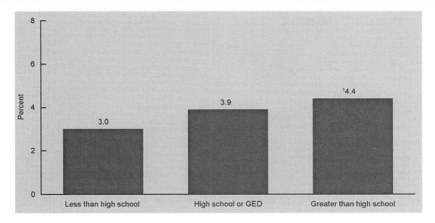

Figure 47.3. *Age-Adjusted Percentage of Adults Aged 20 and over Who Used Prescription Sleep Aids in the Past 30 Days, by Education: United States, 2005 to 2010* (Source: Centers for Disease Control and Prevention (CDC)/National Center for Health (NCHS), National Health and Nutrition Examination Survey (NHANES).)

[1] Significant increasing linear trend by education (p < 0.05).
Note: *GED is General Educational Development high school equivalency diploma. Data are age-adjusted to the 2000 projected U.S. standard population using the age groups 20 to 39, 40 to 59, and 60 and over. Sleep aids include all hypnotic drugs and four antidepressant or sedative medications commonly prescribed for insomnia or depression.*

Prescription Sleep Aid Use in the Past 30 Days Varied by Sleep Duration

The National Sleep Foundation (NSF) suggests that 7 hours of sleep is the minimum amount of sleep that adults need on a regular basis for optimal performance, thus 7 hours is used as the reference point for sleep duration. Compared with those who reported 7 hours of sleep (3.2%), adults with 5 or fewer hours of sleep per night had the highest use of sleep aids in the past 30 days (6.0%). Those with 6 hours of sleep (3.8%) did not significantly differ from the reference group, whereas those with 8 hours (4.1%) or 9 or more hours (5.3%) of sleep showed higher usage of sleep aids. In other words, when sleep duration was greater or less than 7 hours, the use of sleep aids increased.

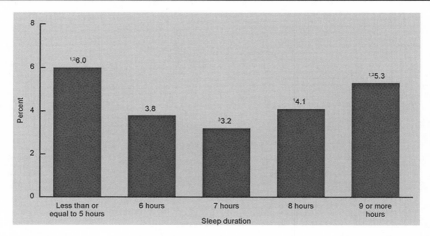

Figure 47.4. *Age-Adjusted Percentage of Adults Aged 20 and over Who Used Prescription Sleep Aids in the Past 30 Days, by Sleep Duration: United States, 2005 to 2010* (Source: Centers for Disease Control and Prevention (CDC)/National Center for Health (NCHS), National Health and Nutrition Examination Survey (NHANES).)

[1] *Significantly different from reference group (p < 0.05).*
[2] *Significant quadratic trend with sleep duration (p < 0.05).*
[3] *Reference group.*
Note: *Data are age-adjusted to the 2000 projected U.S. standard population using the age groups 20 to 39, 40 to 59, and 60 and over. Sleep aids include all hypnotic drugs and four antidepressant or sedative medications commonly prescribed for insomnia or depression.*

Prescription Sleep Aid Use in the Past 30 Days Was Higher among Adults with Diagnosed Sleep Disorders and among Adults with Trouble Sleeping

Over 16 percent of adults who reported a physician's diagnosis of a sleep disorder reported using sleep aids in the past 30 days, which was more than 5 times higher than those who did not report such a diagnosis. About 13 percent of adults who told their doctor that they had trouble sleeping reported sleep aid use, which was nearly 12 times higher than those who did not report any trouble sleeping.

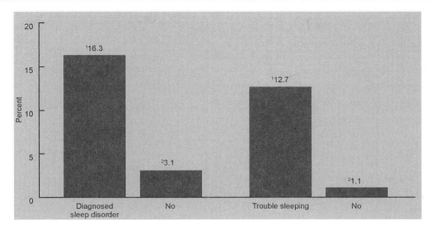

Figure 47.5. *Age-Adjusted Percentage of Adults Aged 20 and over Who Used Prescription Sleep Aids in the past 30 Days, by Physician-Diagnosed Sleep Disorder and Self-Reported Trouble Going to Sleep: United States, 2005 to 2010* (Source: Centers for Disease Control and Prevention (CDC)/National Center for Health (NCHS), National Health and Nutrition Examination Survey (NHANES).)

[1] *Significantly different from reference group (p < 0.05).*
[2] *Reference group.*
Note: *Data are age-adjusted to the 2000 projected U.S. standard population using the age groups 20 to 39, 40 to 59, and 60 and over. Sleep aids include all hypnotic drugs and four antidepressant or sedative medications commonly prescribed for insomnia or depression.*

Summary

According to estimates, 50 to 70 million Americans suffer from sleep disorders or deprivation, which can not only hinder daily functioning, but can also adversely affect their health. Prescription sleep aids are one of the treatment options for trouble going into or maintaining sleep. However, long-term use of sleep aids has been linked to adverse outcomes in health.

So far, studies on sleep aid use are mostly based on administrative claims data, which describe the number of times sleep aid prescriptions are filled rather than how many people have actually used prescription sleep aids. This section provides the first person-based national data on prescription sleep aid use among the noninstitutionalized U.S. adult population. Approximately 4 percent of adults 20 years of age and older reported using a prescription sleep aid in the past month. Use increased with age and was more common among women, non-Hispanic White adults, and those with greater than a high-school education. Use also varied by sleep duration and was significantly higher among adults who reported sleep disorders or trouble sleeping.

Section 47.2

Medicines to Help You Sleep

This section contains text excerpted from "Sleep Problems," U.S. Food and Drug Administration (FDA), April 12, 2019.

Prescription Insomnia Drugs

Prescription sleep medicines work well for many people, but they can cause serious side effects.

- Talk to your doctor about all the risks and benefits of using prescription sleep medicines.

- Sleep drugs taken for insomnia can affect your driving the morning after use.

- Sleep drugs can cause rare side effects, such as:

  - Severe allergic reactions

  - Severe face swelling

  - Behaviors such as making phone calls, eating, having sex or driving while you are not fully awake

Over-the-Counter Insomnia Drugs

Over-the-counter (OTC) sleep drugs have side effects too.

Tips for Better Sleep

Making some changes to your nighttime habits may help you get the sleep you need.

- Go to bed and get up at the same times each day.

- Sleep in a dark, quiet room.

- Avoid caffeine and nicotine.

- Do not drink alcohol before bedtime.

- Do something to help you relax before bedtime.

- Do not exercise before bedtime.

- Do not take a nap after 3 p.m.

- Do not eat a large meal before you go to sleep.

Talk to your healthcare provider if you have trouble sleeping almost every night for more than two weeks.

Section 47.3

Taking Z-Drugs for Insomnia? Know the Risks

This section includes text excerpted from "Taking Z-Drugs for Insomnia? Know the Risks," U.S. Food and Drug Administration (FDA), April 30, 2019.

If you are lying awake night after night, unable to sleep, you may want to talk to your healthcare provider about it. She or he may prescribe insomnia medicines, such as eszopiclone (Lunesta), zaleplon (Sonata), and zolpidem (Ambien, Ambien CR, Edluar, and Zolpimist)—sometimes known as "Z-drugs"—to help you get a good night's sleep. But as with any medication, there are risks.

Prescription-only "Z-drugs" work by slowing activity in the brain. Used properly, they can help you sleep. Quality sleep can have a positive impact on physical and mental health. But, the treatments also carry the risk—though rare—of serious injuries and even death.

The U.S. Food and Drug Administration (FDA) wants you and your healthcare provider to be fully aware of these risks, so the agency is requiring the addition of a new boxed warning—the FDA's most prominent warning—to the prescribing information, known as "labeling," and patient medication guides. In addition, the FDA is adding a contraindication, which is the agency's strongest warning, stating that patients who have experienced an episode of what is known as "complex sleep behavior" should not take these drugs.

What Are Complex Sleep Behaviors?

Complex sleep behaviors (CSBs) occur while you are asleep or not fully awake. Examples include sleepwalking, sleep driving, sleep cooking, or taking other medicines. The FDA has received reports of people taking these insomnia medicines and accidentally overdosing, falling, being burned, shooting themselves, and wandering outside in extremely cold weather, among other incidents. Since Ambien was approved in 1992, the FDA has identified 66 serious cases of complex sleep behaviors after a person has taken a Z-drug, 20 of which resulted in death.

Considering the large number of individuals who take the drugs, the FDA wants people to be aware of the potential dangers that can occur as a result. Patients may not remember these behaviors when they wake up the next morning. Moreover, they may experience these types of behaviors after their first dose of one of these Z-drugs or after continued use.

Your Healthcare Provider Has Prescribed a Z-Drug for You: What Should You Do?

If your healthcare provider prescribes a Z-drug to help you sleep, here are some things to keep in mind:

- Talk with your healthcare provider about all of the benefits and risks of taking this medicine.

- Read the patient medication guide as soon as you get the prescription filled and before you start taking the medicine. If you have any questions, or if there is anything you do not understand, ask your prescriber.

- If, after taking the medication, you experience a complex sleep behavior in which you engage in activities while not fully awake or take actions that you do not remember, stop taking the drug and contact your prescriber immediately.

- These events can occur on the first night you use these medicines or after a much longer period of treatment.

Complex sleep behaviors can occur at lower dosages, as well as high dosages. It is important to carefully follow the dosing instructions in the patient medication guide.

- Do not take these medicines with any other sleep medicines, including those you can buy over-the-counter without a prescription.

- Do not drink alcohol before or while taking these medicines. Together, they may be more likely to cause side effects.

- You may still feel drowsy the day after taking one of these drugs. Keep in mind that all medicines taken for insomnia can impair your ability to drive and activities that require alertness the morning after use.

Section 47.4

Risk of Next-Morning Impairment after Use of Zolpidem and Other Insomnia Drugs

This section includes text excerpted from "Questions and Answers: Risk of Next-Morning Impairment after Use of Insomnia Drugs; FDA Requires Lower Recommended Doses for Certain Drugs Containing Zolpidem (Ambien, Ambien CR, Edluar, and Zolpimist)," U.S. Food and Drug Administration (FDA), February 13, 2018.

The U.S. Food and Drug Administration (FDA) is notifying the public of new information about zolpidem, a widely prescribed insomnia drug. The FDA recommends that the bedtime dose be lowered because new data show that blood levels in some patients may be high enough the morning after use to impair activities that require alertness, including driving. This announcement focused on zolpidem products approved for bedtime use, which are marketed as generics and under the brand names "Ambien," "Ambien CR," "Edluar," and "Zolpimist."

The FDA is also reminding the public that all drugs taken for insomnia can impair driving and activities that require alertness the morning after use. Drowsiness is already listed as a common side effect in the drug labels of all insomnia drugs, along with warnings that patients may still feel drowsy the day after taking these products. Patients who take insomnia drugs can experience an impairment of mental alertness the morning after use, even if they feel fully awake.

The FDA urges healthcare professionals to caution all patients who use these zolpidem products about the risks of next-morning impairment for activities that require complete mental alertness. For zolpidem products, data show the risk for next-morning impairment is highest for patients taking the extended-release forms of these drugs (Ambien CR and generics). Women appear to be more susceptible to this risk because they eliminate zolpidem from their bodies more slowly than men.

Because use of lower doses of zolpidem will result in lower blood levels in the morning, the FDA is requiring the manufacturers of Ambien, Ambien CR, Edluar, and Zolpimist to lower the recommended dose. The FDA has informed the manufacturers that the recommended dose of zolpidem for women should be lowered from 10 mg to 5 mg for immediate-release products (Ambien, Edluar, and Zolpimist) and from 12.5 mg to 6.25 mg for extended-release products (Ambien CR). The FDA also informed the manufacturers that, for men, the labeling should recommend that healthcare professionals consider prescribing the lower doses? 5 mg for immediate-release products and 6.25 mg for extended-release products.

Frequently Asked Questions
What Is Zolpidem?

Zolpidem is a sedative-hypnotic (sleep) medicine that is used in adults for the treatment of insomnia. Zolpidem is available as an oral tablet (Ambien and generics), an extended-release tablet (Ambien CR and generics), a sublingual (under-the-tongue) tablet (Edluar), and an oral spray (Zolpimist).

Zolpidem is also available under the brand name "Intermezzo," a lower dose sublingual tablet that is approved for use as needed for the treatment of insomnia when a middle-of-the-night awakening is followed by difficulty returning to sleep.

Why Is the U.S. Food and Drug Administration Requiring the Manufacturers of Certain Zolpidem-Containing Products to Revise the Labeling to Lower the Recommended Dose of Zolpidem for Women and to Recommend Consideration of the Lower Dose in Men?

The FDA is requiring the manufacturers of certain zolpidem-containing products to revise the labeling to lower the recommended dose of zolpidem-containing medicines for women and to recommend that healthcare professionals consider prescribing the lower dose for men because next-morning blood levels of zolpidem may be high enough to impair activities that require alertness. Patients with high levels of zolpidem can be impaired even if they feel fully awake. Zolpidem is eliminated from the body more slowly in women, so the drug can stay in their systems longer than it does in men.

What Should Patients Currently Taking the 10 mg or 12.5 mg Dose of Zolpidem-Containing Insomnia Medicines Do Now?

If you are taking the 10 mg or 12.5 mg dose of zolpidem-containing insomnia medicine, continue taking your prescribed dose as directed until you have contacted your healthcare professional to ask for instructions on how to safely continue to take your medicine. Each patient and situation is unique, and the appropriate dose should be discussed with your healthcare professional.

Will a Lower Dose of Zolpidem Be Effective in Treating Insomnia?

The FDA has informed the manufacturers that the recommended dose of zolpidem for women should be lowered from 10 mg to 5 mg for immediate-release products (Ambien, Edluar, and Zolpimist) and from 12.5 mg to 6.25 mg for extended-release products (Ambien CR). For men, the FDA has informed the manufacturers that the labeling should recommend that healthcare professionals consider prescribing these lower doses. These lower doses of zolpidem (5 mg for immediate-release products and 6.25 mg for extended-release products) will be effective in most women and many men.

Is the U.S. Food and Drug Administration Requiring the Manufacturer of Intermezzo (Zolpidem Tartrate) Sublingual Tablets to Also Change the Dosing Recommendations?

No. When Intermezzo was FDA-approved in November 2011, the label already recommended a lower dosage in women compared to men. The recommended and maximum dose of Intermezzo is 1.75 mg for women and 3.5 mg for men, taken only once per night as needed if a middle-of-the-night awakening is followed by difficulty returning to sleep.

Do Any Other Factors, Such as a Patient's Age, Weight, or Ethnicity, Have an Effect on Zolpidem Levels?

Based on data from pharmacokinetic trials, no relationship was evident between the zolpidem blood level and patients' body weight or ethnicity. In elderly patients, zolpidem blood levels can be higher, and the lower doses are already recommended. In contrast to younger patients, zolpidem blood levels in elderly patients are not affected by sex.

Why Is the U.S. Food and Drug Administration Informing the Public about This Safety Risk Now, after Zolpidem Has Been on the Market for Nearly 20 Years?

Since the approval of zolpidem, the FDA has been continually monitoring the drug's safety profile. As more data became available, the FDA continued to assess the benefits and risks of zolpidem treatment. Over the years, the FDA has received reports of possible driving impairment and motor vehicle accidents associated with zolpidem; however, in most cases, it was difficult to determine if the driving impairment was related to zolpidem or to specific zolpidem blood levels because information about time of dosing and time of the impairment was often not reported. Data from clinical trials and driving simulation studies have become available that allowed the FDA to better characterize the risk of driving impairment caused by specific blood levels of zolpidem and to recognize the increased risk of driving-impairing blood levels of zolpidem in women. This led the FDA to require the manufacturers of certain zolpidem-containing products to revise the dosing recommendations.

Is Next-Morning Impairment the Same as Complex Sleep-Related Behaviors?

No, they are different. Next-morning impairment occurs when patients are awake the next morning, but levels of the insomnia medicine in their blood remain high enough to impair activities that require alertness. Complex sleep-related behaviors occur when patients get out of bed while not fully awake, and sleepwalk or do an activity, such as drive a car, prepare and eat food, make phone calls, or have sex. Both problems are made worse by high levels of zolpidem.

Is the U.S. Food and Drug Administration Requiring the Manufacturers of Other Insomnia Medicines to Revise Their Dosing Recommendations?

No. At this time, the FDA is only requiring the manufacturers of certain zolpidem-containing products to revise their dosing recommendations. The U.S. Food and Drug Administration is continuing to evaluate ways to lower the risk of next-morning impairment with other insomnia medicines.

Do Other Insomnia Medicines Have the Same Gender Effect as Zolpidem?

The U.S. Food and Drug Administration is evaluating other insomnia medicines to determine if they affect women and men differently.

Do Over-the-Counter Insomnia Medicines That Are Available without a Prescription Have a Risk of Next-Morning Impairment?

Yes. Over-the-counter (OTC) insomnia medicines also have a risk for next-morning impairment. The FDA is not recommending that patients who are taking prescription insomnia medicines switch to OTC insomnia medicines.

Patients who drive or perform activities that require full alertness the next morning should discuss with their healthcare professional if the insomnia medicine they are using is right for them.

What Can Patients Do to Decrease Their Risk of Next-Morning Impairment with Insomnia Medicines?

Patients can decrease their risk of next-morning impairment by taking the lowest dose of their insomnia medicine that treats their symptoms. It is important for patients to take their insomnia medicine exactly as prescribed. Taking a higher dose than prescribed or using more than one insomnia medicine is dangerous if patients drive or perform activities that require full alertness the next morning, even if the drugs are taken at the beginning of the night. In addition, patients should not take insomnia medicine intended for bedtime use if less than a full night's sleep (seven to eight hours) remains. Likewise, patients should not take Intermezzo, a zolpidem product that is approved for use in the middle of the night, if less than four hours of sleep remain.

How Many Reports of Zolpidem and Impaired Driving Has the U.S. Food and Drug Administration Received? Were These Reports Used as Evidence to Support the Proposed New Dosing Recommendations for Certain Zolpidem-Containing Products?

The FDA has received about 700 reports of zolpidem and "impaired driving ability and/or road traffic accident." Following a zolpidem label change in 2007, which added information to the warnings and precautions section of the label about complex sleep-related behaviors, including sleep-driving (patients getting out of bed while not fully awake and driving), there was a great deal of media attention. Since such publicity tends to "stimulate" reporting, this led to the considerable number of reports of zolpidem and impaired driving that were submitted to the FDA's Adverse Event Reporting System (AERS) database.

However, while the adverse event reporting system reports generally can be helpful in evaluating safety concerns, these AERS reports for zolpidem lacked the information necessary to understand whether high morning blood levels of zolpidem were the cause of the reported impaired driving. Specifically, these reports often did not include the dose or time zolpidem was taken, the time of the accident, whether alcohol or other drugs were also taken, and whether and when blood levels of the drug were measured. It was not until the FDA received the new data on next-day blood levels and driving simulation studies that the apparent frequency of next-morning mental impairment was better identified.

Section 47.5

Harmful Effects of CNS Depressants

This section includes text excerpted from "What Classes of Prescription Drugs Are Commonly Misused?" National Institute on Drug Abuse (NIDA), December 2018.

What Are Central Nervous System Depressants?

Central nervous system (CNS) depressants, a category that includes tranquilizers, sedatives, and hypnotics, are substances that can slow brain activity. This property makes them useful for treating anxiety and sleep disorders. The following are among the medications commonly prescribed for these purposes:

- **Benzodiazepines**, such as diazepam (Valium®), clonazepam (Klonopin®), and alprazolam (Xanax®), are sometimes prescribed to treat anxiety, acute stress reactions, and panic attacks. Clonazepam may also be prescribed to treat seizure disorders and insomnia. The more sedating benzodiazepines, such as triazolam (Halcion®) and estazolam (Prosom®), are prescribed for short-term treatment of sleep disorders. Usually, benzodiazepines are not prescribed for long-term use because of the high risk for developing tolerance, dependence, or addiction.

- **Nonbenzodiazepine sleep medications**, such as zolpidem (Ambien®), eszopiclone (Lunesta®), and zaleplon (Sonata®), known as "Z-drugs," have a different chemical structure but act on the same gamma-aminobutyric acid (GABA) type A receptors in the brain as benzodiazepines. They are thought to have fewer side effects and less risk of dependence than benzodiazepines.

- **Barbiturates**, such as mephobarbital (Mebaral®), phenobarbital (Luminal®), and pentobarbital sodium (Nembutal®), are used less frequently to reduce anxiety or to help with sleep problems because of their higher risk of overdose compared to benzodiazepines. However, they are still used in surgical procedures and to treat seizure disorders.

How Do Central Nervous System Depressants Affect the Brain and Body?

Most CNS depressants act on the brain by increasing activity at receptors for the inhibitory neurotransmitter GABA. Although the different classes of CNS depressants work in unique ways, it is through their ability to increase GABA signaling—thereby increasing inhibition of brain activity—that they produce a drowsy or calming effect that is medically beneficial to those suffering from anxiety or sleep disorders.

What Are the Possible Consequences of Central Nervous System Depressant Misuse?

Despite their beneficial therapeutic effects, benzodiazepines and barbiturates have the potential for misuse and should be used only as prescribed. The use of nonbenzodiazepine sleep aids, or Z-drugs, is less well-studied, but certain indicators have raised concern about their misuse potential as well.

During the first few days of taking a depressant, a person usually feels sleepy and uncoordinated, but as the body becomes accustomed to the effects of the drug and tolerance develops, these side effects begin to disappear. If one uses these drugs long term, she or he may need larger doses to achieve the therapeutic effects. Continued use can also lead to dependence and withdrawal when use is abruptly reduced or stopped. Because CNS depressants work by slowing the brain's activity, when an individual stop taking them, there can be a rebound effect, resulting in seizures or other harmful consequences.

Although withdrawal from benzodiazepines can be problematic, it is rarely life-threatening, whereas withdrawal from prolonged use of barbiturates can have life-threatening complications. Therefore, someone who is thinking about discontinuing a CNS depressant or who is suffering withdrawal after discontinuing use should speak with a physician or seek immediate medical treatment.

Chapter 48

Implantable Device for Central Sleep Apnea

The U.S. Food and Drug Administration (FDA) approved a new treatment option for patients who have been diagnosed with moderate to severe central sleep apnea. The remede® System is an implantable device that stimulates a nerve located in the chest that is responsible for sending signals to the diaphragm to stimulate breathing.

"This implantable device offers patients another treatment option for central sleep apnea," said Tina Kiang, Ph.D., acting director of the Division of Anesthesiology, General Hospital, Respiratory, Infection Control, and Dental Devices in the FDA's Center for Devices and Radiological Health. "Patients should speak with their healthcare providers about the benefits and risks of this new treatment compared to other available treatments."

Sleep apnea is a disorder that causes individuals to have one or more pauses in breathing or shallow breaths during sleep. Breathing pauses can last from a few seconds to minutes. Central sleep apnea occurs when the brain fails to send signals to the diaphragm to breathe, causing an individual to stop breathing during sleep for a period of 10 seconds or more before restarting again. According to the National Institute of Health's (NIH) National Center on Sleep

This chapter includes text excerpted from "FDA Approves Implantable Device to Treat Moderate to Severe Central Sleep Apnea," U.S. Food and Drug Administration (FDA), October 6, 2017.

Disorders Research (NCSDR), central sleep apnea can lead to poor sleep quality and may result in serious health issues, including an increased risk for high blood pressure, heart attack, heart failure, stroke, obesity, and diabetes. Common treatment options for moderate to severe sleep apnea include medication, positive airway pressure devices (e.g., continuous positive airway pressure machine), or surgery.

The remede® System is comprised of a battery pack surgically placed under the skin in the upper chest area and small, thin wires that are inserted into the blood vessels in the chest near the nerve (phrenic) that stimulates breathing. The system monitors the patient's respiratory signals during sleep and stimulates the nerve to move the diaphragm and restore normal breathing.

The FDA evaluated data from 141 patients to assess the effectiveness of the remede® System in reducing apnea-hypopnea index (AHI), a measure of the frequency and severity of apnea episodes. After 6 months, AHI was reduced by 50 percent or more in 51 percent of patients with an active remede® System implanted. AHI was reduced by 11 percent in patients without an active remede® System implanted.

The most common adverse events reported included concomitant device interaction, implant site infection, and swelling and local tissue damage or pocket erosion. The remede® System should not be used by patients with an active infection or by patients who are known to require magnetic resonance imaging (MRI). This device is not intended for use in patients with obstructive sleep apnea, a condition in which the patient attempts to breathe, but the upper airway is partially or completely blocked.

The FDA granted approval of the remede® System to Respicardia, Inc.

The FDA, an agency within the U.S. Department of Health and Human Services (HHS), protects the public health by assuring the safety, effectiveness, and security of human and veterinary drugs, vaccines, and other biological products for human use and medical devices. The agency also is responsible for the safety and security of the nation's food supply, cosmetics, dietary supplements, products that give off electronic radiation, and for regulating tobacco products.

Chapter 49

Complementary and Alternative Medicine and Dietary Supplements for Sleep Disorders

Chapter Contents

Section 49.1

Complementary and Alternative Medicine and Sleep Disorders: An Overview

This section includes text excerpted from "Sleep Disorders: In Depth," National Center for Complementary and Integrative Health (NCCIH), October 2015. Reviewed May 2019.

What Are Sleep Disorders and How Important Are They?

There are more than 80 different sleep disorders. This section focuses on insomnia—difficulty falling asleep or difficulty staying asleep. Insomnia is one of the most common sleep disorders. Chronic, long-term sleep disorders affect millions of Americans each year. These disorders and the sleep deprivation they cause can interfere with work, driving, social activities, and overall quality of life, and they can have serious health implications. Sleep disorders account for an estimated $16 billion in medical costs each year, plus indirect costs due to missed days of work, decreased productivity, and other factors.

What the Science Say about Complementary Health Approaches and Insomnia?

Research has produced promising results for some complementary health approaches for insomnia, such as relaxation techniques. However, evidence of effectiveness is still limited for most products and practices, and safety concerns have been raised about a few.

Mind and Body Practices

There is evidence that relaxation techniques can be effective in treating chronic insomnia.

- **Progressive relaxation** may help people with insomnia and nighttime anxiety.

- **Music-assisted relaxation** may be moderately beneficial in improving sleep quality in people with sleep problems, but the number of studies has been small.

- **Various forms of relaxation** are sometimes combined with components of cognitive-behavioral therapy (CBT) (such as sleep restriction and stimulus control), with good results.

- **Using relaxation techniques before bedtime** can be part of a strategy to improve sleep habits that also includes other steps, such as maintaining a consistent sleep schedule; avoiding caffeine, alcohol, heavy meals, and strenuous exercise too close to bedtime; and sleeping in a quiet, cool, dark room.

- **Relaxation techniques are generally safe.** However, rare side effects have been reported in people with serious physical or mental-health conditions. If you have a serious underlying health problem, it would be a good idea to consult your healthcare provider before using relaxation techniques.

In a preliminary study, mindfulness-based stress reduction, a type of meditation, was as effective as a prescription drug in a small group of people with insomnia.

- Several other studies have also reported that mindfulness-based stress reduction improved sleep, but the people who participated in these studies had other health problems, such as cancer.

Preliminary studies in postmenopausal women and women with osteoarthritis (OA) suggest that yoga may be helpful for insomnia.

Some practitioners who treat insomnia have reported that hypnotherapy enhanced the effectiveness of cognitive-behavioral therapy and relaxation techniques in their patients, but very little rigorous research has been conducted on the use of hypnotherapy for insomnia.

A small 2012 study on massage therapy showed promising results for insomnia in postmenopausal women. However, conclusions cannot be reached on the basis of a single study.

Most of the studies that have evaluated acupuncture for insomnia have been of poor scientific quality. The current evidence is not rigorous enough to show whether acupuncture is helpful for insomnia.

Dietary Supplements
Melatonin and Related Supplements

Melatonin may help with jet lag and sleep problems related to shift work.

A 2013 evaluation of the results of 19 studies concluded that melatonin may help people with insomnia fall asleep faster, sleep longer, and sleep better, but the effect of melatonin is small compared to that of other treatments for insomnia.

Dietary supplements containing substances that can be changed into melatonin in the body—L-tryptophan and 5-hydroxytryptophan (5-HTP)—have been researched as sleep aids.

Herbs

Although chamomile has traditionally been used for insomnia, often in the form of a tea, there is no conclusive evidence from clinical trials showing whether it is helpful. Some people, especially those who are allergic to ragweed or related plants, may have allergic reactions to chamomile.

Although kava is said to have sedative properties, very little research has been conducted on whether this herb is helpful for insomnia. More importantly, kava supplements have been linked to a risk of severe liver damage.

Clinical trials of valerian (another herb said to have sedative properties) have had inconsistent results, and its value for insomnia has not been demonstrated. Although few people have reported negative side effects from valerian, it is uncertain whether this herb is safe for long-term use.

Some "sleep-formula" dietary supplements combine valerian with other herbs, such as hops; lemon balm; passionflower; and kava or other ingredients, such as melatonin and 5-HTP. There is little evidence on these preparations from studies in people.

Other Complementary Health Approaches

Aromatherapy is the therapeutic use of essential oils from plants. It is uncertain whether aromatherapy is helpful for treating insomnia because little rigorous research has been done on this topic.

A 2010 systematic review concluded that current evidence does not demonstrate significant effects of homeopathic medicines for insomnia.

If You Are Considering Complementary Health Approaches for Sleep Problems

Talk to your healthcare providers. Tell them about the complementary health approach you are considering, and ask any questions you may have. Because trouble sleeping can be an indication of a more serious condition, and because some prescription and over-the-counter (OTC) drugs can contribute to sleep problems, it is important to discuss your sleep-related symptoms with your healthcare providers before trying any complementary health product or practice.

Be cautious about using any sleep product—prescription medications, over-the-counter medications, dietary supplements, or homeopathic remedies. Find out about potential side effects and any risks from long-term use or combining products.

Keep in mind that "natural" does not always mean safe. For example, kava products can cause serious harm to the liver. Also, a manufacturer's use of the term "standardized" (or "verified" or "certified") does not necessarily guarantee product quality or consistency. Natural products can cause health problems if not used correctly. The healthcare providers you see about your sleep problems can advise you.

Consult with Your Healthcare Provider

If you are pregnant, nursing a child, or considering giving a child a dietary supplement or other natural health product, it is especially important to consult your (or your child's) healthcare provider.

If you are considering a practitioner-provided complementary health practice, check with your insurer to see if the services will be covered, and ask a trusted source (such as your healthcare provider or a nearby hospital or medical school) to recommend a practitioner.

Tell all your healthcare providers about any complementary health approaches you use. Give them a full picture of what you do to manage your health. This will help ensure coordinated and safe care.

Section 49.2

Tai Chi Chih

This section contains text excerpted from the following sources:
Text under the heading "What Are Tai Chi and Qi Gong?" is
excerpted from "Tai Chi and Qi Gong: In Depth," National Center for
Complementary and Integrative Health (NCCIH), October 2016; Text
under the heading "Tai Chi Chih Improves Sleep Quality in Older
Adults" is excerpted from "Tai Chi Chih Improves Sleep Quality in
Older Adults," National Center for Complementary and Integrative
Health (NCCIH), July 1, 2008. Reviewed May 2019.

What Are Tai Chi and Qi Gong?

Tai chi and qi gong are centuries-old, related to mind and body practices. They involve certain postures and gentle movements with mental focus, breathing, and relaxation. The movements can be adapted or practiced while walking, standing, or sitting. In contrast to qi gong, tai chi movements, if practiced quickly, can be a form of combat or self-defense.

Tai Chi Chih Improves Sleep Quality in Older Adults

Poor sleep quality is a common problem among older adults. Many have moderate sleep complaints, where they experience insomnia-like symptoms but are not yet diagnosed with insomnia. Sedative medications are commonly used to treat sleep disorders but can cause harmful side effects, and behavioral interventions, such as cognitive-behavioral therapy (CBT), are not always practical. Few treatments focus on improving sleep quality in people with moderate complaints. Tai chi chih—the Westernized version of the Chinese slow-motion meditative exercise tai chi—may serve as an effective alternative approach.

Researchers at the University of California, Los Angeles conducted a randomized controlled trial, funded in part by the National Center for Complementary and Integrative Health (NCCIH), to determine whether tai chi chih could improve sleep quality in healthy, older adults with moderate sleep complaints. In the study, 112 individuals between the ages of 59 and 86 participated in either tai chi chih training or health education classes for 25 weeks. Participants rated their sleep quality based on the Pittsburgh Sleep Quality Index (PSQI), a self-rated questionnaire that assesses sleep quality, duration, and disturbances.

The results of the study showed that the people who participated in tai chi chih sessions experienced slightly greater improvements in self-reported sleep quality. The researchers concluded that tai chi chih can be a useful nonpharmacologic approach to improving sleep quality in older adults with moderate sleep complaints, and it may also help to prevent the onset of insomnia.

Section 49.3

Melatonin

This section includes text excerpted from "Melatonin: In Depth," National Center for Complementary and Integrative Health (NCCIH), May 2015. Reviewed May 2019.

What Is Melatonin?

Melatonin is a natural hormone that plays a role in sleep. Melatonin production and release in the brain is related to the time of day, rising in the evening and falling in the morning. Light at night blocks its production. Melatonin dietary supplements have been studied for sleep disorders, such as jet lag, disruptions of the body's internal clock, insomnia, and problems with sleep among people who work night shifts. It has also been studied for dementia symptoms.

What the Science Says about the Effectiveness of Melatonin
For Sleep Disorders

Studies suggest that melatonin may help with certain sleep disorders, such as jet lag, delayed sleep phase disorder (a disruption of the body's biological clock in which a person's sleep–wake timing cycle is delayed by three to six hours), sleep problems related to shift work, and some sleep disorders in children. It is also been shown to be helpful for a sleep disorder that causes changes in blind people's sleep and wake times. Study results are mixed on whether melatonin is effective for insomnia in adults, but some studies suggest it may slightly reduce the time it takes to fall asleep.

Jet lag

Jet lag is caused by rapid travel across several time zones; its symptoms include disturbed sleep, daytime fatigue, indigestion, and a general feeling of discomfort.

- In a 2009 research review, results from six small studies and two large studies suggested that melatonin may ease jet lag.
- In a 2007 clinical practice guideline, the American Academy of Sleep Medicine (AASM) supported using melatonin to reduce jet lag symptoms and to improve sleep after traveling across more than one time zone.

Delayed Sleep Phase Disorder

Adults and teens with delayed sleep phase disorder have trouble falling asleep before 2 a.m. and have trouble waking up in the morning.

- In a 2007 review of the literature, researchers suggested that a combination of melatonin supplements, a behavioral approach to delay sleep and wake times until the desired sleep time is achieved, and reduced evening light may even out sleep cycles in people with this sleep disorder.
- In a 2007 clinical practice guideline, the AASM recommended timed melatonin supplementation for this sleep disorder.

Shift Work Disorder

Shift work refers to job-related duties conducted outside of morning to evening working hours. About two million Americans who work afternoon to nighttime or nighttime to early morning hours are affected by shift work disorder.

- A 2007 clinical practice guideline and 2010 review of the evidence concluded that melatonin may improve daytime sleep quality and duration, but not nighttime alertness, in people with shift work disorder.
- The AASM recommended taking melatonin prior to daytime sleep for night shift workers with shift work disorder to enhance daytime sleep.

Insomnia

Insomnia is a general term for a group of problems characterized by an inability to fall asleep and stay asleep.

- **In adults.** A 2013 analysis of 19 studies of people with primary sleep disorders found that melatonin slightly improved time it took to fall asleep, total sleep time, and overall sleep quality. In a 2007 study of people with insomnia that were 55 years of age or older, researchers found that prolonged-release melatonin significantly improved quality of sleep and morning alertness.

- **In children.** There is limited evidence from rigorous studies of melatonin for sleep disorders among young people. A 2011 literature review suggested a benefit with minimal side effects in healthy children, as well as youth with attention deficit hyperactivity disorder (ADHD), autism, and several other populations. There is insufficient information to make conclusions about the safety and effectiveness of long-term melatonin use.

For Other Conditions

While there has not been enough research to support melatonin's use for other conditions:

- Researchers are investigating whether adding melatonin to standard cancer care can improve response rates, survival time, and quality of life.

- Results from a few small studies in people (clinical trials) have led investigators to propose additional research on whether melatonin may help to improve mild cognitive impairment in patients with Alzheimer disease (AD) and prevent cell damage associated with amyotrophic lateral sclerosis (ALS, also known as "Lou Gehrig disease"). An analysis of the research suggested that adding sustained-release melatonin (but not fast-release melatonin) to high blood pressure management reduced elevated nighttime blood pressure.

What the Science Says about Safety and Side Effects of Melatonin

Melatonin appears to be safe when used short term, but the lack of long-term studies means that we do not know if it is safe for extended use.

- In one study, researchers noted that melatonin supplements may worsen mood in people with dementia.

- In 2011, the U.S. Food and Drug Administration (FDA) issued a warning to a company that makes and sells "relaxation brownies," stating that the melatonin in them has not been deemed a safe food additive.

- Side effects of melatonin are uncommon but can include drowsiness, headache, dizziness, or nausea. There have been no reports of significant side effects of melatonin in children.

More to Consider

- If you or a family member has trouble sleeping, see your healthcare provider.

- When you take a melatonin supplement is important because it may affect your biological clock.

- The FDA regulates dietary supplements, such as melatonin, but the regulations for dietary supplements are different and less strict than those for prescription or over-the-counter drugs.

- Some dietary supplements may interact with medications or pose risks if you have medical problems or are going to have surgery.

- Most dietary supplements have not been tested in pregnant women, nursing mothers, or children. If you are pregnant or nursing a child, it is especially important to see your healthcare provider before taking any medication or supplement, including melatonin.

- To use dietary supplements safely, read and follow the label instructions and recognize that "natural" does not always mean "safe."

- Tell all of your healthcare providers about any complementary or integrative health approaches you use. Give them a full picture of what you do to manage your health. This will help ensure safe and coordinated care.

Section 49.4

Valerian

This section includes text excerpted from "Valerian,"
National Center for Complementary and Integrative
Health (NCCIH), September 2016.

Valerian is a plant native to Europe and Asia; it also grows in North America. It has been used medicinally since the times of early Greece and Rome; Hippocrates wrote about its uses. Historically, valerian was used to treat nervousness, trembling, headaches, and heart palpitations.

Now, valerian is used as a dietary supplement for insomnia; anxiety; and other conditions, such as depression and menopause symptoms. The roots and rhizomes (underground stems) of valerian are used to make capsules, tablets, and liquid extracts, as well as teas.

What Is Known about Valerian?

Knowledge about valerian is limited because there have been only a small number of high-quality studies in people. The evidence on whether valerian is helpful for sleep problems is inconsistent. There is not enough evidence to allow any conclusions about whether valerian can relieve anxiety, depression, or menopausal symptoms.

What Is Known about Valerian Safety?

Studies suggest that valerian is generally safe for use by most healthy adults for short periods of time. No information is available about the long-term safety of valerian or its safety in children younger than the age of three, pregnant women, or nursing mothers.

Few side effects have been reported in studies of valerian. Those that have occurred include headache, dizziness, itching, and digestive disturbances. Because it is possible (though not proven) that valerian might have a sleep-inducing effect, it should not be taken along with alcohol or sedatives.

Keep in Mind

Tell all of your healthcare providers about any complementary or integrative health approaches you use. Give them a full picture of what you do to manage your health. This will help ensure coordinated and safe care.

Chapter 50

Continuous Positive Airway Pressure

Continuous positive airway pressure, also known as "CPAP," is a treatment that uses mild air pressure to keep your breathing airways open. It involves using a CPAP machine that includes a mask or other device that fits over your nose or your nose and mouth, straps to position the mask, a tube that connects the mask to the machine's motor, and a motor that blows air into the tube. CPAP is used to treat sleep-related breathing disorders, including sleep apnea. It also may be used to treat preterm infants who have underdeveloped lungs.

If your doctor prescribes CPAP over other treatment options for your sleep apnea, your insurance will work with a medical device company to provide you with a CPAP machine and the disposable mask and tube. Your doctor will set up your machine with certain pressure settings. After using your machine for a while, your doctor and possibly your insurance company will want to check the data card from your machine to confirm that you are using your CPAP device and to see if the machine and its pressure settings are working to reduce or eliminate apnea events while you sleep.

For the treatment to work, you should use your CPAP machine every time you sleep at home, while traveling, and during naps. Getting used to using your CPAP machine can take time and requires

This chapter includes text excerpted from "CPAP," National Heart, Lung, and Blood Institute (NHLBI), December 26, 2012. Reviewed May 2019.

patience. Your doctor may need to adjust your pressure settings for you. You may have to work with your sleep doctor to grow accustomed to your CPAP machine, such as finding the most comfortable mask that works best for you, trying the humidifier chamber in your machine, or using a different CPAP machine that allows multiple or auto-adjusting pressure settings.

Some patients notice immediate improvements after starting CPAP treatment, such as better sleep quality, reduction or elimination of snoring, and less daytime sleepiness. Equally important are the long-term benefits that you cannot notice, such as helping to prevent or control high blood pressure, lowering your risk for stroke, and improving memory and other cognitive function.

Side effects of CPAP treatment may include congestion, runny nose, dry mouth, or nosebleeds. If you experience stomach discomfort or bloating, you should stop using your CPAP machine and contact your doctor immediately. Some masks can cause irritation. Your doctor can help you find ways to relieve these symptoms and adjust to using your CPAP machine. It is important that you clean your mask and tube every day, and refill your medical device prescription at the right time to replace the mask and tube to ensure that the treatment continues to work.

Chapter 51

Treating Sleep Problems of People in Recovery from Substance-Use Disorders

Sleep problems are a common complaint among people with substance-use disorders (SUDs). They can occur during withdrawal, but they can also last months and years into recovery and can be associated with relapse to substance use. This chapter, in brief, alerts healthcare providers to the relationship between sleep disturbances and SUDs, and provides guidance on how to assess for and treat sleep problems in patients in recovery.

Sleep Disturbances and Substance Use

Many Americans suffer from unhealthy sleep-related behaviors. The prevalence of insomnia symptoms (difficulty initiating or maintaining sleep) in the general population is estimated at 33 percent, with an estimated 6 percent having a diagnosis of insomnia. According to a 12-state survey conducted by the Centers for Disease Control and Prevention (CDC):

- 35.3 percent of survey respondents obtain less than 7 hours of sleep on average during a 24-hour period.

This chapter includes text excerpted from "Treating Sleep Problems of People in Recovery from Substance Use Disorders," Substance Abuse and Mental Health Services Administration (SAMHSA), 2014. Reviewed May 2019.

- 48.0 percent snore.

- 37.9 percent unintentionally fall asleep during the day.

Substance use can exacerbate sleep difficulties, which in turn present a risk factor for substance use or relapse to use. The types of sleep problems vary by substance used and can include insomnia, sleep latency (the time it takes to fall asleep), disturbances in sleep cycles and sleep continuity, or hypersomnia (excessive daytime sleepiness). Specific findings on the relationship between sleep disturbances and substance use are presented below.

Alcohol Abuse

Insomnia and other sleep disturbances are common symptoms of alcohol dependence. Many people with alcohol use disorder (AUD) have insomnia before entering treatment. Reported rates of sleep problems among people with AUD in treatment range from 25 to 72 percent. Some people recovering from AUD may continue to have sleep problems, including insomnia or sleep-disordered breathing (such as sleep apnea), for weeks, months, or sometimes years after initiating abstinence.

Illicit-Drug Use

Sleep disturbances are common among people abstaining from chronic substance use. People stopping marijuana use can experience sleep problems in the first days of withdrawal, and these problems can last for weeks. People in detoxification from opioids often report symptoms of insomnia. A study that objectively measured sleep in people who chronically use cocaine found that sleep quality deteriorated during a period of abstinence, even though the subjects perceived their sleep to be improving. Another study of people in withdrawal from cocaine found that three-quarters of the studied population experienced poor sleep quality. In a study of college students, those who reported a history of nonmedical psychostimulant use or current use reported worse subjective and overall sleep quality and more sleep disturbance compared with those who had not used such substances.

The Effects of Sleep Loss during Recovery

Sleep loss can have significant negative effects on the physical, mental, and emotional well-being of people in recovery. It can also interfere with substance-abuse treatment. Persistent sleep complaints after withdrawal are associated with relapse to alcohol use. Poor sleep quality before a quit attempt from cannabis use is a risk factor for lapsing back into use within two days.

Assessing Sleep Disorders

If a patient initiating withdrawal from a substance or recovering from a SUD complains of a sleep disturbance, the healthcare provider should assess for causes by doing the following:

- Determine the duration of recovery and medications used for SUD treatment.

- Ask questions about difficulty falling asleep, waking during the night, amount of sleep per night, snoring, sleep apnea, excessive movements during sleep, uncontrollable movements that are relieved by getting up and walking, and excessive daytime sleepiness. If possible, ask significant others the same questions about the patient.

- Rule out other causes of the sleep problem, such as stress, a life crisis, or side effects of medications the patient is taking.

- Ask the patient to write in a sleep diary or log immediately on awakening. The patient should record total time in bed, time of sleep onset, number of times awakened, and total time spent awake.

- Determine the frequency and duration of symptoms of insomnia. If difficulties occur two or three nights per week and last for one month or more, the patient warrants a diagnosis of insomnia.

Note that some patients tend to overestimate the quality and duration of their sleep on self-report questionnaires and in sleep logs. If warranted, a referral for an objective sleep study in a sleep laboratory can be made.

Treatment for Sleep Disorders

The association between insomnia and relapse calls for treatment that addresses insomnia during recovery. The first step in treating insomnia should focus on the status of the patient's recovery. Patients should be receiving treatment from an appropriate substance-abuse treatment program. It is important to address other psychological, social, and medical problems that may contribute to insomnia, such as co-occurring mental and medical disorders, use of medications that disturb sleep, and nicotine use.

Nonpharmacological Treatments

Nonpharmacological treatments are preferred because many pharmacological treatments for insomnia have the potential for abuse and can interfere with SUD recovery. Research on cognitive-behavioral therapy (CBT) to treat insomnia has shown positive results, generally and also in patients who are alcohol dependent. Combining approaches may be more effective than using one approach.

Healthcare providers can educate patients about simple nonpharmacological techniques that can improve sleep. Sleep education includes teaching about sleep, the effects of recovery from substance use on sleep, and health practices and environmental factors that affect sleep. Sleep can be improved by limiting bedroom activities to sleeping (e.g., refraining from activities, such as reading the newspaper, paying bills, or working on electronic devices) and going to bed only when sleepy and at about the same time each day. These activities help reassociate the bed and bedroom with going to sleep. Establishing a relaxing pre-sleep routine, which can include progressive muscle relaxation, imagery, or a warm bath, also promotes sleep. Some patients may benefit from a referral to a sleep medicine specialist.

Pharmacological Treatments
Over-the-Counter Medications and Dietary Supplements

Some people who have trouble sleeping have tried over-the-counter (OTC) sleep medications or dietary supplements to help them sleep. Patients may ask about these, and care should be taken to explain their safety and efficacy. Many over-the-counter sleep medications contain antihistamines that cause sedation. They are not recommended as a long-term treatment for insomnia because they negatively affect the natural sleep cycle and have side effects, such as morning grogginess, daytime sleepiness, and impaired alertness and judgment. Furthermore, evidence supporting their long-term effectiveness is insufficient.

Popular dietary supplements taken with the intent to promote sleep include valerian and melatonin. Valerian, an herb, is thought to have sedative effects. However, studies of valerian offer mixed results, and evidence supporting the supplement's efficacy is insufficient to warrant its use. In addition, valerian could damage the liver. Melatonin is a brain hormone that helps regulate sleep patterns. Limited evidence shows that it can treat chronic insomnia in some people, and, to date, there is no evidence that it is harmful.

Prescription Medications without Known Abuse Potential

Medications without known abuse potential should be the first treatment option when pharmacotherapy is necessary to treat insomnia during recovery. Ramelteon and doxepin are the only unscheduled prescription medications approved by the U.S. Food and Drug Administration (FDA) for the treatment of insomnia. Ramelteon decreases the amount of time it takes to fall asleep. Doxepin, originally FDA-approved as an antidepressant, has been approved for treating insomnia typified by problems staying asleep. These medications may be suitable for treating insomnia in patients in recovery because they do not appear to have potential for abuse.

Off-Label Medications

Other medications are often prescribed off-label (for purposes other than the medication's FDA-approved use) to treat insomnia. According to a survey of addiction medicine physicians, the sedating antidepressant trazodone is the medication most often prescribed for the management of sleep disorders in patients in early recovery from AUD. One study found that its use among people in recovery from AUD improved sleep efficiency. Studies of its effects on abstinence and relapse in persons with AUD are conflicting. A 2008 study comparing trazodone with placebo for people after detoxification from alcohol showed that the trazodone group had improved sleep quality but had less improvement in the proportion of days abstinent while taking the medication. Furthermore, when the medication was discontinued, the trazodone group experienced less improvement in abstinence days and an increase in the number of drinks per drinking day. In contrast, a study published in 2011 of patients discharged from residential treatment did not find an association between trazodone use and relapse or a return to heavy drinking. A study of patients on methadone maintenance treatment found that trazodone use provided no improvement in sleep.

Other sedating antidepressants that have been used to treat insomnia include amitriptyline, mirtazapine, nefazodone, and nortriptyline. In a study of the use of mirtazapine on subjects with cocaine dependence and co-occurring depression, the medication decreased sleep latency; however, it had no measurable effect on treatment for cocaine dependence and depressive symptoms.

Gabapentin, an anticonvulsant with sedative properties, also has evidence of efficacy for treating insomnia. It has been found to be more effective in promoting sleep than lorazepam (an anxiolytic commonly prescribed to treat insomnia) among people withdrawing from alcohol. It has also been found to be more effective than trazodone in promoting sleep among those in early recovery. Acamprosate, a medication used to maintain alcohol abstinence, may also improve sleep during withdrawal from alcohol.

Prescription Medications with Known Abuse Potential

Sedative-hypnotic medications, such as benzodiazepines and non-benzodiazepines, are commonly prescribed to treat sleep problems. However, these medications should be avoided by people with histories of SUDs, as these individuals are at an increased risk for abusing them. Benzodiazepines, such as alprazolam, diazepam, and triazolam, are especially risky for use with people with SUDs because they are potentially addicting. They can also cause residual daytime sedation, cognitive impairment, motor incoordination, and rebound insomnia. Long-term treatment of insomnia with benzodiazepines may lead to withdrawal symptoms (e.g., anxiety, irritability, seizures) when patients stop taking the medications. A careful clinical evaluation is needed to ensure appropriate prescribing. Measures to prevent abuse include the following:

- Observe closely and perform ongoing evaluations.
- Prescribe a few tablets at a time.
- Schedule frequent office visits.
- Conduct occasional urine screenings.
- Use one source to dispense the medication.
- Occasionally taper the medication.
- Be attentive to risk factors, such as antisocial personality disorder and dependence on multiple substances.

Alternatives to benzodiazepines include sedative-hypnotic medications, such as zaleplon, eszopiclone, and zolpidem. These medications all have the same mechanism of action as benzodiazepines but lack some of the negative side effects. However, some research indicates that, at high doses, they may have the same side effects as benzodiazepines. The three medications are Schedule IV controlled substances, indicating abuse potential. For these reasons, these medications should be used only for short-term treatment of insomnia in people with a history of SUDs.

Part Six

A Special Look at Pediatric Sleep Issues

Chapter 52

Infants and
Sleep-Related Concerns

Chapter Contents

Section 52.1

Babies and Sleep-Related Deaths

This section includes text excerpted from "About 3,500 Babies in the US Are Lost to Sleep-Related Deaths Each Year," Centers for Disease Control and Prevention (CDC), January 9, 2018.

There are about 3,500 sleep-related deaths among U.S. babies each year, including sudden infant death syndrome (SIDS), accidental suffocation, and deaths from unknown causes.

In the 1990s, there were sharp declines in sleep-related deaths following the national "Back to Sleep" safe sleep campaign. However, the declines have slowed since the late 1990s, and data from a Vital Signs report from the Centers for Disease Control and Prevention (CDC) shows the risk for babies persists.

"Unfortunately, too many babies in this country are lost to sleep-related deaths that might be prevented," said the CDC's Director, Brenda Fitzgerald, M.D. "We must do more to ensure every family knows the American Academy of Pediatrics (AAP) recommendations—babies should sleep on their backs, without any toys or soft bedding, and in their own crib. Parents are encouraged to share a room with the baby but not the same bed. These strategies will help reduce the risk and protect our babies from harm."

Unsafe Sleep

For the Vital Signs report, the CDC analyzed Pregnancy Risk Assessment Monitoring System (PRAMS) data to describe sleep practices for babies. PRAMS, a state-based surveillance system, has monitored self-reported behaviors and experiences before, during, and after pregnancy among women with a recent U.S. live birth since the late 1980s.

The Centers for Disease Control and Prevention examined 2015 data reported by mothers about unsafe sleep positioning, any bed sharing, and the use of soft bedding from states with available data. Unsafe sleep positioning means placing the baby on her or his side or stomach to sleep. Soft bedding includes pillows, blankets, bumper pads, stuffed toys, and sleep positioners.

In 2015, within states included in the analysis:

- About 1 in 5 mothers (21.6%) reported placing their baby to sleep on their side or stomach, more than half of the mothers

(61.4%) reported any bed sharing with their baby, and 2 in 5 mothers (38.5%) reported using any soft bedding in the baby's sleep area

- The percentage of mothers who reported placing their baby on her or his side or stomach to sleep varied by state, ranging from 12.2 percent in Wisconsin to 33.8 percent in Louisiana.

- Placing babies on their side or stomach to sleep was more common among mothers who were non-Hispanic Black, younger than 25 years of age, or had 12 or fewer years of education.

Safe Sleep

Safe sleep practices recommended by the AAP include:

- Placing the baby on her or his back at all sleep times—including naps and at night

- Using a firm sleep surface, such as a safety-approved mattress and crib

- Keeping soft objects and loose bedding out of the baby's sleep area

- Sharing a room with baby but not the same bed

"This report shows that we need to do better at promoting and following safe sleep recommendations," said Jennifer Bombard, M.S.P.H., scientist in the CDC's Division of Reproductive Health (DRH) and lead author of the analysis. "This is particularly important for populations where data show infants may be at a higher risk of sleep-related deaths."

In recent years, state public-health agencies have worked with partners to promote safe sleep. These efforts include communication campaigns, messages shared during visits through Women, Infants, and Children (WIC) and through home-visiting programs; safe sleep policies; and quality-improvement initiatives in hospitals and child care centers.

Healthcare providers can increase the likelihood that parents follow AAP recommendations by giving them accurate advice about safe sleep for babies. A previous study shows that only 55 percent of mothers have reported receiving correct advice about safe sleep during pregnancy and baby care visits, while 20 percent say they get no advice and 25 percent report getting incorrect advice.

Section 52.2

Helping Babies Sleep Safely

This section includes text excerpted from "Helping
Babies Sleep Safely," Centers for Disease Control
and Prevention (CDC), October 9, 2018.

Expecting or caring for a baby? Take these steps to help the baby
sleep safely and reduce the risk of sleep-related infant deaths, including sudden infant death syndrome (SIDS).

There are about 3,500 sleep-related deaths among U.S. babies each
year. The Centers for Disease Control and Prevention (CDC) supports the 2016 recommendations issued by the American Academy of
Pediatrics (AAP) to reduce the risk of all sleep-related infant deaths,
including SIDS.

Parents and caregivers can help create a safe sleep area for babies
by taking the following steps:

- **Place your baby on her or his back for all sleep times—
  naps and at night.** Some parents may be concerned that a
  baby who sleeps on her or his back will choke if she or he spits
  up during sleep. However, babies' anatomy and gag reflex will
  prevent them from choking while sleeping on their backs. Babies
  who sleep on their backs are much less likely to die of SIDS than
  babies who sleep on their sides or stomachs.

- **Use a firm, flat sleep surface, such as a mattress in a
  safety-approved crib, covered only by a fitted sheet.** Some
  parents might feel that they should place their baby on a soft
  surface to help her or him to be more comfortable while sleeping.
  However, soft surfaces can increase the risk of sleep-related
  death. A firm sleep surface helps reduce the risk of SIDS and
  suffocation.

- **Keep your baby's sleep area (for example, a crib or
  bassinet) in the same room where you sleep until your
  baby is at least 6 months old, or ideally, until your baby
  is 1 year old.** Some parents may feel they should share their
  bed with their baby to help them feel more connected. However,
  accidental suffocation or strangulation can happen when a
  baby is sleeping in an adult bed or other unsafe sleep surfaces.
  Sharing a room with your baby is much safer than bed sharing
  and may decrease the risk of SIDS by as much as 50 percent.

Also, placing the crib close to your bed so that the baby is within view and reach can also help make it easier to feed, comfort, and monitor your baby.

- **Keep soft bedding, such as blankets, pillows, bumper pads, and soft toys, out of your baby's sleep area.** Additionally, do not cover your baby's head or allow your baby to get too hot. Some parents may feel they should add sheets or blankets to their baby's crib to help keep their baby warm and comfortable while sleeping. However, sheets, comforters, and blankets can increase the risk of suffocation or overheat your baby. If you are worried about your baby getting cold during sleep, you can dress her or him in sleep clothing, such as a wearable blanket.

Section 52.3

Sudden Infant Death Syndrome and Sleep

This section contains text excerpted from the following sources: Text in this section begins with excerpts from "Safe Sleep for Baby," *NIH News in Health*, National Institutes of Health (NIH), December 2018; Text under the heading "Myths and Facts about Sudden Infant Death Syndrome and Safe Infant Sleep" is excerpted from "Myths and Facts about Sudden Infant Death Syndrome and Safe Infant Sleep," *Eunice Kennedy Shriver* National Institute of Child Health and Human Development (NICHD), September 22, 2013. Reviewed May 2019.

Did you know that babies should sleep on their back rather than their belly? Research has revealed many risk factors for sudden infant death, and sleep position is the most important one. Each year in the United States, about 3,500 infants die suddenly and unexpectedly in their sleep. In about half of these deaths, doctors cannot find a medical reason to explain why, even after a complete review. When the doctor does not have answers, the death is called "sudden infant death syndrome" (SIDS).

"All babies are at risk, especially those under one year of age," explains Dr. Marion W. Koso-Thomas, a child health expert at the

National Institutes of Health (NIH). Babies are most vulnerable to SIDS up to four months of age. "One of the critical pieces to SIDS risk reduction is how the baby sleeps," she says. "Babies who are sleeping should be on their back."

Limit a baby's belly time to when they are awake. A baby should not sleep on their belly or side. Why does sleep position matter? Sleeping on the belly lowers an infant's blood pressure and reduces their ability to get oxygen to the brain. Between two and four months of age, especially, the reflex to breathe to get more oxygen is repressed when an infant sleeps on their belly.

Researchers also suspect that a brain condition may be a cause of SIDS. They have been studying the part of the brain that controls breathing and heart rate during sleep. They think that these babies may not have the reflex to awaken when breathing becomes impaired. "More research needs to be done to understand what is going on in those babies and hopefully identify a screening tool to help save their life," Koso-Thomas says.

What causes sudden infant death syndrome may not be known, but several things raise the risk. In addition to sleep position, research shows that soft bedding above or below your infant is a danger. "There is no need to have a blanket," Koso-Thomas says. Instead, dress your baby in sleep clothing, such as a onesie, that is designed to keep them warm. This keeps them safer. Make sure they are dressed appropriately for the environment. But do not overbundle. Check for signs that they are too hot, such as sweating or if their chest is hot to the touch.

It is important to prevent your baby's nose and mouth from becoming covered. "The area around them should not have any clutter—no toys, no bumpers," Koso-Thomas emphasizes. Experts also advise that you keep your baby in the same room, but not in your bed with you. When you are done feeding, place your baby in their safe area, such as a cradle next to your bed. "The safe sleep environment is the biggest factor that is going to reduce or eliminate the SIDS risk for a baby that is less than a year old," Koso-Thomas says.

Myths and Facts about Sudden Infant Death Syndrome and Safe Infant Sleep

Myth: Babies can "catch" SIDS.

Fact: A baby cannot catch SIDS. SIDS is not caused by an infection, so it cannot be caught or spread.

Myth: Cribs cause "crib death" or SIDS.

Fact: Cribs themselves do not cause SIDS. But features of the sleep environment—such as a soft sleep surface—can increase the risk of SIDS and other sleep-related causes of infant death. Find out more about what is a safe sleep environment for your baby.

Myth: Babies who sleep on their backs will choke if they spit up or vomit during sleep.

Fact: Babies automatically cough up or swallow fluid that they spit up or vomit—it is a reflex to keep the airway clear. Studies show no increase in the number of deaths from choking among babies who sleep on their backs. In fact, babies who sleep on their backs might clear these fluids better because of the way the body is built.

Myth: SIDS can be prevented.

Fact: There is no known way to prevent SIDS, but there are effective ways to reduce the risk of SIDS.

Myth: Shots, vaccines, immunizations, and medicines cause SIDS.

Fact: Recent evidence suggests that shots for vaccines may have a protective effect against SIDS. All babies should see their healthcare providers regularly for well-baby checkups and should get their shots on time as recommended by their healthcare provider.

Myth: SIDS can occur in babies at any age.

Fact: Babies are at risk of SIDS only until they are 1 year old. Most SIDS deaths occur when babies are between 1 month and 4 months of age. SIDS is not a health concern for babies older than 1 year of age.

Myth: If parents sleep with their babies in the same bed, they will hear any problems and be able to prevent them from happening.

Fact: Because SIDS occurs with no warning or symptoms, it is unlikely that any adult will hear a problem and prevent SIDS from occurring. Sleeping with a baby in an adult bed increases the risk of suffocation and other sleep-related causes of infant death.

Sleeping with a baby in an adult bed is even more dangerous when:

- The adult smokes cigarettes or has consumed alcohol or medication that causes drowsiness.

- The baby shares a bed with other children.

- The sleep surface is a couch, sofa, waterbed, or armchair.

- There are pillows or blankets in the bed

- The baby is younger than 11 weeks to 14 weeks of age.

- The baby shares a bed with more than one person, especially if sleeping between two adults.

Instead of bed sharing, healthcare providers recommend room sharing—keeping baby's sleep area separate from your sleep area in the same room where you sleep. Room sharing is known to reduce the risk of SIDS and other sleep-related causes of infant death.

Section 52.4

Infant Sleep Positioners and the Risk of Suffocation

This section includes text excerpted from "Do Not Use Infant Sleep Positioners due to the Risk of Suffocation," U.S. Food and Drug Administration (FDA), April 18, 2019.

The U.S. Food and Drug Administration (FDA) is reminding parents and caregivers not to put babies in sleep positioners. These products—sometimes also called "nests" or "antiroll" products—can cause suffocation (a struggle to breathe) that can lead to death.

The FDA regulates baby products as medical devices if, among other things, the manufacturer claims that the product is intended to cure, mitigate, treat, or prevent, or reduce a disease or condition in its labeling, packaging, or advertising. A number of sleep positioners are considered medical devices because of their intended use. (This intended use can be outlined by statements made on the labels, labeling, instructions for use, or promotional materials for the products.)

Sleep positioners that do not meet the definition of a medical device may be regulated by the U.S. Consumer Product Safety Commission (CPSC).

Some types of sleep positioners can feature raised supports or pillows (called "bolsters") that are attached to each side of a mat or a wedge to raise a baby's head. Products called "nests" can feature soft, wall-like structures that surround the base. The positioners claim to keep a baby in a specific position while sleeping and are often used for babies under six months of age.

To reduce the risk of sleep-related infant deaths, including accidental suffocation and sudden infant death syndrome (SIDS), the American Academy of Pediatrics (AAP) recommends that infants sleep on their backs, positioned on a firm, empty surface. This surface should not contain soft objects, toys, pillows, or loose bedding.

About Infant Suffocation and Other Dangers

Each year, about 4,000 infants die unexpectedly during sleep time from accidental suffocation, SIDS, or unknown causes, according to the *Eunice Kennedy Shriver* National Institute of Child Health and Human Development (NICHD).

The federal government has received reports about babies who have died from suffocation associated with their sleep positioners. In most of these cases, the babies suffocated after rolling from their sides to their stomachs.

In addition to reports about deaths, the federal government also has received reports about babies who were placed on their backs or sides in positioners but were later found in other, dangerous positions within or next to these products.

To avoid these dangers, remember:

- The safest crib is a bare crib.

- Always put babies on their backs to sleep.

Safety Advice

The following advice is for putting babies to sleep safely:

- **Never use infant sleep positioners.** Using this type of product to hold an infant on her or his side or back is dangerous.

- **Never put pillows, blankets, loose sheets, comforters, or quilts under a baby or in a crib.** These products also can be dangerous. Babies do not need pillows and adequate clothing—instead of blankets—can keep them warm.

- **Always keep cribs and sleeping areas bare.** That means you should also never put soft objects or toys in sleeping areas.

- **Always place a baby on her or his back at night and during nap time.** An easy way to remember this is to follow the ABCs of safe sleep: "Alone on the Back in a bare Crib."

Beware of Medical Claims about Sleep Positioners

Some manufacturers have advertised that their sleep positioners prevent SIDS; gastroesophageal reflux disease (GERD), in which stomach acids back up into the esophagus; or flat head syndrome (plagiocephaly), a deformation caused by pressure on one part of the skull.
Here are the facts:

- The FDA has never cleared an infant sleep positioner that claims to prevent or reduce the risk of SIDS.

- The FDA had previously cleared some infant positioners for GERD or flat head syndrome.

- In 2010, the FDA became aware of infant positioners being marketed with SIDS claims and notified manufacturers to stop marketing these devices and submit information to support FDA clearance.

The U.S. Food and Drug Administration intends to take action against device manufacturers who make unproven medical claims about their products. You can do your part to keep your baby safe by not using sleep positioners.

You can report an incident or injury from an infant sleep positioner to the FDA's MedWatch program. Finally, if you have questions about how to safely put a baby to sleep or how to avoid or treat certain health issues, talk to your healthcare provider.

Chapter 53

Ways to Reduce the Risk of Sudden Infant Death Syndrome

What Is Sudden Infant Death Syndrome?

Sudden infant death syndrome (SIDS) is the sudden, unexplained death of a baby younger than one year of age that does not have a known cause even after a complete investigation. This investigation includes performing a complete autopsy, examining the death scene, and reviewing the clinical history. When a baby dies, healthcare providers, law enforcement personnel, and communities try to find out why. They ask questions, examine the baby, gather information, and run tests. If they cannot find a cause for the death, and if the baby

This chapter contains text excerpted from the following sources: Text under the heading "What Is Sudden Infant Death Syndrome" is excerpted from "What Is SIDS?" *Eunice Kennedy Shriver* National Institute of Child Health and Human Development (NICHD), September 22, 2013. Reviewed May 2019; Text under the heading "Reducing the Risk of Sudden Infant Death Syndrome: Recommendations" is excerpted from "Ways to Reduce the Risk of SIDS and Other Sleep-Related Causes of Infant Death," *Eunice Kennedy Shriver* National Institute of Child Health and Human Development (NICHD), February 10, 2016.

was younger than one year old, the medical examiner or coroner will call the death "SIDS."

Reducing the Risk of Sudden Infant Death Syndrome: Recommendations

Research shows that there are several ways to reduce the risk of sudden infant death syndrome (SIDS) and other sleep-related causes of infant death. The actions listed here in this chapter are based on recommendations from the American Academy of Pediatrics (AAP) Task Force on SIDS.

Always Place Babies on Their Back to Sleep

The back-sleep position is the safest position for all babies, until they are one year old. Babies who are used to sleeping on their backs but who are then placed to sleep on their stomachs, such as for a nap, are at a very high risk for SIDS.

If a baby rolls over on her or his own from back to stomach or stomach to back, there is no need to reposition the baby. Starting sleep on the back is most important for reducing SIDS risk. Preemies (infants born preterm) should be placed on their backs to sleep as soon as possible after birth.

Can My Baby Choke If Placed on the Back to Sleep?

The short answer is no—babies are not more likely to choke when sleeping on their backs.

Use a Firm and Flat Sleep Surface

Never place baby to sleep on soft surfaces, such as on a couch, sofa, waterbed, pillow, quilt, sheepskin, or blanket. These surfaces can be very dangerous for babies. Do not use a car seat, stroller, swing, infant carrier, infant sling, or similar products as a baby's regular sleep area. Following these recommendations reduces the risk of SIDS and death or injury from suffocation, entrapment, and strangulation.

A crib, bassinet, portable crib, or play yard that follows the safety standards of the Consumer Product Safety Commission (CPSC) is recommended.

Why Should I Not Use Crib Bumpers in My Baby's Sleep Area?

Evidence does not support using crib bumpers to prevent injury. In fact, crib bumpers can cause serious injuries and even death.

Breastfeed Your Baby

Breastfeeding has many health benefits for the mother and her baby. Babies who breastfeed, or are fed breast milk, are at a lower risk for SIDS than are babies who were never fed breast milk. Longer duration of exclusive breastfeeding leads to a lower risk.

If you bring your baby into your bed for feeding, put her or him back in a separate sleep area when finished. This sleep area should be made for infants, such as a crib or bassinet, and close to your bed. If you fall asleep while feeding or while comforting your baby in an adult bed, place her or him back in a separate sleep area as soon as you wake up. Evidence shows that the longer a parent and an infant share a bed, the higher the risk for sleep-related causes of infant death, such as suffocation.

What If I Fall Asleep While Feeding My Baby?

It is less dangerous to fall asleep with an infant in an adult bed than on a sofa or armchair.

Share Your Room with Your Baby

Room sharing reduces the risk of SIDS. Babies should not sleep in an adult bed, on a couch, or on a chair alone, with you, or with anyone else, including siblings or pets. Having a separate safe sleep surface for the baby reduces the risk of SIDS and the chance of suffocation, strangulation, and entrapment.

If you bring your baby into your bed for feeding or comforting, remove all soft items and bedding from the area. When finished, put your baby back in a separate sleep area made for infants, such as a crib or bassinet, and close to your bed.

Couches and armchairs can also be very dangerous for babies if adults fall asleep as they feed, comfort, or bond with the baby while on these surfaces. Parents and other caregivers should be mindful of how tired they are during these times.

There is no evidence for or against devices or products that claim to make bed sharing "safer."

Can I Practice Skin-to-Skin Care as Soon as My Baby Is Born?

Yes, when the mother is stable, awake, and able to respond to her baby.

Baby's Sleep Area Should Be Free of Excess Items

Keeping these items out of baby's sleep area reduces the risk of SIDS and suffocation, entrapment, and strangulation. Because evidence does not support using them to prevent injury, crib bumpers are not recommended. Crib bumpers are linked to serious injuries and deaths from suffocation, entrapment, and strangulation. Keeping these and other soft objects out of the baby's sleep area is the best way to avoid these dangers.

Clothing for Baby

Dress your baby in sleep clothing, such as a wearable blanket designed to keep her or him warm without the need for loose blankets in the sleep area.

Dress your baby appropriately for the environment, and do not over-bundle. Parents and caregivers should watch for signs of overheating, such as sweating or the baby's chest feeling hot to the touch.

Keep the baby's face and head uncovered during sleep.

Can I Swaddle My Baby to Reduce the Risk of Sudden Infant Death Syndrome?

There is no evidence that swaddling reduces SIDS risk. In fact, swaddling can increase the risk of SIDS and other sleep-related causes of infant death if babies are placed on their stomachs for sleep or roll onto their stomachs during sleep.

If you decide to swaddle your baby, always place the baby fully on her or his back to sleep. Stop swaddling the baby once she or he starts trying to roll over.

Give Your Baby Plenty of Tummy Time

Supervised tummy time helps strengthen your baby's neck, shoulders, and arm muscles. It also helps to prevent flat spots on the back of your baby's head.

Limiting the time spent in car seats, once the baby is out of the car, and changing the direction the infant lays in the sleep area from week to week also can help to prevent these flat spots.

Chapter 54

Tonsil Surgery Improves Some Behaviors in Children with Sleep Apnea Syndrome

Children with sleep apnea syndrome who have their tonsils and adenoids removed sleep better, are less restless and impulsive, and report a generally better quality of life (QOL), finds a study funded by the National Institutes of Health (NIH). However, the study found that cognitive abilities did not improve when compared with children who did not have surgery, and researchers say that the findings do not mean surgery is an automatic first choice.

"This is the first rigorous, controlled evaluation of a commonly performed treatment for childhood sleep apnea, in terms of looking at functional outcomes," said Susan Shurin, M.D., a pediatrician and deputy director of the NIH's National Heart, Lung, and Blood Institute (NHLBI). "This study provides additional data that can help parents and providers make more informed decisions about treating children with this disorder, and it identifies additional areas of research."

Obstructive sleep apnea (OSA) syndrome is a common disorder in which the airway becomes blocked during sleep, causing shallow

This chapter includes text excerpted from "Tonsil Surgery Improves Some Behaviors in Children with Sleep Apnea Syndrome," National Heart, Lung, and Blood Institute (NHLBI), May 21, 2013. Reviewed May 2019.

breathing or breathing pauses. The sleep disturbances that result can lead to many issues in children, including learning difficulties and behavioral problems.

Enlarged or swollen tonsils are a major risk factor for pediatric sleep apnea syndrome, and surgery to remove them and the nearby adenoid can help open up blocked airways. Over 500,000 adenotonsillectomies are performed annually on children, primarily for sleep apnea. However, the extent that surgery can improve cognition and behavior previously had not been rigorously studied.

The Childhood Adenotonsillectomy Trial (CHAT) enrolled 464 children between the ages of 5 and 9 with OSA syndrome from 7 sleep centers across the United States and randomly assigned them into 2 groups. One received adenoid and tonsil surgery within a month after enrolment, while the other received supportive medical care and careful monitoring, or watchful waiting. At enrolment, both groups of children were evaluated by psychometricians—people trained to administer and interpret psychological tests—on their cognition (primarily attention and organizational skills); they were also evaluated by caregivers and teachers on their behavior and QOL, and they had sleep studies to assess their breathing and sleep parameters. After 7 months, the children were reevaluated.

The researchers found no differences in cognitive skills between the two groups, but the children who underwent surgery showed improved sleep quality; behavioral regulation; and QOL measures, such as being more active and experiencing less daytime sleepiness. Beneficial effects were observed even among overweight children, in whom there has been particular uncertainty about the role of surgery for sleep apnea treatment.

Overall, 79 percent of children in the surgery group had resolution of their sleep apnea after 7 months, compared to 46 percent in the watchful waiting group.

"While more of the children who underwent early surgery had improvements in their sleep apnea measures, nearly half of the children without surgery also had improvements during the seven months of observation," said senior author Susan Redline, M.D., M.P.H., of Brigham and Women's Hospital and Beth Israel Deaconess Medical Center, both in Boston. "This and the lack of significant cognitive decline in the watchful waiting group suggest that reassessing a child after a period of observation may be a valid therapeutic option for some children, especially those with mild symptoms."

Redline added that these results should not be applied to children with the most severe sleep apnea syndrome or very young children, who were not included in this study.

The study was funded by NIH grants.

Chapter 55

Bed-Wetting

Children may have a bladder control problem—also called "urinary incontinence" (UI)—if they leak urine by accident and are past the age of toilet training. A child may not stay dry during the day (called "daytime wetting") or through the night (called "bed-wetting.")

Children normally gain control over their bladders somewhere between the ages of two and four—each in their own time. Occasional wetting is common even in children between the ages of four and six. By four years of age, when most children stay dry during the day, daytime wetting can be very upsetting and embarrassing. By five or six years of age, children might have a bed-wetting problem if the bed is wet once or twice a week over a few months.

Most bladder control problems disappear naturally as children grow older. When needed, a healthcare professional can check for conditions that may lead to wetting.

Loss of urine is almost never due to laziness, a strong will, emotional problems, or poor toilet training. Parents and caregivers should always approach this problem with understanding and patience.

Children usually have one of two main bladder control problems:

This chapter contains text excerpted from the following sources: Text in this chapter begins with excerpts from "Definition and Facts for Bladder Control Problems and Bedwetting in Children," National Institute of Diabetes and Digestive and Kidney Diseases (NIDDK), September 2017; Text beginning with the heading "How Common Is Urinary Incontinence in Children?" is excerpted from "Urinary Incontinence in Children," National Institute of Diabetes and Digestive and Kidney Diseases (NIDDK), June 2012. Reviewed May 2019.

- Daytime wetting, also called "diurnal enuresis"
- Bed-wetting, also called "nocturnal enuresis"

Some children may have trouble controlling their bladders both day and night.

Children and Bed-Wetting

Children who wet the bed falls into two groups: those who have never been dry at night and those who started wetting the bed again after staying dry for six months. Bed-wetting that is never treated during childhood can last into the teen years and adulthood, causing emotional distress.

How Common Is Urinary Incontinence in Children?

By 5 years of age, more than 90 percent of children can control urination during the day. Nighttime wetting is more common than daytime wetting in children, affecting 30 percent of 4-year-olds. The condition resolves itself in about 15 percent of children each year; about 10 percent of 7-year-olds, 3 percent of 12-year-olds, and 1 percent of 18-year-olds continue to experience nighttime wetting.

What Causes Nighttime Urinary Incontinence

The exact cause of most cases of nighttime urinary incontinence is not known. Though a few cases are caused by structural problems in the urinary tract, most cases probably result from a mix of factors including slower physical development, an overproduction of urine at night, and the inability to recognize bladder filling when asleep. Nighttime UI has also been associated with attention deficit hyperactivity disorder (ADHD), obstructive sleep apnea (OSA), and anxiety. Children also may inherit genes from one or both parents that make them more likely to have nighttime urinary incontinence.

Slower Physical Development

Between the ages of 5 and 10, bed-wetting may be the result of a small bladder capacity, long sleeping periods, and an underdevelopment of the body's alarms that signal a full or emptying bladder. This form of UI fades away as the bladder grows, and the natural alarms become operational.

Overproduction of Urine at Night

The body produces antidiuretic hormone (ADH), a natural chemical that slows down the production of urine. More ADH is produced at night, so the need to urinate lessens. If the body does not produce enough ADH at night, the production of urine may not slow down, leading to bladder overfilling. If a child does not sense the bladder filling and awaken to urinate, wetting will occur.

Structural Problems

A small number of UI cases are caused by physical problems in the urinary tract. Rarely, a blocked bladder or urethra may cause the bladder to overfill and leak. Nerve damage associated with the birth defect spina bifida can cause UI. In these cases, UI can appear as a constant dribbling of urine.

Attention Deficit Hyperactivity Disorder

Children with attention deficit hyperactivity disorder are three times more likely to have nighttime UI than children without ADHD. The connection between ADHD and bed-wetting has not been explained, but some experts theorize that both conditions are related to delays in central nervous system (CNS) development.

Obstructive Sleep Apnea

Nighttime urinary incontinence may be one sign of OSA. Other symptoms of OSA include snoring, mouth breathing, frequent ear and sinus infections, sore throat, choking, and daytime drowsiness. Experts believe that when the airway in people with OSA closes, a chemical may be released in the body that increases water production and inhibits the systems that regulate fluid volume. Successful treatment of OSA often resolves the associated nighttime UI.

Anxiety

Anxiety-causing events that occur between two and four years of age—before total bladder control is achieved—might lead to primary enuresis. Anxiety experienced after the age of four might lead to secondary enuresis in children who have been dry for at least six months. Events that cause anxiety in children include physical or sexual abuse; unfamiliar social situations, such as moving or starting at a new school; and major family events, such as the birth of a sibling, a death, or divorce. UI itself is an anxiety-causing event. Strong bladder contractions resulting in daytime leakage can cause embarrassment and anxiety that lead to nighttime wetting.

Genetics

Certain genes have been found to contribute to UI. Children have a 30 percent chance of having nighttime UI if one parent was affected as a child. If both parents were affected, there is a 70 percent chance of bed-wetting.

How Is Bed-Wetting Cured?

Most urinary incontinence fades away naturally as a child grows and develops and does not require treatment. When treatment is needed, options include bladder training and related strategies, moisture alarms, and medications.

As children mature:

- Bladder capacity increases.

- Natural body alarms become activated.

- An overactive bladder settles down.

- Production of ADH becomes normal.

- Response to the body's signal that it is time to void improves.

Bladder Training and Related Strategies

Bladder training consists of exercises to strengthen the bladder muscles to better control urination. Gradually lengthening the time between trips to the bathroom can also help by stretching the bladder so it can hold more urine. Additional techniques that may help control daytime UI include:

- Urinating on a schedule—timed voiding—such as every two hours

- Avoiding food or drinks with caffeine

- Following suggestions for healthy urination, such as relaxing muscles and taking enough time to allow the bladder to empty completely

Waking children up to urinate can help decrease nighttime UI. Ensuring children drink enough fluids throughout the day so they do not drink a lot of fluids close to bedtime may also help. A healthcare provider can give guidance about how much a child needs to drink each day, as the amount depends on a child's age, physical activity, and other factors.

Moisture Alarms

At night, moisture alarms can wake children when they begin to urinate. These devices use a water-sensitive pad connected to an alarm that sounds when moisture is first detected. A small pad can clip to the pajamas, or a larger pad can be placed on the bed. For the alarm to be effective, children must awaken as soon as the alarm goes off, stop the urine stream, and go to the bathroom. Children using moisture alarms may need to have someone sleep in the same room to help wake them up.

Medications

Nighttime UI may be treated by increasing ADH levels. The hormone can be boosted by a synthetic version known as "desmopressin" (DDAVP), which is available in pill form, nasal spray, and nose drops. DDAVP is approved for use in children. Another medication, called "imipramine" (Tofranil), is also used to treat nighttime UI, though the way this medication prevents bed-wetting is not known. Although both of these medications may help children achieve short-term success, relapse is common once the medication is withdrawn. UI resulting from an overactive bladder may be treated with oxybutynin (Ditropan), a medication that helps calm the bladder muscle and control muscle spasms.

Chapter 56

Bruxism and Sleep

Bruxism is a type of movement disorder characterized by the grinding, gnashing, and clenching of the teeth. Many people may unconsciously grind or clench their teeth, but whether or not it qualifies as a case of bruxism depends largely on such factors as frequency, physical damage, and discomfort. The marked absence of clinical symptoms makes it difficult to estimate the prevalence of bruxism. Most cases go unreported, since the majority of "bruxers" remain unaware of their problem until a diagnosis can be made on the basis of visible signs of teeth wear. Bruxism is thought to affect an estimated 30 to 40 million people in the United States and tends to occur episodically during certain periods of a person's life. Bruxism can be either diurnal (daytime) or nocturnal (night). When people unconsciously clench their jaws during the day, it is called "awake bruxism," and when they grind or clench their teeth while they are asleep, it is called "sleep bruxism" (SB).

Prevalence of Sleep Bruxism

Since sleep bruxism is a type of parasomnia disorder that takes place during the night, it is consequently harder to control. While many people who grind their teeth during the night are not even aware of it, severe cases of sleep bruxism can have serious health consequences. According to reports, SB is more common in children than in adults. In most cases, the onset of SB is around one year of age, soon after the

"Bruxism and Sleep," © 2016 Omnigraphics. Reviewed May 2019.

appearance of the primary incisors. The prevalence among adults is nearly 12 percent, dropping to 3 percent in older individuals. Although, awake bruxism is more common among females, there does not appear to be any gender difference in SB prevalence.

Risk Factors for Sleep Bruxism

Sleep bruxism has been shown to have a wide range of causes. But, long-term studies linking bruxism to its causal factors are still ongoing. Among the peripheral factors studied, the most important one is dental occlusion, which refers to the misalignment of the teeth in the upper and lower jaws. Certain pathophysiological factors have also been linked to SB, the most significant one being sleep arousal disorder. This condition is characterized by a sudden shift in the brain wave pattern during the transition from rapid eye movement (REM) sleep to non-REM sleep, or wakefulness, and is accompanied by an increase in respiratory rate and muscle activity. Bruxism has been shown to be a part of this arousal response.

Among all the factors that may contribute to sleep bruxism, the ones most extensively studied have been the psychosocial factors, which include stress and anxiety. Bruxing in children may often be traced to their emotional and psychological state. For instance, anxiety in children stemming from such causes as school exams, bullying, scolding from parents, or moving to a new neighborhood, may be a significant risk factor for SB. Some small children may grind their teeth as part of the teething process or due to frequent earaches. Among children, SB may disappear on its own at puberty.

For adults, common sources of stress include workplace tensions, family problems, relationship issues, or anxiety about health conditions. Certain personality types tend to be more vulnerable to stress-related bruxism, including those who are highly aggressive, competitive, or hyperactive. The risk of developing bruxism can be increased by certain lifestyle factors, such as smoking, alcohol consumption, and drug use. Bruxism may also develop as a side effect of certain medications or as a symptom of neurological disorders, such as Huntington disease (HD) and Parkinson disease (PD). Studies have also shown that bruxism is often related to other sleep disorders, such as excessive snoring, pauses in breathing, or obstructive sleep apnea.

Symptoms and Diagnosis of Sleep Bruxism

The most common symptom of SB is rhythmic masticatory muscle activity (RMMA), or repetitive jaw muscle contractions. While mild to moderate muscle activity in bruxers may not cause any issues, severe cases could lead to dental problems, such as premature wearing of the teeth and dental implants, as well as temporomandibular dysfunction, which is pain and atrophy of the muscles and joints associated with chewing.

Bruxism is usually diagnosed through a visit to a dentist. During a regular checkup, the dentist will look for and inquire about the following symptoms:

- Damaged teeth

- Unusual teeth sensitivity

- Swelling and pain in the jaw or facial muscles around the mouth

- Tongue indentations

- Headaches or earaches

- Frequent awakening or poor quality of sleep

Treatment of Sleep Bruxism

Treatments for bruxism should be selected to best fit the individual patient and the underlying cause of the disorder. When a dental problem is determined to be the cause of bruxism, a dental appliance, such as a splint or mouth guard, might alleviate the condition. These devices help prevent the teeth from grinding together and also protect the tooth enamel from further damage. Various dental procedures can also be performed to correct misalignment of the teeth and jaw, or address damage to the teeth from clenching and grinding. Cognitive behavioral therapy (CBT) can also help patients deal with improper mouth and jaw alignment. Correcting the position and placement of the tongue, teeth, and lips can bring about a significant improvement in the condition. Biofeedback is another treatment method used to assess and alter the movement of the muscles around the mouth and jaw. The doctor may use monitoring equipment to help guide the patient toward overcoming the habit of clenching the jaw or grinding the teeth.

If the primary cause of bruxism is determined to be psychological in nature, a number of behavioral and related therapies may help alleviate the condition. Stress management is the foremost issue to be addressed in people with bruxism. Counseling sessions with experts can help patients develop coping strategies. Other common means of reducing stress include meditation, relaxation, exercise, and music. Hypnosis has also proven to be an effective treatment for people who grind their teeth at night. Most patients with bruxism tend to respond well with proper treatment prescribed by the appropriate professional.

References

1. "Causes of Bruxism," The Bruxism Association, n.d.

2. "Bruxism," The Nemours Foundation/KidsHealth®, n.d.

3. Shilpa Shetty et al. "Bruxism: A Literature Review," *The Journal of Indian Prosthodontic Society* Volume 10 (3): 141–148, National Center for Biotechnology (NCBI).

Chapter 57

Pediatric Movement Disorders in Sleep

Babies between the ages of six and nine months sometimes begin to exhibit repetitive, rhythmic movements as part of the process of going to sleep. Some of the most common movements include body rocking, head rolling, and headbanging. Children who exhibit these behaviors may roll their heads forcefully from side to side; rise up on their hands and knees, and rock back and forth vigorously; or bang their heads repeatedly on a mattress, pillow, headboard, or side rail.

Although these violent movements can be alarming for parents and caregivers to witness, they are quite common, usually harmless, and tend to disappear gradually by the age of two or three. Parents often express concerns that headbanging or body rocking will result in injury or brain damage, but this is rarely the case. In addition, many parents worry that these repetitive behaviors may indicate a developmental disability, yet they occur frequently among normal children. Parents should consult a pediatrician if the behaviors persist for more than a few months or if the child nods or shakes their head frequently at other times, does not interact with other people, or shows evidence of developmental delays.

Researchers are not certain why children engage in body rocking, head rolling, and headbanging. They have determined that the

"Pediatric Movement Disorders in Sleep," © 2016 Omnigraphics. Reviewed May 2019.

behaviors occur three times more often in boys than in girls, and most children outgrow the habit before they reach three years of age. Some experts believe that rocking offers babies comfort or pleasure because it simulates being carried in the womb or in a parent's arms. Others theorize that the behaviors are part of the natural process of mastering movement and gaining control of the body. Some claim that rhythmic motion helps babies to release stress, tension, or unspent energy and relax before going to sleep. For other children, headbanging may provide a distraction from teething pain or an outlet for frustration or anger.

Coping with Repetitive Movements

Body rocking, headbanging, and head rolling can be distressing for parents and caregivers. In addition to feeling concern for the child's well-being, they may also feel frustrated or irritated by the noise or damage to furniture or walls. It is important to remember that babies who rock or bang their heads will usually fall asleep within a short time. Since most children simply outgrow the behavior over time, the easiest approach may be to do nothing and wait for it to go away. Reacting to the repetitive movements—even in a negative way—sometimes tends to reinforce the behavior. Other tips for dealing with body rocking, head rolling, and headbanging at bedtime include the following:

- Engage in a relaxing bedtime routine that includes quiet time, cuddling, songs, nursery rhymes, or a story.

- Place a mobile above the bed or an activity center on the side of the crib to provide interest and distraction.

- Play soft, soothing music or white noise in the bedroom to promote relaxation.

- Ensure that the child does not spend too much time in bed before it is time to sleep.

- Check to make sure the child is not experiencing pain from teething, an ear infection, allergies, or other sources.

- Use a padded bumper on crib rails or headboards.

- Pull the bed away from the wall, and put a thick carpet or rubber pad under the legs—or put the mattress on the floor—to reduce movement and noise.

- Try changing the bedroom in which the child sleeps.

References

1. "Body-Rocking, Head-Rolling, and Head-Banging," Raising Children Network, August 25, 2014.

2. "Body-Rocking, Head-Rolling, and Head-Banging in Babies," World of Moms, October 10, 2014.

3. "Guide to Your Child's Symptoms: Rocking/Head Banging," American Academy of Pediatrics (AAP), 2001.

Chapter 58

Sleepwalking in Children

Sleepwalking, also known as "somnambulism," is a behavior disorder that involves getting up and walking around while sleeping. It originates during deep sleep. Sleepwalking is more common in children between the ages of four and eight, and it is usually outgrown by the teen years. Typically, sleepwalking incidents do not require any treatment; however, recurrent sleepwalking may be a sign of an underlying sleep disorder.

Causes of Sleepwalking

The most common causes of sleepwalking are as follows:

- Heredity
- Lack of sleep
- Irregular sleep schedule
- Stress

An underlying medical condition may also be the cause of sleepwalking, such as:

- Fever
- Heart rhythm problems
- Nighttime seizures

- Nighttime asthma
- Obstructive sleep apnea (OSA)
- Restless legs syndrome (RLS)
- Psychiatric disorders
- Use of drugs or medications

Symptoms of Sleepwalking

Sleepwalking occurs one or two hours after falling asleep, during the nonrapid eye movement (non-REM) sleep or deep sleep. The most obvious symptom of sleepwalking is getting out of bed and walking around. The sleepwalker may be partially aroused during the episode. Sleepwalking can last up to several minutes, but it may last longer. During sleepwalking, the person may:

- Be difficult to wake up
- Not respond or communicate
- Be confused for a short time after awakening
- Not remember the sleepwalking episode

Other events that may occur while sleepwalking are as follows:
- Talking while asleep
- A glassy-eyed expression
- Leaving the house
- Driving a car
- Engaging in unusual behavior
- Injuring oneself

Complications of Sleepwalking

Sleepwalking may co-occur with night terrors. The complications of sleepwalking are:

- **Injury.** The sleepwalking person may hurt themselves or others during the episode.
- **Embarrassment.** Due to sleepwalking, the affected individual may feel embarrassed, or they may experience problems with

relationships. This can lead to depression or anxiety if left untreated for a long time.

- **Sleep deprivation.** Excess daytime sleepiness and tiredness may be a result of sleepwalking.

When to See a Doctor

Sleepwalking is usually normal if it occurs periodically, and it typically resolves on its own. However, consult your doctor if sleepwalking episodes:

- Cause daytime symptoms (sleepiness)

- Lead to dangerous events, such as using fragile objects, injuring oneself or others, etc.

- Occur often and/or last longer than usual

- Prevails after teenage years

Diagnosis of Sleepwalking

To diagnose sleepwalking, the doctor reviews your child's medical history, which is typically followed by:

- **A physical examination.** The doctor conducts a physical examination in order to identify any conditions that may be confused with sleepwalking, such as nighttime seizures or panic attacks.

- **A discussion of your symptoms.** The doctor may ask you or your child to fill out a questionnaire that helps you describe the sleepwalking episodes; provides health information, including past sleeping problems; documents the first notice of the sleepwalking, etc.

- **A nocturnal sleep study (polysomnography).** In some cases, the doctor may recommend an overnight stay in order to conduct a sleep study. Through the use of sensors, a person's blood oxygen level, heart rate, breathing, and eye and leg movements will be monitored.

It is recommended to inform your doctor if your family members have a history of sleepwalking.

Treatment for Sleepwalking

Treatment options for sleepwalking include the following;

- **Treating any underlying condition.** If sleepwalking is associated with an underlying condition, treatment is focused on that medical condition.

- **Adjusting medication.** If medications are found to be the cause of sleepwalking, those medications are adjusted accordingly.

- **Resolving stress.** Relaxation therapies, biofeedback, hypnosis, and cognitive behavioral therapy (CBT) are recommended to reduce stress or any other mental-health condition for improving sleep quality.

- **Anticipatory awakenings.** This treatment option involves waking a person 15 minutes before she or he sleepwalks.

- **Medications.** Medications are not initially recommended; however, the doctor may recommend them after diagnosis.

Prevention of Sleepwalking

Sleepwalking and its complications can be prevented by:

- **Get adequate sleep.** Fatigue can lead to sleepwalking. Put your child to bed early in order to avoid sleepwalking.

- **Establish a relaxing activity.** Complete calming activities before sleep, such as reading a book, taking a warm bath, meditating, solving puzzles, or completing relaxing exercises.

- **Find a pattern.** Take note of the time when sleepwalking occurs. If there is a pattern within the timings, it may be used for anticipatory awakenings.

- **Make a quiet bedroom.** A calm atmosphere can improve your child's quality of sleep.

- **Avoid caffeine.** It is recommended to avoid caffeine and sugar before bedtime.

What to Do if Your Child Sleepwalks

When your child sleepwalks, do the following:

- **Do not wake your child.** Try not to wake your child during a sleepwalking episode; waking your child from sleepwalking may cause them to feel confused and disorientated.

- **Get your child back to bed.** Guide your child safely back to bed by repeating soothing statements and reassuring them that they are at home.

- **Offer comfort.** Provide them with physical comfort.

- **Take safety measures.** Make the environment safe by locking doors and windows, and putting fragile objects away in order to prevent any injuries during sleepwalking episodes.

References

1. "Sleepwalking," Mayo Clinic, July 21, 2017.

2. "Sleep Disorders: Sleepwalking Basics," WebMD, October 25, 2018.

3. "Sleepwalking," The Nemours Foundation/KidsHealth®, August 2018.

4. "Sleepwalking," Cleveland Clinic, May 9, 2014.

5. "Kids and Sleepwalking," CHOC Children's, February 3, 2016.

Chapter 59

Myalgic Encephalomyelitis/ Chronic Fatigue Syndrome in Children

Myalgic encephalomyelitis (ME)/chronic fatigue syndrome (CFS) is a disabling and complex illness. Scientists do not know what causes it, and there is no cure or approved treatment for the illness. ME/CFS is often thought of as a problem in adults, but children (both adolescents and younger children) can also get ME/CFS.

- Not as much is known about ME/CFS in children because there have been few studies in this age group.

- Scientists estimate that up to 2 in 100 children suffer from ME/ CFS.

- ME/CFS is more common in adolescents than in younger children.

Symptoms and Diagnosis of Myalgic Encephalomyelitis/Chronic Fatigue Syndrome in Children

Children and adolescents with ME/CFS mostly have the same symptoms as adults. Some differences are:

This chapter includes text excerpted from "ME/CFS in Children," Centers for Disease Control and Prevention (CDC), July 12, 2018.

- Children, especially adolescents, with ME/CFS have orthostatic intolerance (dizziness and light-headedness and other symptoms that are triggered when standing up and sometimes also sitting upright) more often than adults. It is often the most unbearable symptom and may make other symptoms of ME/CFS worse.

- Sleep problems in young children may show up as a lack of their usual energy. In adolescents with ME/CFS, sleep problems may be hard to detect, as sleep cycles change during puberty. Many adolescents begin to stay up late and often have trouble waking up early. The demands of classes, homework, after-school jobs, and social activities also affect sleep. Common sleep complaints in children and adolescents with ME/CFS include:

  - Difficulty falling or staying asleep

  - Daytime sleepiness

  - Intense and vivid dreaming

- Unlike adults with ME/CFS, children and adolescents with ME/CFS do not usually have muscle and joint pain. Yet, headaches and stomach pain may be more common in this age group. Younger children may not be able to describe the pain well.

- In children, particularly in adolescents, ME/CFS is more likely to start after an acute illness, such as the flu or mononucleosis. Sometimes, ME/CFS in children might begin gradually.

Diagnosis of Myalgic Encephalomyelitis/Chronic Fatigue Syndrome in Children

As in adults, symptoms of ME/CFS in children and adolescents may appear similar to many other illnesses, and there is no test to confirm ME/CFS. This makes ME/CFS difficult to diagnose. The illness can be unpredictable. Symptoms may come and go, or there may be changes in how bad they are over time.

A diagnosis of ME/CFS requires at least six months of illness. However, children and other patients should be seen by doctors and get support as soon as they become ill. In other words, a child with some or all of the symptoms of ME/CFS should not wait for months to see a doctor. This six-month period is used to complete laboratory tests and other activities, including follow-up appointments, to check for other illnesses that have symptoms similar to ME/CFS. The six-month period also allows time for improvement for children with illnesses that have symptoms such as ME/CFS, but that do not usually last as long as ME/CFS. It is also important that management of symptoms begins before six months have passed, and that support and accommodations for children in school are considered and implemented during this time.

To diagnose ME/CFS, the child's doctor may undertake the following:

- Ask about child's and family's medical history, including a review of any medications and recent illnesses

- Do a thorough physical and mental status examination

- Order blood, urine, or other tests

To get a better idea about the child's illness, the doctor may ask many questions. Depending on the age of the child, the questions might be asked of the patient, parent/guardian, or both (together or independently). Questions might include:

- What is the child able to do now? How does it compare to what the child was able to do before?

- How long has the child been ill?

- Does the child feel better after sleeping or resting?

- What makes the child feel worse? What helps the child feel better?

- What symptoms keep the child from doing what she/he needs or wants to do?

- Does the child ever feel dizzy or lightheaded? Has the child been falling more often than before?

- Does the child seem to have trouble remembering or focusing on tasks?

- What happens when the child tries to do activities that used to be normal?

Parents or guardians and patients may want to keep a journal for their ill child. This could help patients and families remember important details during their healthcare visit. Keeping track of child's activities and what leads to worsening of child's symptoms can help identify the effects of the illness on daily activities.

Doctors might refer patients to see a specialist, such as a neurologist, rheumatologist, or a sleep specialist, to check for other conditions that can cause similar symptoms. These specialists might find other conditions that could be treated. Patients can have other conditions and still have ME/CFS. However, getting treatment for other conditions might help patients with ME/CFS feel better.

A number of factors can make diagnosing ME/CFS more difficult. For example:

- There is no laboratory test to confirm ME/CFS.

- Fatigue and other symptoms of ME/CFS are common to many illnesses.

- The illness is unpredictable and symptoms may come and go.

- The type, number, and severity of ME/CFS symptoms vary from person to person.

When diagnosing ME/CFS in children and adolescents, it is useful to remember that:

- Children and adolescents cannot always accurately describe their symptoms or how they feel.

- Parents may describe their child's symptoms differently from how the child describes her/his symptoms.

Children with ME/CFS may miss school, which may be mistaken for school phobia. But unlike those with school phobia, children with ME/CFS are still ill and inactive on weekends and holidays. They may not be able to do their hobbies and take part in social activities as they did before the illness. They also may have a problem completing school assignments within the usual time. This might be a result of problems with thinking, learning, and memory caused by the illness.

Treatment of Myalgic Encephalomyelitis/Chronic Fatigue Syndrome in Children

As for adults, there is no cure or approved treatment for ME/CFS in children. However, some symptoms can be treated or managed. Treating these symptoms might provide relief for some patients with ME/CFS but not others. Other strategies, such as learning new ways to manage activity, can also be helpful.

Patients, their families, and healthcare providers need to work together to decide which symptom causes the most problems. They should discuss the possible benefits and harms of any treatment plans, including medicines and other therapies. A treatment plan for a child who might have ME/CFS should focus on the most disruptive symptoms first.

Symptoms that healthcare providers might try to address are:

Sleep Problems

Good sleep habits are important for all people, including those with ME/CFS. When children try these tips but are still unable to sleep, their doctor might recommend taking medicine to help with sleep.

Children might continue to feel unrefreshed even after the medications help them to get a full night of sleep. If so, they should consider seeing a sleep specialist. Most people with sleep disorders, such as sleep apnea (symptoms include brief pausing in breathing during sleep) and narcolepsy symptoms include excessive daytime sleepiness, respond to therapy. However, for children with ME/CFS, not all symptoms may go away.

Postexertional Malaise

Postexertional malaise (PEM) is the worsening of symptoms after even minor physical, mental or emotional exertion. The symptoms typically get worse 12 to 48 hours after the activity and can last for days, weeks, or even longer.

Postexertional malaise can be addressed by activity management, also called "pacing." The goal of pacing is for children with ME/CFS to learn to balance rest and activity to avoid PEM flare-ups caused by exertion that they cannot tolerate. To do this, patients need to find their individual limits for mental and physical activity. Then they need to plan activity and rest to stay within these limits. Some patients and doctors refer to staying within these limits as staying within the "energy envelope." The limits may be different for each patient. Keeping activity and symptom diaries may help patients find their personal limits, especially early on in the illness.

Patients with ME/CFS need to avoid "push-and-crash" cycles through carefully managing activity. Push-and-crash cycles are when someone with ME/CFS is having a good day and tries to push to do more than they would normally attempt (do too much, crash, rest, start to feel a little better, do too much once again). This can then lead to a "crash" (worsening of ME/CFS symptoms).

Any activity or exercise plan for children with ME/CFS needs to be carefully designed with input from each patient. While vigorous aerobic exercise is beneficial for many chronic illnesses, patients with ME/CFS do not tolerate such exercise routines. Standard exercise recommendations for healthy people can be harmful for patients with ME/CFS. However, it is important that patients with ME/CFS undertake activities that they can tolerate.

For patients with ME/CFS, it is important to find a balance between inactivity and excessive activity, which can make symptoms worse. This means a new way of thinking about daily activities. For example, daily chores and school activities may need to be broken down into smaller steps.

A symptom diary can be very helpful for managing ME/CFS. Keeping daily track of how patients feel and what patients do may help to find ways to make activities easier.

Rehabilitation specialists or exercise physiologists who know ME/CFS may help patients with adjusting to life with ME/CFS. Patients who have learned to listen to their bodies might benefit from carefully increasing exercise to improve fitness and avoid deconditioning. However, exercise is not a cure for ME/CFS.

Parents/guardians and doctors of children with ME/CFS can work with teachers and school administrators to adjust the school load for children with ME/CFS. While it is true that exercise can benefit children with certain chronic illnesses, children with ME/CFS should avoid activity that makes their symptoms worse.

Dizziness and Light-Headedness or Orthostatic Intolerance

Some children and adolescents with ME/CFS might also have symptoms of orthostatic intolerance that are triggered when-or made worse by-standing or sitting upright. These symptoms can include:

- Frequent dizziness and light-headedness

- Changes in vision (blurred vision, seeing white or black spots)

- Weakness

- Feeling such as your heart is beating too fast or too hard, fluttering, or skipping a beat

For patients with these symptoms, their doctor will check their heart rate and blood pressure, and may recommend they see a specialist, such as a cardiologist or neurologist.

For children with ME/CFS who do not have heart or blood vessel disease, their doctor might suggest patients increase daily fluid and salt intake and use support stockings. If symptoms do not improve, prescription medication can be considered.

Problems Concentrating, Thinking, and Remembering

Children with ME/CFS may have problems paying attention, thinking, remembering, and responding. For instance, after becoming ill it may be hard for children to take notes and listen to their teacher at the same time.

For children with ME/CFS who have concentration problems, some doctors have prescribed stimulant medications, such as those typically used to treat attention deficit hyperactivity disorder (ADHD). While stimulants might help improve concentration for some patients with ME/CFS, they might lead to the push-and-crash cycle and worsen symptoms. Push-and-crash cycles are when someone with ME/CFS is having a good day and tries to push to do more than they would normally attempt (do too much, crash, rest, start to feel a little better, do too much once again).

Depression, Stress, and Anxiety

Adjusting to any chronic illness can sometimes lead to symptoms of depression and anxiety. Anxiety in children with ME/CFS is not caused by the illness itself. It can happen because of the changes the child must make to live with the illness. When healthcare providers are concerned about a patient's psychological condition, they may recommend seeing a mental-health professional.

Counseling may help to reduce stress and some symptoms of depression and anxiety, such as sleep problems and headaches. Some children might benefit from antidepressants and anti-anxiety medications. However, doctors should use caution in prescribing these medications. Some drugs used to treat depression have other effects that might worsen other ME/CFS symptoms and cause side effects.

Some children with ME/CFS might benefit from trying techniques, such as deep breathing and muscle relaxation, massage, and movement therapies (stretching, yoga, and tai chi). These can reduce stress and anxiety, and promote a sense of well-being.

Although treating depression and anxiety can ease mental and emotional distress in some patients and can be very beneficial, it is not a cure for ME/CFS.

409

Pain

Children with ME/CFS often have headaches and stomach pains. Doctors may want to check for food allergies and vision problems.

Gentle massage and heat may relieve pain for some patients. Parents/guardians should always talk to their child's healthcare provider before trying any medication. Doctors may recommend trying over-the-counter (OTC) pain-relievers, such as acetaminophen or ibuprofen.

It is important that healthcare providers talk with family members and children about the child's lifestyle and behaviors to find out how the illness impacts the child's daily life. For example, the child's lack of energy may be because of ME/CFS or caused by normal changes in sleep cycles that often happen in puberty. Trying to understand what is causing the symptoms is important because it affects the treatment plan for the child.

Chapter 60

Caffeine and Teens' Sleep

Caffeine is a bitter substance that occurs naturally in more than 60 plants including:

- Coffee beans

- Tea leaves

- Kola nuts, which are used to flavor soft drink colas

- Cacao pods, which are used to make chocolate products

There is also synthetic caffeine, which is added to some medicines, foods, and drinks. For example, some pain relievers, cold medicines, and over-the-counter (OTC) medicines for alertness contain synthetic caffeine. So do energy drinks and "energy-boosting" gums and snacks.

Most people consume caffeine from drinks. The amounts of caffeine in different drinks can vary a lot, but it is generally:

- An 8-ounce cup of coffee: 95–200 mg

- A 12-ounce can of cola: 35–45 mg

This chapter contains text excerpted from the following sources: Text in this chapter begins with excerpts from "Caffeine," MedlinePlus, National Institutes of Health (NIH), April 30, 2019; Text under the heading "Do You Need to Stay Away from Caffeine?" is excerpted from "The Buzz on Caffeine," National Institute on Drug Abuse (NIDA) for Teens, June 25, 2014. Reviewed May 2019.

- An 8-ounce energy drink: 70–100 mg
- An 8-ounce cup of tea: 14–60 mg

What Are Caffeine's Effects on the Body?

Caffeine has many effects on your body's metabolism. It:

- Stimulates your central nervous system, which can make you feel more awake and give you a boost of energy
- Is a diuretic, meaning that it helps your body get rid of extra salt and water by urinating more
- Increases the release of acid in your stomach, sometimes leading to an upset stomach or heartburn
- May interfere with the absorption of calcium in the body
- Increases your blood pressure

Within one hour of eating or drinking caffeine, it reaches its peak level in your blood. You may continue to feel the effects of caffeine for four to six hours.

What Are the Side Effects from Too Much Caffeine?

For most people, it is not harmful to consume up to 400 mg of caffeine a day. If you do eat or drink too much caffeine, it can cause health problems, such as:

- Insomnia
- Restlessness and shakiness
- Headaches
- Dizziness
- Rapid or abnormal heart rhythm
- Dehydration
- Anxiety
- Dependency, so you need to take more of it to get the same results

Some people are more sensitive to the effects of caffeine than others.

What Are Energy Drinks, and Why Can They Be a Problem?

Energy drinks are beverages that have added caffeine. The amount of caffeine in energy drinks can vary widely, and sometimes the labels on the drinks do not give you the actual amount of caffeine in them. Energy drinks may also contain sugars, vitamins, herbs, and supplements.

Companies that make energy drinks claim that the drinks can increase alertness and improve physical and mental performance. This has helped make the drinks popular with American teens and young adults. There is limited data showing that energy drinks might temporarily improve alertness and physical endurance. There is not enough evidence to show that they enhance strength or power. But what we do know is that energy drinks can be dangerous because they have large amounts of caffeine. And since they have lots of sugar, they can contribute to weight gain and worsen diabetes.

Sometimes, young people mix their energy drinks with alcohol. It is dangerous to combine alcohol and caffeine. Caffeine can interfere with your ability to recognize how drunk you are, which can lead you to drink more. This also makes you more likely to make bad decisions.

Who Should Avoid or Limit Caffeine?

You should check with your healthcare provider about whether you should limit or avoid caffeine if you:

- Are pregnant, since caffeine passes through the placenta and to the fetus

- Are breastfeeding, since a small amount of caffeine that you consume is passed along to your baby

- Have sleep disorders, including insomnia

- Have migraines or other chronic headaches

- Have anxiety

- Have gastroesophageal reflux disease (GERD) or ulcers

- Have fast or irregular heart rhythms

- Have high blood pressure

- Take certain medicines or supplements, including stimulants, certain antibiotics, asthma medicines, and heart medicines. Check with your healthcare provider about whether there might be interactions between caffeine and any medicines and supplements that you take.

- Are a child or teen. Neither should have as much caffeine as adults. Children can be especially sensitive to the effects of caffeine.

What Is Caffeine Withdrawal?

If you have been consuming caffeine on a regular basis and then suddenly stop, you may have caffeine withdrawal. Symptoms can include:

- Headaches

- Drowsiness

- Irritability

- Nausea

- Difficulty concentrating

These symptoms usually go away after a couple of days.

Do You Need to Stay Away from Caffeine?

Drinking a cup of coffee or eating a bar of chocolate is usually not a big deal. But, there are alternatives to caffeine if you are looking for an energy burst but do not want to get that jittery feeling caffeine sometimes causes. Here are a few alternatives you can try to feel energized without overdoing the caffeine:

- **Sleep.** This may sound obvious, but getting enough sleep is important. Teens need nine hours of sleep a night.

- **Eat regularly.** When you do not eat, your glucose (sugar) levels drop, making you feel drained. Some people find it helpful to eat four or five smaller meals throughout the day instead of fewer big meals.

- **Drink enough water.** Since our body has more than two-thirds of water, we need at least 64 ounces of water a day.

- **Take a walk.** If you are feeling drained in the middle of the day, it helps to move around. Do sit-ups or jumping jacks. Go outside for a brisk walk or ride your bike.

Part Seven

Research and Clinical Studies on Sleep and Sleep Disorders

Chapter 61

Research on Sleep and Sleep Disorders

Chapter Contents

Section 61.1

Research Overview

This section includes text excerpted from "Your Guide to
Healthy Sleep," National Heart, Lung, and Blood
Institute (NHLBI), August 2011. Reviewed May 2019.

Researchers have learned a lot about sleep and sleep disorders in recent years. That knowledge has led to a better understanding of the importance of sleep to our lives and our health. Research supported by the National Heart, Lung, and Blood Institute (NHLBI) has helped identify some of the causes of sleep disorders and their effects on the heart, brain, lungs, and other body systems.

Many questions remain about sleep and sleep disorders. The researchers have been focusing on:

- Gaining a better understanding of how a lack of sleep increases the risk for obesity, diabetes, heart disease, and stroke

- New ways to diagnose sleep disorders

- Genetic, environmental, and social factors that lead to sleep disorders

- The adverse effects from a lack of sleep on body and brain

Much of this research depends on the willingness of volunteers to participate in clinical research. If you would like to help researchers advance science on sleep or about a sleep disorder you have and possible treatments, talk to your doctor about participating in clinical research.

Researchers can learn quite a bit about sleep and sleep disorders by studying animals. However, to fully understand sleep and its effect on health and functioning, as well as how best to diagnose and treat sleep disorders, researchers need to do clinical research on people. This type of research is called "clinical research" because it is often conducted in clinical settings, such as hospitals or doctors' offices.

The two types of clinical research are clinical trials and clinical studies.

- **Clinical trials** test new ways to diagnose, prevent, or treat various disorders. For example, treatments (such as medicines, medical devices, surgery, or other procedures) for a disorder need to be tested in people who have the disorder. A trial helps determine whether a treatment is safe and effective in humans before it is made available for public use. In a clinical trial, participants are randomly assigned to groups. One group receives the new treatment being tested. Other groups may receive a different treatment or a placebo (an inactive substance resembling a drug being tested). Comparing results from the groups gives researchers confidence that changes in the test group are due to the new treatment and not to other factors.

- **Other types of clinical studies** are done to discover the factors, including environmental, behavioral, or genetic factors, that cause or worsen various disorders. Researchers may follow a group of people over time to learn what factors contribute to becoming sick.

Clinical studies and trials may be relatively brief, or they may last for years and require many visits to the study sites. These sites usually are university hospitals or research centers, but they can include private doctors' offices and community hospitals.

If you participate in clinical research, the research will be explained to you in detail, you will be given a chance to ask questions, and you will be asked to provide written permission. You may not directly benefit from the results of the clinical research you participate in, but the information gathered will help others and add to scientific knowledge. Taking part in clinical research has other benefits as well. You will learn more about your disorder, you will have the support of a team of healthcare providers, and your health will likely be monitored closely. However, participation also can have risks, which you should discuss with your doctor. No matter what you decide, your regular medical care will not be affected.

If you are thinking about participating in a clinical study, you may have questions about the purpose of the study, the types of tests and treatment involved, how participation will affect your daily life, and whether any costs are involved. Your doctor may be able to answer some of your questions and help you find clinical studies in which you can participate. You also can visit the following websites to learn about being in a study and to search for clinical trials being done on your disorder:

- www.clinicaltrials.gov

- www.clinicalresearch.nih.gov

- www.nhlbi.nih.gov/studies/index.htm

Section 61.2

Sweet Dreams: Researchers Explore the Link between Sleep and Health

This section includes text excerpted from "Sweet Dreams: Researchers Explore Link between Sleep and Health," National Heart, Lung, and Blood Institute (NHLBI), November 5, 2018.

Feeling sleepy during the day? You are not alone.

Insufficient sleep is a common and fast-growing problem, with almost a third of U.S. adults reporting they get less than the recommended amount of shuteye. But while some people experience occasional restless nights that still allow them to be alert and productive during the day, many others experience something quite different: a prolonged pattern of irregular, insufficient, and poor-quality sleep that experts say can pose a danger to your heart and to your overall health.

Researchers have associated a persistent lack of sleep with conditions such as heart disease, high blood pressure, diabetes, obesity, and even certain types of cancer. To learn more about why sleep deficiency causes this constellation of problems, researchers funded by the National Heart, Lung, and Blood Institute (NHLBI) are looking at how the body regulates breathing during sleep, how sleep deficiencies affect the whole body, and what biomarkers can help assess sleep health. What the researchers discover, they said, could one day lead to better ways to reduce the health risks associated with sleep disorders.

"There are many unanswered scientific questions about how and why people have sleep disorders," said Michael Twery, Ph.D., Director of the NHLBI's National Center on Sleep Disorders Research (NCSDR). "The good news is that while researchers search for answers, there are many steps you can take to improve the quality and duration of your sleep, which can make you happier and more productive during the day."

The NCSDR supports and coordinates sleep science and disorders research, training, and awareness across the National Institutes of Health (NIH), other federal agencies, and partner organizations. Based on some of its research, they have come up with the following ways to get better sleep.

Establish a Regular, Relaxing Bedtime Routine

It pays to periodically take stock of your "sleep hygiene"—the sleep environment you have created and the nighttime habits you have adopted over the years. A good place to start: computer screens. Artificial light from computer screens, whether cell phones, laptops, or televisions, can signal the brain that it is time to be awake. This light exposure can translate into a loss in sleep duration and irregular sleep schedules in both children and adults. In a study partly funded by the NHLBI, researchers showed that smartphone use before bed is associated with shorter sleep duration than normal and worse sleep quality during the night. Studies by other researchers have found similar links. Experts suggest that sleep quality can be enhanced by powering down devices at least 30 minutes before getting in bed. Other tips for getting a good night's sleep include avoiding strenuous exercise just before bedtime and abstaining from alcoholic drinks immediately before turning in for the night.

Commit to Getting the Recommended Seven to Eight Hours of Sleep

Getting the recommended seven to eight hours of sleep each night can be tough for many, but experts say if you create a more relaxing sleeping environment, stick to a regular sleep schedule, and avoid caffeine and other stimulants before bed, you may be able to hit the mark better.

For many teenagers who often stay up late and wake up early, getting the eight to ten hours recommended for them can be even more challenging. Yet, without proper sleep, an NHLBI-funded study recently showed that teenagers may have a higher likelihood of developing risk factors for heart disease, such as high blood pressure and excess body fat.

In one of the largest and most comprehensive studies of its kind, scientists tracked the sleep and daytime activity of 829 adolescents for 7 to 10 days. They evaluated the quantity and quality of sleep, as well as factors related to cardiovascular health—including blood pressure, cholesterol levels, and abdominal fat distribution. The researchers found that the teens who slept less than 7 hours a night (nearly a third of the participants) tended to have more body fat, elevated blood pressure, and less healthy cholesterol levels.

Establish a Regular Time to Go to Bed and Wake Up Every Day

Daily schedules can sometimes be unpredictable, but your health will get a boost if you can stick to a consistent sleep pattern. In a recent study funded by the NHLBI, researchers reported that having regular go-to-bed and wake-up times can especially benefit the heart. The study of 1,978 older adults found that those who slept and woke at the same times every day weighed less, had lower blood sugar levels, lower blood pressure, and a lower risk of developing a heart attack or stroke within 10 years than those with irregular sleep patterns.

How do you get on a healthy schedule and stay on it? Decide what time you need to get up each weekday morning, count 7 to 8 hours backward, then make that your bedtime. Following that schedule may feel odd and undoable at first, but you can "train" yourself over a period of weeks, by going to bed a few minutes earlier (or later) every night, until you have established the habit you want. Then try to keep that same schedule on weekends. If you need to change it up, limit the difference to no more than about an hour. Staying up late and sleeping in late on weekends can disrupt your body's circadian rhythm, the 24-hour internal body clock which controls your sleep-wake cycle.

Spend Time Outside Every Day When Possible

Scientists have discovered that daylight is as essential to optimal health as food and exercise. It is also a key player in optimal sleep. Natural light delivers the entire spectrum of light needed by your eyes and brain to associate daytime with being awake and nighttime with preparing for sleep. However, traditional indoor lighting produces artificial light that deprives the brain of the type needed to properly prepare our bodies for sleep at night. Similarly, light from TV screens and digital devices can confuse the brain and impede the natural process of preparing for sleep. If you cannot get plenty of exposure to daylight, consider this: scientists are developing next-generation light-emitting diode (LED) lighting that could help improve human sleep cycles. In the future, this new artificial lighting will mimic natural sunlight in a way that is better for your sleep.

Experts suggest that you should just go outside for at least 30 minutes each day. If possible, wake up with the sun or use very bright lights in the morning. Sleep experts recommend that, if you have problems falling asleep, you should get a full hour of exposure to morning sunlight, then start dimming the lights inside even before it is time to go to bed.

See a Health Professional If Your Sleep Does Not Improve or Worsens

Sleep problems should not be taken lightly and could be a sign of major underlying health issues, including heart disease or cancer. (They can also put you—and others—at risk while driving or working machinery.) Talk to your doctor if you constantly wake up feeling sluggish and listless, feel sleepy during the day, or cannot adapt to night shift work.

Doctors can diagnose some sleep disorders by asking questions about sleep schedules and habits (such as your use of caffeine, tobacco, alcohol, and any medicines) and by getting information from sleep partners or parents. To diagnose other sleep disorders, doctors also use the results from sleep studies and other medical tests. If a sleep problem is suspected, doctors can prescribe medicines and other health interventions or even rule out other health or psychiatric problems that may be disturbing your sleep. In some cases, they can refer a patient to a sleep specialist or sleep center for further evaluation.

Section 61.3

Dancing to the Circadian Rhythm: Researcher from the National Heart, Lung, and Blood Institute Finds New Genes for the Body's Internal Clock

This section includes text excerpted from "Dancing to the Circadian Rhythm: NHLBI Researcher Finds New Genes for Body's Internal Clock," National Heart, Lung, and Blood Institute (NHLBI), November 6, 2017.

If you feel energized or tired around the same time each day, or routinely get up early or stay up late—the familiar "early riser" or "night owl" syndrome—you are witnessing, in real time, your circadian rhythm at work. That is the 24-hour internal body clock which controls your sleep–wake cycle.

Circadian rhythms have long fascinated researchers—decades ago three of them marked a critical milestone when they discovered the molecular components behind that mysterious timing cycle. For this game-changing finding, the trio was awarded the 2017 Nobel Prize in Physiology or Medicine. Since their discovery, researchers have come to know that the circadian clock affects not just sleep, but hormone production, eating habits, body temperature, heart rate, and other biological functions as well.

Yet, for all these advances, scientists still know relatively little about the clock's genetic underpinnings. Now, a team of researchers from the National Heart, Lung, and Blood Institute (NHLBI) is working to change that with the discovery of scores of new genes they say have a profound impact on the circadian rhythm. These researchers say these genes could hold the key to a new understanding of a wide range of health conditions, from insomnia to heart disease, and perhaps pave the way for new treatments for them.

"We all 'dance' to the circadian rhythm," said Susan Harbison, Ph.D., an investigator in the NHLBI's Laboratory of Systems Genetics, who is among an elite cadre of scientists studying the complex genetics of the biological clock. "Quietly, this clock influences our body and our health in ways that are just now being understood."

The studies are slowly unfolding. For example, long-term night shift work has been associated with an increased risk of high blood pressure, obesity, and heart disease. Some studies have shown a link between circadian rhythm changes and cancer. And a recent study by researchers in France found that heart surgery is safer in the afternoon than in the morning, a phenomenon they attribute to the body's circadian clock having a better repair mechanism in the afternoon than in the morning.

Now, thanks to Harbison and her research team, new insights into why some people experience longer or shorter periods of wakefulness or sleepiness than others—and what it might mean for a host of health conditions—could be on the horizon.

To explore this line of research more deeply, Harbison is working with a favorite laboratory model of sleep researchers: Drosophila melanogaster, the common fruit fly. While this little fly may seem like an unlikely choice, it turns out to be an appropriate stand-in for humans.

"The clock mechanisms regulating circadian rhythm in humans and fruit flies are remarkably similar," Harbison said. "They both have biological rhythms of about 24 hours. In fact, the genes involved in mammalian circadian rhythms were first identified in flies."

Previous studies by other researchers had identified approximately 126 genes for circadian rhythms in fruit flies. In recent studies using a natural population of flies, Harbison's group estimates that there are more than 250 new genes associated with the circadian clock, among the largest number identified to date. Many of the genes appear to be associated with nerve cell development—not surprising, she said, given the wide-ranging impact of circadian rhythms on biological processes.

In addition to finding this treasure trove of clock-related genes, Harbison's group also found that the circadian patterns among the flies were highly variable and that some of the genes code for variability in the circadian clock. Some flies had unusually long circadian periods—up to 31 hours—while others had extremely short circadian periods of 15 hours. In other words: just like people, there were "early risers" and "night owls" and long sleepers and short sleepers among the fruit flies.

"Before we did our studies, there was little attention paid to the genes responsible for variability in the circadian period," noted Harbison, who is also looking at environmental factors that might influence these genes, such as drugs like alcohol and caffeine. "We now have new details about this variability, and that opens up a whole new avenue of research in understanding what these genes do and how they influence the circadian clock."

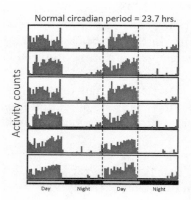 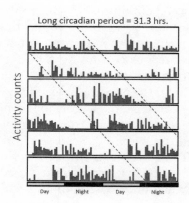

Figure 61.1. *Rest and Activity Patterns for Two Different Fruit Flies*

This graph shows rest and activity patterns for two different fruit flies. The graph on the left shows the rest and activity of a fly with a normal circadian period (about 24 hours). Vertical bars show the fly's activity during the day and night. The graph on the right shows the rest and activity of a fly with an abnormal circadian period (about 31 hours). The abnormal pattern is similar to an individual with a circadian rhythm disorder.

Harbison says that for most people, disruptions to the circadian clock have a temporary effect, as occurs with daylight saving time or jet lag from overseas travel, when a person may experience short-term fatigue as they adjust to a time change or new time zone. But for some, disruptions to the clock are associated with chronic health effects, as occurs with night shift workers. Others who suffer from certain circadian rhythm disorders—such as delayed sleep phase disorder—may find it extremely difficult to fall asleep at the desired time.

"The clock architecture is not set in stone and is not a 'one size fits all' device," she noted. "What we are finding is that the effect of disrupting the circadian clock differs depending on the genetic makeup of the individual. Just as the human height and other traits are variable, the same is true of circadian traits among different individuals."

In the future, Harbison hopes that these newly identified genes might ultimately be linked to specific disease processes in humans. Her findings could lead to the discovery of new biomarkers for diagnosing circadian disorders and lay the groundwork for new treatments for sleep and circadian disorders in humans.

Section 61.4

The Brain's Internal Clock Continually Takes Its Temperature

This section includes text excerpted from "The Brain's Internal Clock Continually Takes Its Temperature," News and Events, National Institutes of Health (NIH), March 7, 2018.

Circuits in the brain act as an internal clock to tell us it is time to sleep and to control how long we then stay asleep. A new study in flies suggests that a part of that clock constantly monitors changes in external temperature and integrates that information into the neural network controlling sleep. The study was published in *Nature* and was supported by the National Institute of Neurological Disorders and Stroke (NINDS), a part of the National Institutes of Health (NIH).

"This study takes advantage of the powerful model system of the fly's circadian clock network to demonstrate how temperature cues from the environment are used to control the time and duration of sleep," said Janet He, Ph.D., Program Director, at the NINDS.

The circadian clock is a fundamental process found in nearly every living organism that coordinates sleep behavior with changes in the environment. The link between the light–dark cycle and the onset of sleep is well recognized; however, changes in temperature also appear to affect sleep patterns in humans.

"The clock discovered in flies more than 30 years ago is essentially the same one found in the human brain," said Orie Shafer, Ph.D., associate professor at the University of Michigan, Ann Arbor and senior author of this study. "Circadian clock studies are beautiful examples of how the fly has important things to tell us about how our bodies work."

By using a special fluorescent protein that changes from green to red when neurons fire, Dr. Shafer and his team watched the activity of different parts of the fly brain's circadian clock while they increased or decreased the surrounding temperature. To their surprise, an area in the fly brain's circadian clock called the "DN1p" increased its activity when cooled and became less active when heated.

"We knew that light excites the circadian clock overall and that light and heat typically increase at the same time, so it was completely unexpected to find a region of the clock that increased its activity in response to cooling," said Dr. Shafer.

As experienced by anyone who has traveled across time zones, the circadian clock can be "reset" over time in response to new day-light cycles. The clock of flies can be retrained to new cycles of either light or temperature, so Dr. Shafer and his colleagues next looked at whether the DN1p is involved in resetting the clock to the new heating-cooling cycle.

Because DN1p neurons are thought to be sleep-promoting, the researchers blocked their activity or eliminated them genetically. Both affected the flies' ability to retrain their sleep cycle in response to changes in temperature, highlighting the importance of the DN1p for the control of sleep behavior.

"Because flies' bodies are translucent, their clock neurons can respond to light directly," said Dr. Shafer. "We next asked whether temperature worked in the same way or required external organs."

In flies, temperature could be sensed directly by neurons in the brain or via nerve impulses from sensory organs in the body. To distinguish between the two, the investigators genetically manipulated or physically removed the sensory organs and found that the DN1p neurons no longer responded to changes in temperature. This meant that the clock interprets temperature signals from the body rather than sensing temperature changes directly.

The circadian clock of larger animals and humans is also sensitive to changes in temperature, and because of their larger size, it would require input from external sensory organs. The fact that, despite its small size, the fly clock also relies on temperature sensors outside the brain suggests that the findings of this study could have broad implications in the control of sleep in humans.

Funding for this study was provided by the NINDS, the National Science Foundation (NSF), and the Damon Runyon Cancer Foundation.

Section 61.5

Study Shows How Memories Ripple through the Brain

This section includes text excerpted from "Study Shows How Memories Ripple through the Brain," News and Events, National Institutes of Health (NIH), October 31, 2017.

Using innovative NeuroGrid technology, scientists showed that sleep boosts communication between two brain regions whose connection is critical for the formation of memories. The work, published in *Science*, was partially funded by the Brain Research through Advancing Innovative Neurotechnologies (BRAIN) Initiative, a project of the National Institutes of Health (NIH) devoted to accelerating the development of new approaches to probing the workings of the brain.

"Using new technologies advanced by the BRAIN Initiative, these researchers made a fundamental discovery about how the brain creates and stores new memories," said Nick Langhals, Ph.D., Program Director at the NIH's National Institute of Neurological Disorders and Stroke (NINDS).

A brain structure called the "hippocampus" is widely thought to turn new information into permanent memories while we sleep. Previous work by the new study's senior author, New York University School of Medicine professor György Buzsáki, M.D., Ph.D., revealed high-frequency bursts of neural firing called "ripples" in the hippocampus during sleep and suggested they play a role in memory storage. The current study confirmed the presence of ripples in the hippocampus during sleep and found them in certain parts of association neocortex, an area on the brain's surface involved in processing complex sensory information.

"When we first observed this, we thought it was incorrect because it had never been observed before," said Dion Khodagholy, Ph.D., the study's co-first author and assistant professor at Columbia University in New York.

Using a cutting-edge NeuroGrid system they invented, along with recording electrodes placed deeper into the brain, the researchers examined activity in several parts of rats' brains during nonrapid eye movement (non-REM) sleep, the longest stage of sleep. Their NeuroGrid consists of a collection of tiny electrodes linked together like the threads of a blanket, which is then laid across an area of the brain so

431

that each electrode can continuously monitor the activity of a different set of neurons.

"This particular device allows us to look at multiple areas of the brain at the same time," said Jennifer Gelinas, M.D., Ph.D., the study's co-first author and assistant professor at Columbia University.

The team was also surprised to find that the ripples in the association neocortex and hippocampus occurred at the same time, suggesting that the two regions were communicating as the rats slept. Because the association neocortex is thought to be a storage location for memories, the researchers theorized that this neural dialogue could help the brain retain information.

To test that idea, they examined brain activity during non-REM sleep in rats trained to locate rewards in a maze and in rats that explored the maze in a random fashion. In the latter group of animals, the ripples in the hippocampus and cortex were no more synchronized before exploring the maze than afterward. In the trained rats, the learning task increased the cross-talk between those areas, and a second training session boosted it even more, further suggesting that such communication is important for the creation and storage of memories.

The group hopes to use the NeuroGrid in people undergoing brain surgery for other reasons to determine if the same ripples occur in the human brain. The researchers also plan to investigate if manipulating that neural firing in animals can boost or suppress memory formation in order to confirm that ripples are important for that process.

"Identifying the specific neural patterns that go along with memory formation provides a way to better understand memory and potentially even address disorders of memory," said Dr. Gelinas.

The study was funded by the NINDS and the National Institute of Mental Health (NIMH).

Section 61.6

Sleep Loss Encourages the Spread of a Toxic Alzheimer Protein

This section includes text excerpted from "Sleep Loss Encourages Spread of Toxic Alzheimer's Protein," National Institutes of Health (NIH), February 5, 2019.

In addition to memory loss and confusion, many people with Alzheimer disease (AD) have trouble sleeping. Now, a team of researchers funded by the National Institutes of Health (NIH) has evidence that the reverse is also true: a chronic lack of sleep may worsen the disease and its associated memory loss.

The new findings center on a protein called "tau," which accumulates in abnormal tangles in the brains of people with Alzheimer disease. In a healthy brain, active neurons naturally release some tau during waking hours, but it normally gets cleared away during sleep. Essentially, your brain has a system for taking the "garbage" out while you are off in dreamland.

The latest findings in studies of mice and people further suggest that sleep deprivation upsets this balance, allowing more tau to be released, accumulate, and spread in toxic tangles within brain areas that are important for memory. While more research is needed, the findings suggest that regular and substantial sleep may play an unexpectedly important role in helping to delay or slow down Alzheimer disease.

It is long been recognized that AD is associated with the gradual accumulation of beta-amyloid peptides and tau proteins, which form plaques and tangles that are considered hallmarks of the disease. It has only more recently become clear that, while beta-amyloid is an early sign of the disease, tau deposits track more closely with disease progression and a person's cognitive decline.

Such findings have raised hopes among researchers, including David Holtzman at the Washington University School of Medicine, St. Louis, that tau-targeting treatments might slow this devastating disease. Though much of the hope has focused on developing the right drugs, some has also focused on sleep and its nightly ability to reset the brain's metabolic harmony.

In the new study published in *Science*, Holtzman's team set out to explore whether tau levels in the brain naturally are tied to the sleep–wake cycle. Earlier studies had shown that tau is released in small amounts by active neurons. But when neurons are chronically activated, more tau gets released. So, do tau levels rise when we are awake and fall during slumber?

The Holtzman team found that they do. The researchers measured tau levels in brain fluid collected from mice during their normal waking and sleeping hours. (Since mice are nocturnal, they sleep primarily during the day.) The researchers found that tau levels in brain fluid nearly double when the animals are awake. They also found that sleep deprivation caused tau levels in brain fluid to double yet again.

These findings were especially interesting because Holtzman's team had already made a related finding in people. The team found that healthy adults forced to pull an all-nighter had a 30 percent increase on average in levels of unhealthy beta-amyloid in their cerebrospinal fluid (CSF).

The researchers went back and reanalyzed those same human samples for tau. Sure enough, the tau levels were elevated on average by about 50 percent.

Once tau begins to accumulate in brain tissue, the protein can spread from one brain area to the next along with neural connections. So, Holtzman's team wondered whether a lack of sleep over longer periods also might encourage tau to spread.

To find out, mice engineered to produce human tau fibrils in their brains were made to stay up longer than usual and get less quality sleep over several weeks. Those studies showed that, while less sleep did not change the original deposition of tau in the brain, it did lead to a significant increase in tau's spread. Intriguingly, tau tangles in the animals appeared in the same brain areas affected in people with Alzheimer disease.

Another report by Holtzman's team appearing early in January 2019, *Science Translational Medicine* found yet another link between tau and poor sleep. That study showed that older people who had more tau tangles in their brains by positron emission tomography (PET) scanning had less slow-wave, deep sleep.

Together, these new findings suggest that AD and sleep loss are even more intimately intertwined than had been realized. The findings suggest that good sleep habits and/or treatments designed to encourage plenty of high-quality sleep might play an important role in slowing Alzheimer disease. On the other hand, poor sleep also might worsen the condition and serve as an early warning sign of Alzheimer disease.

For now, the findings come as an important reminder that all of us should do our best to get a good night's rest on a regular basis. Sleep deprivation really is not a good way to deal with overly busy lives. It is not yet clear if better sleep habits will prevent or delay Alzheimer disease, but it surely cannot hurt.

Section 61.7

Poor Sleep Habits in Adolescence Correlated with Cardiovascular Risk

This section includes text excerpted from "Poor Sleep Habits in Adolescence Correlated with Cardiovascular Risk," National Institutes of Health (NIH), June 19, 2018.

Just ask any parent or teacher, most of today's teens and preteens do not seem to get enough sleep. And what sleep they do get is often poor quality—no great surprise, given that smartphones and other electronic devices are usually never far from their reach. Now, a National Institutes of Health (NIH) funded team has uncovered the strongest evidence yet that this lack of quality sleep may be setting our kids up for some serious health issues later in life.

The team's study of more than 800 adolescents, between the ages of 11 and 13, confirmed that many are getting an insufficient amount of undisturbed, restful sleep each night. While earlier studies had found a link between sleep duration and obesity, the new work shows that a wide range of other cardiovascular risk factors are affected by both too little sleep and poor sleep quality. When compared to well-rested kids, sleep deprived youth were found to have higher blood pressure, bigger waistlines, and lower levels of high-density lipoprotein (HDL) cholesterol, which is associated with a lower risk of cardiovascular disease (CVD).

These findings, published in the journal *Pediatrics*, come from a study led by Elsie Taveras from the Massachusetts General Hospital for Children and Harvard T.H. Chan School of Public Health, Boston. Taveras and her team worked with a large group of kids participating in Project Viva, a long-term research study of more than 2,000 women and their children. They asked the adolescents to wear a wrist-watch-like device that recorded their sleep times for at least 7 days, which is long enough to get an idea of their sleep patterns.

The results were certainly nothing to snooze about. The adolescents got on average less than 7½ hours of sleep each night. 1 in 3 regularly slept less than 7 hours per night, while only 2 percent met or exceeded the minimum sleep recommendations for their age. The American Academy of Sleep Medicine (AASM) recommends that teens sleep 8 to 10 hours per night. Preteens should have a minimum of 9 hours of sleep nightly.

More than half of the participants also showed poor sleep efficiency. That is measured as the proportion of nighttime sleep during which a person is actually asleep. A sleep efficiency of less than 85 percent is generally considered insufficient and an indicator of poor sleep quality.

The researchers wondered how this lack of sleep might affect their cardiovascular health. To get the answer, the researchers calculated for each participant a combined risk score, which incorporated waist circumference; blood pressure; cholesterol; insulin resistance; and triglycerides, the main constituent of body fat.

The researchers' analyses showed that adolescents who got the least sleep each night also had the highest risk scores. It was the same story for poor sleep efficiency. In fact, shorter sleep duration and poorer sleep efficiency were negatively associated with waist size, blood pressure, and HDL levels. Those correlations with sleep deprivation and/or disturbance also persisted even when potentially confounding factors were accounted for, including socioeconomic status, race, and puberty, as well as body mass index (BMI), how much time the adolescents spent watching television, and how often they ate fast food.

Obesity and cardiovascular risk factors in childhood often lead to cardiovascular disease later in life. So, the findings suggest that a lack of good sleep is sending far too many of our kids off to an unhealthy future well before they have graduated from high school.

Of course, epidemiologists will remind that correlation does not equal causation. So, it is still possible that some other factors are driving both the poor sleep and the cardiovascular risk factors in these young people. But, these results are certainly a wake-up call to take adolescent sleep patterns more seriously.

In addition to a sleep efficiency of 85 percent or more, good sleep generally includes falling asleep within 30 minutes of going to bed and waking no more than once during the night for an "awake" time of no more than 20 minutes. To get more and better sleep, the Centers for

Diseases Control and Prevention (CDC) recommends a consistent bedtime in a dark, quiet, and comfortable room free of electronic devices. Parents might consider finding ways to make sure their kids eat a balanced diet, get lots of exercises, and, put down their cell phones at night to get the right amounts of sleep that their bodies truly need.

Section 61.8

Study Helps Solve Mystery of How Sleep Protects against Heart Disease

This section includes text excerpted from "Study Helps Solve Mystery of How Sleep Protects against Heart Disease," News and Events, National Institutes of Health (NIH), February 13, 2019.

Researchers say that they are closer to solving the mystery of how a good night's sleep protects against heart disease. In studies using mice, they discovered a previously unknown mechanism between the brain, bone marrow, and blood vessels that appears to protect against the development of atherosclerosis, or hardening of the arteries—but only when sleep is healthy and sound. The study, funded by the National Heart, Lung, and Blood Institute (NHLBI), part of the National Institutes of Health (NIH).

The discovery of this pathway underscores the importance of getting enough quality sleep to maintain cardiovascular health and could provide new targets for fighting heart disease, the leading cause of death among women and men in the United States, the researchers said.

"We have identified a mechanism by which a brain hormone controls the production of inflammatory cells in the bone marrow in a way that helps protect the blood vessels from damage," explained Filip Swirski, Ph.D., the study's lead author who also is an associate professor at Harvard Medical School (HMS) and Massachusetts General Hospital (MGH), Boston. "This anti-inflammatory mechanism is regulated by sleep, and it breaks down when you frequently disrupt sleep or experience poor sleep quality. It is a small piece of to a larger puzzle."

Swirski noted that while other similar mechanisms may exist, the findings are nonetheless exciting. Recent research has linked sleep deficiency and certain sleep disorders, such as sleep apnea, to an increased risk of obesity, diabetes, cancer, as well as heart disease. But scientists have known little about the cellular and molecular underpinnings that could help explain the link between sleep and cardiovascular health.

Poor or insufficient sleep is a major public health problem affecting millions of people of all ages. Studies show that getting enough quality sleep at the right times is vital for health, but fewer than half of adults in the United States get the recommended seven to eight hours per day.

To learn more about the impact of this deficiency on cardiovascular disease, the researchers focused on a group of mice that were genetically engineered to develop atherosclerosis. They disrupted the sleep patterns of half the mice and allowed the other half to sleep normally.

Over time, the mice with disrupted sleep developed progressively larger arterial lesions when compared to the other mice. Specifically, the sleep-disrupted mice developed arterial plaques, or fatty deposits, that were up to one-third larger than the mice with normal sleep patterns. The sleep-disrupted mice also produced twice the level of certain inflammatory cells in their circulatory system than the control mice—and also lower amounts of hypocretin, a hormone made by the brain that is thought to play a key role in regulating sleep and wake states.

The researchers also showed that sleep-deficient, atherosclerotic mice that received hypocretin supplementation tended to produce fewer inflammatory cells and develop smaller atherosclerotic lesions when compared to mice that did not get the supplementation. These results, they said, demonstrate that hypocretin loss during disrupted sleep contributes to inflammation and atherosclerosis. But they cautioned that more studies are needed, particularly in humans, to validate these findings and especially before experimenting with hypocretin therapeutically.

Still, health experts say, targeting the newly discovered biological mechanism—a so-called "neuro-immune axis"—could be a breakthrough that one day leads to new treatments for heart disease, sleep, and other disorders.

"This appears to be the most direct demonstration yet of the molecular connections linking blood and cardiovascular risk factors to sleep health," said Michael Twery, Ph.D., Director of the National Center on Sleep Disorders Research (NCSDR) at the NHLBI. Circadian biology refers to the 24-hour internal body clock that governs the expression of many genes in almost every tissue and the regulation of sleep and wake cycles.

"Understanding the potential impact of poor sleep and circadian health on blood cell formation and vascular disease opens new avenues for developing improved treatments," Twery added.

Section 61.9

Sleep Apnea: The National Heart, Lung, and Blood Institute Sheds Light on an Underdiagnosed Disorder

This section includes text excerpted from "Sleep Apnea: NHLBI Sheds Light on an Underdiagnosed Disorder," National Heart, Lung, and Blood Institute (NHLBI), August 22, 2017.

Mounting scientific evidence about the health dangers of sleep apnea—a common disorder which causes people to stop breathing during sleep—is spurring new and important studies that could lead to improved diagnosis and treatment. Researchers funded by the National, Heart, Lung, and Blood Institute (NHLBI) are sifting through everything from the genetic codes of sleep apnea patients to medications currently on the market, searching for ways to minimize the impact of this potentially deadly disorder.

Millions of Americans suffer from sleep apnea, but many go undiagnosed and untreated, mainly because some of the tell-tale symptoms occur during sleep—frequent snoring, gasping for air, and silent breathing pauses that can last seconds to minutes. Yet, as NHLBI-funded studies have found, sleep apnea can have severe health consequences over time if left untreated. The disorder has been associated with an increased risk of high blood pressure, heart attack, stroke, obesity, diabetes, and glaucoma. And new findings indicate that pregnant women with sleep apnea have a higher chance of developing high blood pressure and giving birth prematurely.

The fallout is not just on individuals but the public at large: because many with the disorder feel persistent sleepiness even after a full night's sleep, untreated sleep apnea has been associated with lower work performance and a higher risk of accidents on the highway and at job sites.

"The good news is that several treatments are currently available, and even more are in the pipeline," said Michael Twery, Ph.D., Director of the National Center on Sleep Disorders Research (NCSDR) at the NHLBI, part of the National Institutes of Health (NIH). But, he added, "a convenient blood test still needs to be developed so that apnea diagnosis is available to all communities and economic groups."

In recent years, researchers have been scurrying to try to make that happen—and they are looking not just at developing blood tests, but also urine and saliva tests that could be done quickly in a doctor's office. "These medical tests are needed to improve the diagnosis of sleep apnea and sleep disorders in general," Twery said.

To help accelerate that effort, the NHLBI's Trans-Omics for Precision Medicine (TOPMed) initiative has been analyzing blood samples from thousands of study volunteers participating in medical research. Over 2,000 adults with sleep apnea already have been studied in TOPMed. For example, the NHLBI-funded researchers have been looking to find new diagnostic markers—clues that indicate the presence of disease—by studying changes in the genetic code, gene expression, and metabolism of those with sleep apnea. Twery said this line of research discovery is promising. "Potential candidate markers have been found," he said, "but it's going to take some time to sort out the best measures."

In the meantime, Twery said, the more familiar people become with the symptoms and dangers of sleep apnea—and what they can do to help minimize their risks—the better off they likely will be. The Centers for Disease Control and Prevention (CDC) estimates that 50 to 75 percent of adults with symptoms of sleep apnea have not discussed their condition with a physician.

Section 61.10

Sleep Apnea Is Common but Largely Undiagnosed in African Americans

This section contains text excerpted from the following sources: Text
in this section begins with excerpts from "Sleep Apnea," National
Heart, Lung, and Blood Institute (NHLBI), December 10, 2018;
Text beginning with the heading "Sleep Apnea Common in African
Americans" is excerpted from "Study: Sleep Apnea Common but
Largely Undiagnosed in African-Americans," National Heart,
Lung, and Blood Institute (NHLBI),
September 5, 2018.

Sleep apnea is a common condition in the United States. It can
occur when the upper airway becomes blocked repeatedly during sleep,
reducing or completely stopping airflow. This is known as "obstructive
sleep apnea" (OSA). If the brain does not send the signals needed to
breathe, the condition may be called "central sleep apnea" (CSA).

Healthcare providers use sleep studies to diagnose sleep apnea.
They record the number of episodes of slow or stopped breathing and
the number of CSA events detected in an hour. They also determine
whether oxygen levels in the blood are lower during these events.

Breathing devices, such as continuous positive air pressure (CPAP)
machines, and lifestyle changes are common sleep apnea treatments.
Undiagnosed or untreated sleep apnea can lead to serious complications, such as heart attack, glaucoma, diabetes, cancer, and cognitive
and behavioral disorders.

There are many risk factors for sleep apnea. Some risk factors,
such as unhealthy lifestyle habits and environments, can be changed.
Other risk factors, such as age, family history and genetics, race and
ethnicity, and sex, cannot be changed. Healthy lifestyle changes can
decrease your risk for developing sleep apnea. In the United States,
sleep apnea is more common among Blacks, Hispanics, and Native
Americans than among Whites.

Sleep Apnea Common in African Americans

Researchers are reporting a high prevalence of sleep apnea in a
large population of African Americans but note that the majority,
nearly 95 percent, were undiagnosed and untreated. Sleep apnea is
associated with an increased risk of heart disease, high blood pressure,
and other chronic health disorders. The study underscores the need

441

to improve sleep apnea screening and diagnosis in this population, which has been underrepresented in sleep apnea research, they say.

The study used data from 852 participants in the Jackson Heart Study, the largest study of cardiovascular disease (CVD) in African Americans. Researchers explored sleep apnea predictors—including habitual snoring, higher body mass index (BMI), and larger neck size—and estimated the proportion of undiagnosed cases. The researchers found a high prevalence of sleep apnea among this large sample of African American men and women. Although about 24 percent had moderate or severe sleep apnea, only 5 percent of these had been diagnosed by a doctor. The article, partly funded by the National Heart, Lung, and Blood Institute (NHLBI), appears in the journal *Sleep*, a publication of the Sleep Research Society (SRS).

"These findings in the Jackson Heart Study reveal that sleep apnea is underdiagnosed and a potential threat to the health and safety of African Americans," said Michael Twery, Ph.D., director of the National Center on Sleep Disorders Research (NCSDR) at the NHLBI. "Further studies are needed to develop the tools and systems required to facilitate diagnosis and treatment of sleep apnea in African Americans and other communities."

Section 61.11

Moderate or Severe Sleep Apnea Doubles the Risk of Hard-to-Treat Hypertension in African Americans

This section includes text excerpted from "Moderate or Severe Sleep Apnea Doubles Risk of Hard-to-Treat Hypertension in African-Americans," National Heart, Lung, and Blood Institute (NHLBI), December 10, 2018.

African Americans with moderate or severe sleep apnea are twice as likely to have hard-to-control high blood pressure when their sleep apnea goes untreated, according to a new study funded mainly by the National Heart, Lung, and Blood Institute (NHLBI), part of the

National Institutes of Health (NIH). The findings, which researchers say may partially explain why African Americans suffer hypertension at rates higher than any other group, point to screening and treatment of sleep apnea as another important strategy for keeping uncontrolled high blood pressure at bay.

A common disorder that blocks the upper airways and causes people to stop breathing during sleep, sleep apnea already has been linked to an increased risk of high blood pressure in White individuals, but the association in Blacks has been largely understudied. This new research demonstrates this link in a large population of African Americans. The results were published in *Circulation*, a journal of the American Heart Association (AHA).

"This is an example of how NHLBI-funded research is making important advances to our basic understanding of cardiovascular risk and sleep health," said Michael Twery, Ph.D., Director of the National Center on Sleep Disorders Research (NCSDR) at the NHLBI. "This report underscores the need for studies to determine whether screening groups at high risk for sleep apnea, such as African Americans, would facilitate early medical intervention and reduce the risk or severity of heart disease."

"This study identifies a risk factor for hard-to-control hypertension that until now has gone underrecognized in African Americans," said study leader Dayna Johnson, Ph.D., an assistant professor in the Department of Epidemiology at Rollins School of Public Health at Emory University in Atlanta. Johnson added that the disproportionately high rate of uncontrolled hypertension among African Americans makes the study results even more consequential. A recent NIH-funded study showed that about 75 percent of African American men and women are likely to develop high blood pressure by the age of 55, compared to 55 percent of White men and 40 percent of White women of the same age.

Johnson noted that the current findings could provide more of an impetus for African Americans with the condition to get evaluated for sleep apnea, which also appears to affect them more than it does Whites. An estimated one in four African Americans in the United States have moderate or severe sleep apnea, but most have not been diagnosed or treated by a doctor, according to a 2018 study led by Johnson when she worked at Brigham and Women's Hospital in Boston.

In the study, the researchers followed 664 African Americans with hypertension who were participants in the Jackson Heart Study, the largest investigation of causes of cardiovascular disease (CVD) in African Americans. The researchers tested the participants for obstructive sleep apnea (OSA), the most common kind, with a special device used overnight in the home. Researchers classified sleep apnea as unaffected, mild, moderate, or severe based on the number of times a person either partially or completely stopped breathing during sleep. The tests revealed that more than a quarter of the participants had moderate or severe sleep apnea and that the condition had gone undiagnosed in almost all of them—i.e., 94 percent of the cases. The remaining participants had either no sleep apnea or a milder form of it.

The researchers also took blood pressure measurements and found that 48 percent of the participants had "uncontrolled" high blood pressure, meaning they had the condition even though they took 1 or 2 antihypertensive medications. About 14 percent had "resistant" hypertension, meaning they had the condition while on 3 or more antihypertensive medications. "Resistant" hypertension is more severe than "uncontrolled" and carries a higher risk for heart disease and death, the researchers said.

The researchers then compared measures of sleep apnea to categories of blood pressure control. Study participants with moderate or severe sleep apnea were twice as likely to have resistant hypertension when compared to participants without sleep apnea. Those with severe sleep apnea were three and a half times as likely to have resistant hypertension when compared to participants without sleep apnea. Somewhat unexpectedly, the researchers found no association between milder forms of sleep apnea and uncontrolled or resistant hypertension.

The results suggest that African Americans with more severe forms of sleep apnea are at a higher risk of having hard-to-treat hypertension, the researchers said. The current study did not explore what proportion of resistant hypertension is attributable to sleep apnea.

The study did not examine the mechanisms by which sleep apnea increases blood pressure. But Susan Redline, M.D., senior physician at Brigham and Women's Hospital and the study's senior author, said that earlier studies indicate that untreated sleep apnea can cause blood pressure to surge during sleep and remain high during the day when a patient is awake. Her earlier research showed that treatment of sleep apnea with continuous positive air pressure (CPAP) lowers blood pressure, especially during the night. CPAP and other breathing devices deliver slight air pressure through a mask and are highly effective for the treatment of sleep apnea.

Section 61.12

Explaining the Traveler's First-Night Sleep Problem

This section includes text excerpted from "Explaining the
Traveler's First-Night Sleep Problem," National Institutes
of Health (NIH), April 26, 2016.

This past weekend, you may have attended a scientific meeting in
New York. As often seems to happen to you in a hotel, you might have
tossed and turned and woke up feeling not very rested. The second
night you did a bit better. Why is this? Using advanced neuroimaging
techniques to study volunteers in a sleep lab, the National Institutes
of Health (NIH) funded researchers have come up with a biological
explanation for this phenomenon, known as the "first-night effect."

As it turns out, the first night when a person goes to sleep in a
new place, a portion of the left hemisphere of her or his brain remains
unusually active, apparently to stay alert for any signs of danger. The
findings not only provide important insights into the function of the
human brain, but they also suggest methods to prevent the first-night
effect and thereby help travelers like you in your ongoing quest to get
a good night's sleep.

The study, presented in an issue of the journal *Current Biology*, was
led by Yuka Sasaki at Brown University, Providence, RI. In the first
experiment, Sasaki and her colleagues recruited 11 young and healthy
people with normal sleep habits to monitor slow-wave brain activity,
a characteristic that reflects the depth of sleep. For 3 days before the
start of the study, participants stuck to their usual sleep schedules,
avoiding alcohol and any unusual activity.

The researchers monitored each participant's brain activity for up
to three hours on the first and second nights in the sleep lab on two
separate occasions. That allowed them to record brain waves and eye
movements, and they could track each person's stage of sleep. They
also used an advanced neuroimaging method called "magnetoenceph-
alography" (MEG) to measure slow-wave brain activity. Because MEG
is not well suited to identify detailed brain structures, the researchers
also used functional magnetic resonance imaging (fMRI) to examine
the brains of study participants while they were awake.

Sasaki and her colleagues focused their attention on four brain
regions and found something intriguing. During the first night of sleep,

445

a portion of the brain that the researchers call the "default-mode network" (DMN) showed a higher-than-normal level of activity on the left side, suggesting it was sleeping less deeply. The DMN has been described as an interconnected neural network that spans several regions of the brain. It is said to be associated with wakeful rest, such as daydreaming and just letting our minds wander.

That a portion of the brain might serve as a "night watch" is not without precedent in nature. In some animals, including marine mammals and some birds, half of the brain can be asleep, while the other half remains alert. Sasaki says that the new findings suggest that the DMN might have a similar ability, although to a lesser extent than in animals, to disengage from the primary task of sleeping and react quickly if needed.

Interestingly, this increased activity in the DMN occurred only in the brain's left hemisphere. In 2 follow-up experiments, the researchers asked whether this lighter sleep in the left side of the DMN allowed people to be more vigilant and responsive to high-pitched beeping alarms played against a background of faint beeps that they had been instructed to ignore. And, indeed, it did. A new group of 13 study participants showed bigger jumps in brain activity in response to those alarms played to their right ears (corresponding to activity in the brain's left hemisphere) on the first night of sleep when compared to the second. In a third experiment, another new group of 11 people was instructed to tap their fingers when a sound woke them. Those individuals woke up enough to tap more often and more quickly on the first night compared to the second.

All three experiments demonstrated a similar pattern of disturbed sleep on the first night in the lab compared to the second. The asymmetry in activity between the left and right brain hemispheres might explain in part why researchers had never noticed this role for the DMN. This phenomenon has likely also been missed because researchers often deal with the first-night effect by simply throwing out that early data.

Sasaki says that she is now curious to know whether this disruptive DMN activity can be knocked out to improve the first night of sleep using transcranial magnetic stimulation (TMS), a noninvasive method of brain stimulation sometimes used to improve mood and treat pain, or some other means. She would also like to look for similar asymmetries in the brain activity of people who suffer from sleep disorders, including insomnia.

Section 61.13

Sleep Duration and Injury-Related Risk Behaviors among the U.S. High-School Students

This section includes text excerpted from "Sleep Duration and Injury-Related Risk Behaviors among High School Students—United States, 2007–2013," Centers for Disease Control and Prevention (CDC), August 25, 2017.

Insufficient sleep is common among high-school students and has been associated with an increased risk for motor vehicle crashes, sports injuries, and occupational injuries. To evaluate the association between self-reported sleep duration on an average school night and several injury-related risk behaviors (infrequent bicycle helmet use, infrequent seatbelt use, riding with a driver who had been drinking, drinking and driving, and texting while driving) among U.S. high-school students, the Centers for Disease Control and Prevention (CDC) analyzed data from 50,370 high-school students (grades 9 to 12) who participated in the national Youth Risk Behavior Surveys (YRBSs) in 2007, 2009, 2011, or 2013. The likelihood of each of the 5 risk behaviors was significantly higher for students who reported sleeping less than 7 hours on an average school night; infrequent seatbelt use, riding with a drinking driver, and drinking and driving were also more likely for students who reported sleeping more than 10 hours compared with 9 hours on an average school night. Although insufficient sleep directly contributes to injury risk, some of the increased risk associated with insufficient sleep might be caused by engaging in injury-related risk behaviors. Intervention efforts aimed at these behaviors might help reduce injuries resulting from sleepiness, as well as provide opportunities for increasing awareness of the importance of sleep.

The national YRBS monitors health-risk behaviors among students in public and private high schools and is conducted by the CDC in the spring of odd-numbered years. Each national YRBS uses an independent, 3-stage cluster sample design to obtain a nationally representative sample of students in grades 9 to 12. The overall response rates were 68 percent in 2007, 71 percent in 2009, 71 percent in 2011, and 68 percent in 2013, and sample sizes ranged from 13,583 (2013) to 16,410 (2009). Students completed the anonymous, self-administered questionnaires during a single class period.

447

The combined analytic sample was composed of 50,370 high-school students who responded to questions about sleep duration on an average school night (less than 4 hours, 5 hours, 6 hours, 7 hours, 8 hours, 9 hours, more than 10 hours); demographic characteristics (sex, grade, and race/ethnicity); and how frequently they used a bicycle helmet (among students who had ridden a bicycle during the past 12 months; responses of never or rarely versus sometimes, most of the time, or always); wore a seatbelt when riding in a car driven by someone else (never or rarely versus sometimes, most of the time, or always); rode in a car or other vehicle with a driver who had been drinking alcohol (i.e., rode with a drinking driver; at least 1 time during the past 30 days versus 0 times); drove a car or other vehicle when they had been drinking alcohol (i.e., drinking and driving; at least 1 time during the past 30 days versus 0 times); or texted or emailed while driving a car or other vehicle (i.e., texting while driving; at least 1 day during the past 30 days versus 0 days). The percentage reporting insufficient sleep duration (less than 7 hours according to the Healthy People 2020 sleep objective for adolescents) and distribution of hours of sleep were calculated by survey year, sex, grade, and race/ethnicity; pairwise t-tests and analysis of variance (ANOVA) (i.e., linear trend) were used to assess crude significant differences.

Because no differences were found in mean sleep duration or prevalence of insufficient sleep duration by survey year, data from all 4 survey years were aggregated for subsequent analyses. Aggregating the data from 4 survey years provided an adequate sample size for the calculation of low prevalence risk behaviors among students reporting each category of sleep duration. The unadjusted prevalence of each risk behavior was calculated by sleep duration. Pairwise t-tests were used to assess significant differences compared with 9 hours, the median of the sleep duration recommendation for teens by the National Sleep Foundation (NSF). Logistic regression analyses were used to calculate adjusted prevalence ratios (APRs) and 95 percent confidence intervals (CIs) for the likelihood of each injury-related behavior with a referent sleep duration of 9 hours and were adjusted for sex, grade, and race/ethnicity. All analyses accounted for the sampling weights and complex survey design. P-values of less than 0.05 were defined to be statistically significant.

Reported sleep duration during an average school night was less than 4 hours for 6.3 percent of respondents, 5 hours (10.5%), 6 hours (21.9%), 7 hours (30.1%), 8 hours (23.5%), 9 hours (5.8%), and more than 10 hours (1.8%). Sleep duration varied by sex, grade, and race/ethnicity. Female students reported a higher prevalence of insufficient sleep (less than 7 hours) than did male students (71.3% versus 66.4%, p<0.001). The percentage reporting insufficient sleep ranged from 59.7 percent of students in 9th grade to 76.6 percent of students in 12th grade (p<0.001 for linear trend). Among racial/ethnic groups, the prevalence of insufficient sleep was lowest for American Indian/Alaska Native students (60.3%) and highest for Asian students (75.7%).

Overall, 86.1 percent of students reported infrequent bicycle helmet use and 8.7 percent reported infrequent seatbelt use. 26 percent of students reported riding with a drinking driver at least 1 time during the past 30 days; 8.9 percent of students reported drinking and driving; and 30.3 percent reported texting while driving during the past 30 days. Unadjusted prevalence of all 5 injury-related risk behaviors varied by sleep duration. The likelihood of each of the 5 risk behaviors was significantly higher (APR >1.0) among students with sleep durations less than 7 hours; infrequent seatbelt use, riding with drinking driver, and drinking and driving were also more likely among students reporting sleeping more than 10 hours when compared with those sleeping 9 hours. The likelihood of drinking and driving was also significantly higher among students sleeping 8 hours when compared with those sleeping 9 hours.

Section 61.14

The Concerning Link between Inadequate Sleep and Adolescent Substance Use

This section includes text excerpted from "The Concerning Link between Inadequate Sleep and Adolescent Substance Use," National Institute on Drug Abuse (NIDA), July 10, 2017.

Children and adolescents require more sleep than adults. The American Academy of Pediatrics (AAP) defines a sufficient night's sleep for an adolescent as 8.5 to 9.5 hours per night. But according to data from the national Youth Risk Behavior Survey (YRBS), just over a quarter of middle- and high-school students (27.5%) got 8 hours or more of sleep on an average night in 2015, and most got much less. Researchers have found striking links between insufficient sleep and a range of adverse outcomes in adolescents, including obesity; poor-school performance; and behavioral problems, including substance use.

For instance, a 2012 longitudinal study of youth (the average age being 14.7 years) participating in 2 Minnesota cohort studies found that less sleep—both weekday and total—at baseline was associated with more past-month cigarette and marijuana use 2 years later. An analysis of data on eighth graders from the 2010 and 2012 Fairfax County Youth Survey—an annual survey of middle- and high-school students in one of the largest school systems of the country—clearly showed that shorter sleep duration correlates with a higher incidence in several risky behaviors. For example, students who reported getting 6 hours of sleep per night were 3 times as likely to have initiated drug use than those who got 8 or 9 hours of sleep per night.

Given this striking correlation, it is important to study the neurobiological mechanisms that link insufficient sleep and substance use. Sleep-deprivation—induced impairment of emotion regulation and executive function, such as inhibitory control, is likely involved. Researchers have found that adults who are sleep deprived show reduced availability (down-regulation) of dopamine D2 receptors in part of the brain's reward circuit, the ventral striatum. Reduced availability of D2 receptors in the ventral striatum could be expected to increase the risk for behaviors such as drug use that produce large surges of dopamine to compensate for this deficit.

The researchers have also shown that reduced hours of sleep mediated the low levels of D2 receptors in individuals suffering from the cocaine-use disorder, which the laboratory and others' have shown are associated with a higher risk for compulsive drug use. The down-regulation of dopamine D2 receptors in the striatum has also been associated with impairment in prefrontal regions necessary for exerting self-control and other executive functions.

The impact of lack of sleep on dopamine receptors suggests that stimulant misuse and impaired sleep could be a vicious cycle: stimulants impair sleep, and reduced sleep produces changes in the brain that predispose to further drug use and addiction. Two-way interactions between reduced sleep and substance use are also possible with other substances. The Minnesota study, for instance, identified a bidirectional relationship between greater cigarette use and greater weekend oversleep (sleeping late on weekends to compensate for less weekday sleep) and between greater marijuana use and less total sleep.

The mechanisms underlying these relationships are still unknown, but a new longitudinal study in late-elementary schoolchildren found relationships between sleep patterns (reduced total sleep and later bedtimes and wake times on weekends) in fourth grade and cigarette or alcohol use in sixth grade, mediated by sleep-related deficits in inhibitory control.

Further research will be needed to shed more light on the links between sleep and substance use versus nonuse. For example, the 10-year longitudinal Adolescent Brain Cognitive Development (ABCD) study, now underway at 20 research sites across the country, will gather data on teens' sleep patterns, as well as substance use and other behaviors, and should be able to provide valuable insight into this issue.

From school start times that are too early to the nighttime use of computers and cell phones, today's adolescents face many challenges to getting a good night's sleep. The clear links between lack of quality sleep and risk behaviors, such as substance use, make this a crucial target for prevention efforts. Recognizing the many health risks known to be linked to poor or insufficient sleep, the AAP has pressed for later start times (no earlier than 8:30 a.m.) in middle school and high schools. Parents should be aware of how important it is for their teenage children to get a full night's sleep every night as a protective factor against substance use, as well as other adverse impacts on their health and success.

Chapter 62

Clinical Studies on Sleep and Sleep Disorders

Chapter Contents

Section 62.1

Clinical Studies Overview

This section includes text excerpted from "Learn about
Clinical Studies," ClinicalTrials.gov, National
Institutes of Health (NIH), March 2019.

What Is a Clinical Study?

A clinical study involves research using human volunteers (also
called "participants") that is intended to add to medical knowledge.
There are two main types of clinical studies: clinical trials (also called
"interventional studies") and observational studies.

Clinical Trials

In a clinical trial, participants receive specific interventions according to the research plan or protocol created by the investigators. These
interventions may be medical products, such as drugs or devices; procedures; or changes to participants' behavior, such as diet. Clinical
trials may compare a new medical approach to a standard one that is
already available, to a placebo that contains no active ingredients, or
to no intervention. Some clinical trials compare interventions that are
already available to each other. When a new product or approach is
being studied, it is not usually known whether it will be helpful, harmful, or no different than available alternatives (including no intervention). The investigators try to determine the safety and efficacy of the
intervention by measuring certain outcomes in the participants. For
example, investigators may give a drug or treatment to participants
who have high blood pressure to see whether their blood pressure
decreases.

Clinical trials used in drug development are sometimes described
by phase. These phases are defined by the U.S. Food and Drug Administration (FDA). Some people who are not eligible to participate in a
clinical trial may be able to get experimental drugs or devices outside
of a clinical trial through expanded access.

Observational Studies

In an observational study, investigators assess health outcomes in
groups of participants according to a research plan or protocol. Participants may receive interventions (which can include medical products,

such as drugs or devices) or procedures as part of their routine medical care, but participants are not assigned to specific interventions by the investigator (as in a clinical trial). For example, investigators may observe a group of older adults to learn more about the effects of different lifestyles on cardiac health.

Who Conducts Clinical Studies

Every clinical study is led by a principal investigator, who is often a medical doctor. Clinical studies also have a research team that may include doctors, nurses, social workers, and other healthcare professionals.

Clinical studies can be sponsored, or funded, by pharmaceutical companies, academic medical centers, voluntary groups, and other organizations, in addition to federal agencies, such as the National Institutes of Health (NIH), the U.S. Department of Defense (DoD), and the U.S. Department of Veterans Affairs (VA). Doctors, other healthcare providers, and other individuals can also sponsor clinical research.

Where Are Clinical Studies Conducted?

Clinical studies can take place in many locations, including hospitals, universities, doctors' offices, and community clinics. The location depends on who is conducting the study.

How Long Do Clinical Studies Last?

The length of a clinical study varies, depending on what is being studied. Participants are told how long the study will last before they enroll.

Reasons for Conducting Clinical Studies

In general, clinical studies are designed to add to medical knowledge related to the treatment, diagnosis, and prevention of diseases or conditions. Some common reasons for conducting clinical studies include:

- Evaluating one or more interventions (for example, drugs, medical devices, approaches to surgery or radiation therapy) for treating a disease, syndrome, or condition

- Finding ways to prevent the initial development or recurrence of a disease or condition. These can include medicines, vaccines, or lifestyle changes, among other approaches.

- Evaluating one or more interventions aimed at identifying or diagnosing a particular disease or condition

- Examining methods for identifying a condition or the risk factors for that condition

- Exploring and measuring ways to improve the comfort and quality of life (QOL) through supportive care for people with a chronic illness

Participating in Clinical Studies

A clinical study is conducted according to a research plan known as the "protocol." The protocol is designed to answer specific research questions and safeguard the health of participants. It contains the following information:

- The reason for conducting the study

- Who may participate in the study (the eligibility criteria)

- The number of participants needed

- The schedule of tests, procedures, or drugs and their dosages

- The length of the study

- What information will be gathered about the participants

Who Can Participate in a Clinical Study?

Clinical studies have standards outlining who can participate. These standards are called "eligibility criteria" and are listed in the protocol. Some research studies seek participants who have the illnesses or conditions that will be studied, other studies are looking for healthy participants, and some studies are limited to a predetermined group of people who are asked by researchers to enroll.

Eligibility. The factors that allow someone to participate in a clinical study are called "inclusion criteria," and the factors that disqualify someone from participating are called "exclusion criteria." They are based on characteristics, such as age, gender, the type and stage of a disease, previous treatment history, and other medical conditions.

How Are Participants Protected?

Informed consent is a process used by researchers to provide potential and enrolled participants with information about a clinical study.

This information helps people decide whether they want to enroll or continue to participate in the study. The informed consent process is intended to protect participants and should provide enough information for a person to understand the risks of, potential benefits of, and alternatives to the study. In addition to the informed consent document, the process may involve recruitment materials, verbal instructions, question-and-answer sessions, and activities to measure participant understanding. In general, a person must sign an informed consent document before joining a study to show that she or he was given information on the risks, potential benefits, and alternatives and that she or he understands it. Signing the document and providing consent is not a contract. Participants may withdraw from a study at any time, even if the study is not over.

Institutional review boards. Each federally supported or conducted clinical study and each study of a drug, biological product, or medical device regulated by FDA must be reviewed, approved, and monitored by an institutional review board (IRB). An IRB is made up of doctors, researchers, and members of the community. Its role is to make sure that the study is ethical and that the rights and welfare of participants are protected. This includes making sure that research risks are minimized and are reasonable in relation to any potential benefits, among other responsibilities. The IRB also reviews the informed consent document.

In addition to being monitored by an IRB, some clinical studies are also monitored by data monitoring committees (also called "data safety and monitoring boards").

Various federal agencies, including the Office of Human Subjects Research Protection (OHRP) and the FDA, have the authority to determine whether sponsors of certain clinical studies are adequately protecting research participants.

Relationship to Usual Healthcare

Typically, participants continue to see their usual healthcare providers while enrolled in a clinical study. While most clinical studies provide participants with medical products or interventions related to the illness or condition being studied, they do not provide extended or complete healthcare. By having her or his usual healthcare provider work with the research team, a participant can make sure that the study protocol will not conflict with other medications or treatments that she or he receives.

Considerations for Participation

Participating in a clinical study contributes to medical knowledge. The results of these studies can make a difference in the care of future patients by providing information about the benefits and risks of therapeutic, preventative, or diagnostic products or interventions.

Clinical trials provide the basis for the development and marketing of new drugs, biological products, and medical devices. Sometimes, the safety and the effectiveness of the experimental approach or use may not be fully known at the time of the trial. Some trials may provide participants with the prospect of receiving direct medical benefits, while others do not. Most trials involve some risk of harm or injury to the participant, although it may not be greater than the risks related to routine medical care or disease progression. (For trials approved by IRBs, the IRB has decided that the risks of participation have been minimized and are reasonable in relation to anticipated benefits.) Many trials require participants to undergo additional procedures, tests, and assessments based on the study protocol. These requirements will be described in the informed consent document. A potential participant should also discuss these issues with members of the research team and with her or his usual healthcare provider.

Questions to Ask

Anyone interested in participating in a clinical study should know as much as possible about the study and feel comfortable asking the research team questions about the study, the related procedures, and any expenses. The following questions may be helpful during such a discussion. Answers to some of these questions are provided in the informed consent document. Many of the questions are specific to clinical trials, but some also apply to observational studies.

- What is being studied?
- Why do researchers believe the intervention being tested might be effective? Why might it not be effective? Has it been tested before?
- What are the possible interventions that I might receive during the trial?
- How will it be determined which interventions I receive (for example, by chance)?

- Who will know which intervention I receive during the trial? Will I know? Will members of the research team know?

- How do the possible risks, side effects, and benefits of this trial compare with those of my current treatment?

- What will I have to do?

- What tests and procedures are involved?

- How often will I have to visit the hospital or clinic?

- Will hospitalization be required?

- How long will the study last?

- Who will pay for my participation?

- Will I be reimbursed for other expenses?

- What type of long-term follow-up care is part of this trial?

- If I benefit from the intervention, will I be allowed to continue receiving it after the trial ends?

- Will results of the study be provided to me?

- Who will oversee my medical care while I am participating in the trial?

- What are my options if I am injured during the study?

Section 62.2

Evaluation of the Reliability and Validity of a Diagnostic Sleep Disorders Questionnaire

This section includes text excerpted from "Evaluation of
the Reliability and Validity of a Diagnostic Sleep Disorders
Questionnaire," ClinicalTrials.gov, National Institutes
of Health (NIH), May 17, 2019.

Purpose

The study aims to develop and test a user-friendly, accessible approach to sleep assessment which can function as an initial "triage" of targeted sleep conditions, such as insomnia, insufficient sleep syndrome, sleep apnea syndromes/snoring, and circadian sleep-wake disorders, within the clinical and community population. Specifically, this study will test the validity and reliability of a self-rated, digitized, and cost-effective diagnostic measure with sufficient sensitivity to accurately assess/diagnose common sleep conditions and/or risk for these conditions. Such an approach, would allow for faster assessment of common sleep conditions and disorders, and provide clinical knowledge to the individual, the physician, and if required insurance companies, as to those persons who need more immediate attention or treatment for their sleep condition.

Eligibility Criteria

1. Ages eligible for study: 21 years to 65 years (adult, older adult)

2. Sexes eligible for study: All

3. Accepts healthy volunteers: Yes

4. Sampling method: Nonprobability sample

Study Population

A general community population and clinical population physician-referred for diagnosis and assessment of sleep disorders at a sleep clinic within a large medical center.

Criteria
Inclusion Criteria

Patients aged 21 to 65 years who are referred to the sleep clinic at Carmel Medical Center and who are capable of filling out an electronic questionnaire in Hebrew.

Exclusion Criteria

1. Patient age younger than 21 years or older than 65 years

2. Women who are pregnant or breastfeeding

3. Nighttime shift-workers

4. Persons who are unable to provide consent due to mental incapacity

5. Persons referred for evaluation by Ministry of Transportation (for licensing purposes)

Section 62.3

Physiologic Effects of Sleep Restriction

This section includes text excerpted from "Physiologic Effects of Sleep Restriction," ClinicalTrials.gov, National Institutes of Health (NIH), March 22, 2019.

Purpose

Evidence suggests a relationship between sleep deprivation and cardiovascular disease. Voluntary sleep restriction is common, with 28 percent of the U.S. adult population reports getting six or fewer hours of sleep per night, and those who do are 24 percent more likely to have cardiovascular disease and have twice the risk of hypertension. Insufficient sleep may conceivably be one of the most common, and most preventable, cardiovascular risk factors. The investigators wish to determine whether 9 nights of modest sleep restriction results in activation of cardiovascular disease mechanisms, thus potentially increasing the risk of cardiovascular disease. The investigators will combine our cardiovascular studies with state-of-the-art sleep monitoring and neurocognitive tests to provide unambiguous data on the physiologic effects of sleep restriction. Together, the investigators findings will help explain whether the reduced sleep duration in the general population may be contributing to the current epidemic of cardiovascular disease, and suggest strategies to reduce this risk.

Eligibility Criteria

1. Ages eligible for study: 18 to 40 years (adult)
2. Sexes eligible for study: All
3. Accepts healthy volunteers: Yes

Criteria
Inclusion Criteria

- Age 18 to 40 years

- No chronic medical conditions other than seasonal or environmental allergies

- On no prescription medications other than second generation antihistamines (Cetirizine, Fexofenadine, Desloratadine, Loratadine, etc.), oral contraceptive pills, or intrauterine devices.

- Body mass index (BMI) of 18.5 to 35 kg/m^2

- Both normotensive and prehypertensive people are eligible and will be studied

- Not a current smoker or tobacco user

- Not pregnant or breastfeeding and not intending to become pregnant or breastfeed

Exclusion Criteria

- The investigators will exclude subjects who have any medical or psychiatric disorders.

- History of anxiety or depression, and those taking any medications other than nonsedating antihistamines or oral contraceptives.

- Those found to have depression on a depression screening tool (BDI-II) will be excluded. Current smokers will be excluded.

- All female subjects will undergo a screening pregnancy test and excluded if positive.

- Subjects found to have significant sleep disorders will be excluded.

Section 62.4

Changes in Sleep Duration and Blood Pressure across School Holiday in Teenagers

This section includes text excerpted from "Changes in Sleep Duration and Blood Pressure across School Holiday in Teenagers," ClinicalTrials.gov, National Institutes of Health (NIH), March 29, 2019.

Purpose

In this study, the investigators will take advantage of changes in sleep duration that occur during school holidays in adolescents who are sleep deprived (more than 6 months' history of sleeping, less than 8 hours per night during school term). The investigators will monitor the changes in ambulatory BP and sleep duration over a period of 3 weeks which consist of a week at school, followed by a week of holiday when natural sleep extension takes place, and then another week of school after the holiday. The sleep–wake cycle will be recorded throughout the whole study period with actigraphy and sleep diary. 24-hour ambulatory BP monitoring will be performed on the same weekday during each study week, when salivary cortisol will also be collected. The primary outcome measure is the difference in ambulatory BP parameters between school term and holiday. A control group without sleep deprivation (history of sleeping more than 8 hours per night) will also be studied concurrently.

It is hypothesized that changes in sleep duration are negatively associated with changes in BP. If this study confirms this hypothesis, sleep extension can be used as a relatively inexpensive and simple behavioral intervention in the management and prevention of blood pressure abnormalities. More importantly positive results from this project will provide background information on which government and local school policy can be based and altered for the betterment of our youths.

Eligibility Criteria

1. Ages eligible for study: 10 to 18 years (child, adult)
2. Sexes eligible for study: All
3. Accepts healthy volunteers: Yes
4. Sampling method: Nonprobability sample

Study Population

Subjects will be recruited from local primary and secondary schools. The invitation letters will be sent to Principals to ask them for their help with screening questionnaire distribution and assessment arrangements in their school. The screening questionnaire asks about children sleep pattern during school terms and holidays, sleep-related symptoms (e.g., snoring), and medical history to see whether they are eligible to participate. Eligible subjects will receive the study factsheet and written informed consent form. Subjects with parental consent will be enrolled in the study.

Criteria
Inclusion Criteria

General Inclusion Criteria

- Adolescents aged between 10 to 18 years
- Written informed consent and assent obtained from parents and adolescents

Inclusion Criteria Specific for the Sleep Deprived Group

- Self-reported time in bed (period from bedtime to get-up time) during school days of less than 8 hours per day
- Self-perceived insufficient sleep during school days

Inclusion Criteria Specific for the Normal Sleep Group

- Self-reported time in bed during school days of more than or equal to 8 hours per day

- Self-perceived sufficient sleep during school days

Exclusion Criteria

- Obesity, which is defined as a body mass index (BMI) ≥95th percentile (corresponding to a z score of 1.645) of the local reference

- Subjects who have a sleep disorder, for example insomnia, and/ or currently receiving treatment for sleep problems

- Known medical or psychiatric conditions or use of current medication that may affect sleep and blood pressure

Section 62.5

Aspects Associated with Sleep Quality

This section includes text excerpted from "Aspects Associated with Sleep Quality," ClinicalTrials.gov, National Institutes of Health (NIH), December 6, 2018.

Purpose

This study will evaluate the correlation between sleep bruxism and sleep quality diagnoses obtained using the application of the smartphone (APP-Sleep Cycle®), polysomnography and questionnaires (Pittsburgh Sleep Quality Index-IQSP and Johansson). Subjects (n=40) between 19 and 60 years old will be submitted to polysomnography from January to December 2019. The questionnaires will be applied before the polysomnography, and the APP will be used together with the polysomnography. The data will be tabulated and a descriptive statistical analysis performed. Specific statistical tests will be determined after preliminary analysis of the data ($\alpha=0.05$).

Eligibility Criteria

1. Ages eligible for study: 20 to 60 years (adult)

2. Sexes eligible for study: All

3. Accepts healthy volunteers: Yes

4. Sampling method: Probability sample

Study Population

All adults (aged 20 to 60 years) and elderly (60 years of age or older) who had undergone PSG at the Pelotas Sleep Institute (ISP), a private medical outpatients clinic, from January to December 2019, will be invited to participate in the study.

Eligibility criteria include adequate cognitive capacity to understand and answer the questionnaire. Written consent will be given by all participants who agreed to participate in the study.

Criteria
Inclusion Criteria

• Adults (aged 20 to 60 years) and elderly (60 years of age or older) (WHO-World Health Organization, 2015) who will be undergone PSG at the Pelotas Sleep Institute (ISP)

• Adequate cognitive capacity to understand and answer the questionnaire

Exclusion Criteria

• Those which the participants were unable to answer the questionnaires and who presented a history of epilepsy that could interfere in the results of PSG.

Section 62.6

The Poweroff Sleep Study

This section includes text excerpted from "The Poweroff
Sleep Study," ClinicalTrials.gov, National Institutes of
Health (NIH), May 22, 2018.

Purpose

The primary objective is to explore the relationship between experimental condition (placebo or Poweroff) and sleep quality between pre- and post-study. In addition, volunteers will wear actigraphy watches that collect objective measures of sleep, such as total sleep time, and these data points will be compared pre- and post-study.

Eligibility Criteria

1. Ages eligible for study: 18 years to 65 years (adult, older adult)

2. Sexes eligible for study: All

3. Accepts healthy volunteers: Yes

Criteria
Inclusion Criteria

- **Sleep-wake history.** Participants must currently maintain a regular sleep/wake schedule (±2 hr average bedtime) and express willingness to continue to follow a regular sleep–wake schedule.

- **Drug/alcohol use.** Participants must be drug-free (including nicotine). No medications (prescription or over the counter) that significantly affect circadian rhythms or sleep are allowed. Subjects must report no history of drug or alcohol dependency to be included in the study.

- **Evaluation of medical suitability.** Only healthy men and women are to be selected for this study. Subjects will be free from any acute, chronic, or debilitating medical conditions. Normality will be established on the basis of self-report clinical history and diagnoses/. Any subject with symptoms of active illness, such as fever, infection, or hypertension, will be excluded.

- **Evaluation of psychiatric/psychological suitability.**
  Individuals with a history of psychiatric illnesses or psychiatric
  disorders will be excluded. Individuals who are unaware of
  specific psychiatric diagnoses but had a history of treatment
  with antidepressant, neuroleptic medications, or major
  tranquilizers will be excluded from the study. Subjects will also
  be questioned to demonstrate their full understanding of the
  requirements, demands, and risks of the study and informed of
  the option to withdraw at any time.

Exclusion Criteria

- Older adults are known to experience decreased depth of
  nonrapid eye movement sleep (non-REM), as well as lesser
  amounts of deep sleep (NREM3), They, therefore, spend greater
  amounts of their sleep time in less protected lighter sleep stages.
  For these reasons, older adults (above age 65) will be excluded
  from the study.

- Individuals whom have had a negative or paradoxical response
  to an over-the-counter (OTC) sleep supplement or OTC sleep
  medication (Nyquil zzz's, Benadryl, melatonin, valerian, etc.).

- Individuals who are or are planning to become pregnant in the
  next 60 days

Section 62.7

Characterizing Sleep Disorders in Children and Adults with Tuberous Sclerosis Complex

This section includes text excerpted from "Characterizing Sleep Disorders in Children and Adults with Tuberous Sclerosis Complex (TSC)," ClinicalTrials.gov, National Institutes of Health (NIH), October 17, 2018.

Purpose

The proposed research project is aimed at further characterization of sleep problems and evaluation of their impact in children and adults with TSC, excluding epilepsy as contributing factor. Questionnaire-based studies have shown that sleep problems occur in up to half of the children and a third of adults with tuberous sclerosis complex (TSC). However, there is only limited information on the nature of sleep problems and their impact on patients with TSC and their families.

Questionnaire-based studies have shown that sleep problems occur in up to half of the children and a third of adults with tuberous sclerosis complex (TSC). However, there is only limited information on the nature of sleep problems and their impact on patients with TSC and their families. It is known from a questionnaire-based study in children with TSC that they often wake early or wake frequently during the night, and that they can be more tired during the day. In some children, sleep-problems seem to be related to the presence of seizures during the night. This has been confirmed in a study on 10 children with TSC and epilepsy by a combination of polysomnography (sleep study) and electroencephalography (EEG). A questionnaire-based study in adults also revealed the association with epilepsy features, and showed influence of mental-health complaints on sleep.

Sleep structure and quality will be assessed through formal sleep studies (polysomnography and actigraphy). The influence of abnormal brain activity on sleep will be mapped by simultaneous recording of brain activity by means of EEG. The impact of sleep disorders will be determined through interviews with individuals with TSC and their relatives. The investigators will also use questionnaires and diaries to supplement their findings.

It is expected that the results of this study will:

* Improve the understanding of sleep problems in TSC.

- Provide additional information on the influence of TSC on sleep.

- Give a more in-depth view on the impact of sleep problems on the lives of individuals with TSC and their families.

- Increase awareness about sleep problems in TSC.

- Contribute to a better management of sleep problems by patients and families.

Eligibility Criteria

Ages eligible for study: Up to 70 years (child, adult, older adult)
Sexes eligible for study: All
Accepts healthy volunteers: Yes

Criteria
Inclusion Criteria

Children and adults with definite TSC, based on the 2012 Consensus Conference Diagnostic

Exclusion Criteria

- Daily alcohol intake

- Pregnancy

- Caffeine abuse (more than four cups a day)

- Shift work

- Drug abuse

- Antidepressive therapy

- Medications, such as benzodiazepine, melatonin, phenobarbital and antihistamines

- The presence of clinical or electrographic

Section 62.8

Sleep Disorders in Transient Ischemic Attack and Stroke: SOMN'AIC Study

This section includes text excerpted from "Sleep Disorders in Transient Ischemic Attack and Stroke: SOMN'AIC Study (SOMN'AIC)," ClinicalTrials.gov, National Institutes of Health (NIH), February 5, 2018.

Purpose

Sleep disorders in the setting of stroke are numerous, including sleep-related breathing disorders, insomnia, excessive daytime sleepiness and restless legs syndrome. Consequences of these sleep disturbances include impaired functional outcome and quality of life, anxious and depressive troubles and increased cardiovascular morbi-mortality. Mechanisms underlying sleep disorders in the setting of stroke are complex and still partly elucidated. They probably involve the consequences of the ischemic lesion and of the handicap, but also of associated vascular risk factors and more generally preexistent medical history, or they could represent themselves a risk factor for stroke. Transient ischemic attack (TIA) is a particular condition in which risk factors and background of patients are similar to that observed in stroke, without any cerebral lesion and no persistent neurological deficit. The main objective of the SOMN'AIC study is to compare the prevalence of sleep disorders in stroke and in transient ischemic attack (TIA). The study hypothesis is that the prevalence of sleep disorders may be higher in stroke than in TIA patients, reflecting the consequences of the lesion and the associated handicap.

Eligibility Criteria

1. Ages eligible for study: 18 years and older (adult, older adult)

2. Sexes eligible for study: All

3. Accepts healthy volunteers: No

4. Sampling method: Nonprobability sample

Study Population

Stroke and transient ischemic attack (TIA) patients

471

Criteria

Inclusion Criteria

- Stroke group: patients with a diagnosis of stroke and seen at the routine poststroke three month' rehabilitation examination
- TIA group: diagnosis of a TIA by a stroke specialist at the "SOS TIA" examination
- Older than 18 years of age

Exclusion Criteria

- Refusal to participate
- Severe cognitive impairment leading to inability to fulfill questionnaires
- For the TIA group: presence of an ischemic lesion on CT scan or MRI

Part Eight

Additional Help and Information

Chapter 63

Glossary of Terms Related to Sleep Disorders

acupuncture: A technique in which practitioners stimulate specific points on the body—most often by inserting thin needles through the skin. It is one of the practices used in traditional Chinese medicine.

alcohol: A chemical substance found in drinks such as beer, wine, and liquor. It is also found in some medicines, mouthwashes, household products, and essential oils (scented liquid taken from certain plants). It is made by a chemical process called "fermentation" that uses sugars and yeast.

allergy: A condition in which the body has an exaggerated response to a substance (e.g., food or drug). Also known as hypersensitivity.

addiction: A chronic, relapsing disease characterized by compulsive drug seeking and use despite serious adverse consequences, and by long-lasting changes in the brain.

antibiotic: A drug that kills or stops the growth of bacteria. Antibiotics are a type of antimicrobial. Penicillin and ciprofloxacin are examples of antibiotics.

anticonvulsant: A drug or other substance used to prevent or stop seizures or convulsions. Also called antiepileptic.

This glossary contains terms excerpted from documents produced by several sources deemed reliable.

antidepressant: A name for a category of medications used to treat depression.

antigen: Any substance that causes the body to make an immune response against that substance. Antigens include toxins, chemicals, bacteria, viruses, or other substances that come from outside the body.

antihistamine: Drugs that are used to prevent or relieve the symptoms of hay fever and other allergies by preventing the action of a substance called histamine, which is produced by the body. Histamine can cause itching, sneezing, runny nose, watery eyes, and sometimes can make breathing difficult. Some of these drugs are also used to prevent motion sickness, nausea, vomiting, and dizziness. Since they may cause drowsiness as a side effect, some of them may be used to help people go to sleep.

apnea: Cessation of breathing.

arthritis: A term used to describe more than 100 rheumatic diseases and conditions that affect joints, the tissues which surround the joint and other connective tissue.

assessment: The process of gathering evidence and documentation of a student's learning.

asthma: A chronic disease in which the bronchial airways in the lungs become narrowed and swollen, making it difficult to breathe.

benzodiazepine: A central nervous system depressant.

biological clock: It times and controls a person's sleep–wake cycle will attempt to function according to a normal day/night schedule even when that person tries to change it.

biomarkers: A biological molecule found in blood, other body fluids, or tissues that is a sign of a normal or abnormal process, or of a condition or disease.

bladder: The organ in the human body that stores urine. It is found in the lower part of the abdomen.

bruxism: A movement disorder characterized by grinding and clenching of teeth.

calcium: A mineral that is an essential nutrient for bone health. It is also needed for the heart, muscles, and nerves to function properly and for blood to clot.

calorie: A unit of energy in food. Carbohydrates, fats, protein, and alcohol in the foods and drinks we eat provide food energy or "calories."

cancer: A term for diseases in which abnormal cells in the body divide without control. Cancer cells can invade nearby tissues and can spread to other parts of the body through the blood and lymphatic system, which is a network of tissues that clears infections and keeps body fluids in balance.

cataplexy: A sudden loss of motor tone and strength.

central sleep apnea: It is caused by irregularities in the brain's normal signals to breathe.

central nervous system (CNS): Comprised of the nerves in the brain and spinal cord. These nerves are used to send electrical impulses throughout the body, resulting in voluntary and reflexive movement. Information about the environment is received by the senses and sent to the central nervous system, which causes the body to respond appropriately.

chronic insomnia: A condition in which sleep problems occur at least 3 nights a week for more than a month.

circadian rhythms: Are physical, mental and behavioral changes that follow a roughly 24-hour cycle, responding primarily to light and darkness in an organism's environment.

clinical trial: A research study in which one or more human subjects are prospectively assigned to one or more interventions (which may include placebo or other control) to evaluate the effects of those interventions on health-related biomedical or behavioral outcomes.

cognitive-behavioral therapy: A blend of two therapies cognitive therapy (CT) and behavioral therapy. It focuses on a person's thoughts and beliefs, and how they influence a person's mood and actions, and aims to change a person's thinking to be more adaptive and healthy.

complementary and alternative medicine (CAM): It is the term for medical products and practices that are not part of standard medical care.

continuous positive airway pressure: A treatment that uses mild air pressure to keep the airways open.

corticosteroids: Powerful anti-inflammatory hormones made naturally in the body or human-made for use as medicine. Corticosteroids may be injected into the affected joints to temporarily reduce inflammation and relieve pain.

culture: A test to see whether there are tuberculosis (TB) bacteria in your phlegm or other body fluids. This test can take 2 to 4 weeks in most laboratories.

diabetes: A disease in which blood glucose (blood sugar) levels are above or below normal.

diet: What a person eats and drinks. Any type of eating plan.

dopamine: A neurotransmitter present in regions of the brain that regulate movement, emotion, motivation, and feelings of pleasure.

enuresis: Involuntary urination during sleep.

enzyme: A protein that speeds up chemical reactions in the body.

exercise: A type of physical activity that involves planned, structured, and repetitive bodily movement done to maintain or improve one or more components of physical fitness.

exposure: Contact with infectious agents (bacteria or viruses) in a manner that promotes transmission and increases the likelihood of disease.

genes: Genes, which are made up of deoxyribonucleic acid (DNA), are the basic units that define the characteristics of every organism. Genes carry information that determine traits, such as eye color in humans and resistance to antibiotics in bacteria.

genetics: The study of particular genes, deoxyribonucleic acid (DNA), and heredity.

genome: A genome is an organism's complete set of genes that carry the genetic instructions for building and maintaining that organism.

hormone: Substance produced by one tissue and conveyed by the bloodstream to another to affect a function of the body, such as growth or metabolism.

hypersomnia: A complaint of excessive daytime sleep or sleepiness.

hypertension: Also called high blood pressure, it is having blood pressure greater than 140 over 90 mmHg (millimeters of mercury). Long-term high blood pressure can damage blood vessels and organs, including the heart, kidneys, eyes, and brain.

hypnosis: A trance-like state in which a person becomes more aware and focused on particular thoughts, feelings, images, sensations, or behaviors.

hypothalamus: The area of the brain that controls body temperature, hunger, and thirst.

immune system: A complex system of cellular and molecular components having the primary function of distinguishing self from not self and defense against foreign organisms or substances.

immunity: Protection against a disease. Immunity is indicated by the presence of antibodies in the blood and can usually be determined with a laboratory test.

inflammation: Redness, swelling, heat, and pain resulting from injury to tissue (parts of the body underneath the skin). Also known as swelling.

insomnia: Not being able to sleep.

jet lag: A sleep disorder caused by traveling across different time zones.

Kleine-Levin syndrome: Is characterized by recurring but reversible periods of excessive sleep.

lesion: An area of abnormal tissue. A lesion may be benign (not cancer) or malignant (cancer).

light therapy: It is used treat seasonal affective disorder.

melatonin: A natural hormone that plays a role in sleep.

metabolism: The chemical changes that take place in a cell or an organism. These changes make energy and the materials cells and organisms need to grow, reproduce, and stay healthy. Metabolism also helps get rid of toxic substances.

multiple sleep latency test (MSLT): A daytime sleep study measures how sleepy you are. It typically is done the day after a PSG.

muscles: Bundles of specialized cells that contract and relax to produce movement when stimulated by nerves.

mutation: A change in a DNA sequence that can result from DNA copying mistakes made during cell division, exposure to ionizing radiation, exposure to chemical mutagens, or infection by viruses.

narcolepsy: A disorder that causes periods of extreme daytime sleepiness. The disorder also may cause muscle weakness.

neuron: A nerve cell that is the basic, working unit of the brain and nervous system, which processes and transmits information.

nightmare: A bad dream that brings out strong feelings of fear, terror, distress, or anxiety.

nocturia: Frequent urination of 2 or more times per night.

non-REM sleep: Stages of sleep ranging from light sleep to deep sleep.

nutrition: The taking in and use of food and other nourishing material by the body. Nutrition is a three-part process. First, food or drink is consumed. Second, the body breaks down the food or drink into nutrients.

obesity: Obesity refers to excess body fat. Because body fat is usually not measured directly, a ratio of body weight to height is often used instead.

obstructive sleep apnea (syndrome): In this condition, the airway collapses or becomes blocked during sleep.

organ: A part of the body that performs a specific function. For example, the heart is an organ.

organism: Any living thing, including humans, animals, plants, and microbes.

osteoarthritis: The most common form of arthritis. It is characterized by the breakdown of joint cartilage, leading to pain, stiffness, and disability.

over-the-counter (OTC): Diseases, including ulcerative colitis (UC) and Crohn disease, that cause swelling in the intestine and/or digestive tract, which may result in diarrhea, abdominal pain, fever, and weight loss. People with inflammatory bowel disease (IBD) are at an increased risk for osteoporosis.

overweight: Overweight refers to an excessive amount of body weight that includes muscle, bone, fat, and water. A person who has a body mass index (BMI) of 25 to 29.9 is considered overweight.

parasomnia: It is defined as undesirable behavioral, physiological, or experiential events that accompany sleep.

perception (hearing): Process of knowing or being aware of information through the ear.

periodic limb movement disorder: Causes repetitive jerking movements of the limbs, especially the legs. These movements occur every 20 to 40 seconds and cause repeated awakening and severely fragmented sleep.

physical activity: Any bodily movement that is produced by the contraction of skeletal muscle and that substantially increases energy expenditure.

polysomnogram: A sleep study that records brain activity, eye movements, heart rate, and blood pressure.

pregnancy: The condition between conception (fertilization of an egg by a sperm) and birth, during which the fertilized egg develops in the uterus. In humans, pregnancy lasts about 288 days.

prevalence: The number of disease cases (new and existing) within a population over a given time period.

prevention: Actions that reduce exposure or other risks, keep people from getting sick, or keep disease from getting worse.

prognosis: The likely outcome or course of a disease; the chance of recovery or recurrence.

protein: A molecule made up of amino acids. Proteins are needed for the body to function properly. They are the basis of body structures, such as skin and hair, and of other substances such as enzymes, cytokines, and antibodies.

quarantine: The isolation of a person or animal who has a disease (or is suspected of having a disease) in order to prevent further spread of the disease.

radiation: Energy moving in the form of particles or waves. Familiar radiations are heat, light, radio, and microwaves.

REM sleep: It is the active or paradoxic phase of sleep in which the brain is active.

restless legs syndrome: A disorder that causes a powerful urge to move your legs. Your legs become uncomfortable when you are lying down or sitting. Some people describe it as a creeping, crawling, tingling or burning sensation. Moving makes your legs feel better, but not for long.

rheumatoid arthritis: A form of arthritis in which the immune system attacks the tissues of the joints, leading to pain, inflammation, and eventually joint damage and malformation. It typically begins at a younger age than osteoarthritis does, causes swelling and redness in joints, and may make people feel sick, tired, and feverish. Rheumatoid arthritis may also affect skin tissue, the lungs, the eyes, or the blood vessels.

seasonal affective disorder (SAD): A type of depression that occurs at a certain time of the year, usually in winter.

sedative: A drug that calms a person and allows her or him to sleep.

seizure: The sudden onset of a jerking or staring spell. Many seizures following a vaccination are caused by fever. Seizures are also known as convulsions.

serotonin: A neurotransmitter that regulates many functions, including mood, appetite, and sleep.

sleep apnea: A disorder involving brief interruptions of breathing during sleep.

sleep cycle: It is defined by a segment of nonrapid eye movement (non-REM) sleep followed by a period of rapid eye movement (REM) sleep.

sleep debt: It develops when daily sleep time is less than an individual needs.

sleep deprivation: Sleep deprivation is a condition that occurs if you do not get enough sleep.

sleep hygiene: The promotion of regular sleep is known as sleep hygiene.

sleep medicine: The specialty concerned with conditions characterized by disturbances of usual sleep patterns or behaviors.

sleepwalking: Refers to doing other activities when you are asleep like eating, talking, or driving a car.

snoring: Snoring is an example of sleep-disordered breathing – a condition that makes it more difficult to breathe during sleep.

sodium: A mineral and an essential nutrient needed by the human body in relatively small amounts (provided that substantial sweating does not occur).

stage 2 sleep: When we enter stage 2 sleep, our eye movements stop and our brain waves (fluctuations of electrical activity that can be measured by electrodes) become slower, with occasional bursts of rapid waves called sleep spindles.

stage 3 sleep: In stage 3, extremely slow brain waves called delta waves begin to appear, interspersed with smaller and faster waves.

steroid: Any of a group of lipids (fats) that have a certain chemical structure. Steroids occur naturally in plants and animals or they may be made in the laboratory.

stimulant: Stimulants increase alertness, attention, and energy, as well as elevate blood pressure, heart rate, and respiration.

stroke: Also known as a cerebrovascular accident (CVA); caused by a lack of blood to the brain, resulting in the sudden loss of speech, language, or the ability to move a body part, and, if severe enough, death.

tobacco: A plant with leaves that have high levels of the addictive chemical nicotine. After harvesting, tobacco leaves are cured, aged, and processed in various ways. The resulting products may be smoked (in cigarettes, cigars, and pipes), applied to the gums (as dipping and chewing tobacco), or inhaled (as snuff).

vaccine: A product made from very small amounts of weak or dead germs that can cause diseases — for example, viruses, bacteria, or toxins. It prepares your body to fight the disease faster and more effectively so you won't get sick. Vaccines are administered through needle injections, by mouth, and by aerosol.

yoga: A mind and body practice with origins in ancient Indian philosophy. The various styles of yoga typically combine physical postures, breathing techniques, and meditation or relaxation.

Chapter 64

Web-Based Resources for People with Sleep Problems

Baby Sleep Basics

BabyCenter
BabyCenter provides parents with trusted information, advice from peers, and support that is Remarkably Right® at every stage of their child's development. Products include websites, mobile apps, online communities, e-mail series, social programs, print publications, and public-health initiatives.
Website: www.babycenter.com/baby-sleep-basics

Basics of Sleep Problems in Children

American Sleep Association
The American Sleep Association (ASA) is a group of sleep professionals seeking to improve public health by increasing awareness of the importance of sleep in ensuring a high quality of life, as well as the dangers of sleep disorders.
Website: www.sleepassociation.org/about-sleep

Resources in this chapter were compiled from multiple sources deemed reliable. This list is intended as a starting point only, and it is not comprehensive. Inclusion does not constitute endorsement and there is no implication associated with omission. All website information was verified and updated in May 2019.

Can't You Sleep?

Sleep Psychologist and Insomnia Therapy
Stephanie Silberman, Ph.D., FAASM, is a licensed psychologist who is a Fellow of the American Academy of Sleep Medicine. She is active in professional organizations and legislative activities affecting psychology and sleep disorders, including two terms as President of the Broward Chapter of the Florida Psychological Association (FPA) and past co-chair of the Legislative Affairs and Public Policy Board for FPA. She has appeared on television news and in national magazines regarding sleep-related issues.
Website: www.sleeppsychology.com

Delayed Sleep Phase Disorder

Circadian Sleep Disorders Network
Circadian Sleep Disorders Network (CSD-N) is an independent nonprofit organization dedicated to improving the lives of people with chronic circadian rhythm disorders.
Website: www.circadiansleepdisorders.org/docs/DSPS-QandA.php

Get Enough Sleep

Healthfinder.gov
The healthfinder.gov has resources on a wide range of health topics selected from approximately 1,400 government and nonprofit organizations to bring the best, most reliable health information on the Internet.
Website: healthfinder.gov/healthtopics/population/men/mental-health-and-relationships/ get-enough-sleep

How Depression Affects Your Sleep

Sleep.org
Sleep.org, by the National Sleep Foundation (NSF), is dedicated to starting a movement about the positive benefits of sleep health. Sleep health is an emerging field of research focused on how we sleep and the benefits it provides to our minds, bodies, and lives.
Website: sleep.org/articles/depression-affects-sleep

How Does Anxiety Affect Sleep?

HealthStatus
HealthStatus, an Internet-based health risk assessment, along with several calculators to take a quick snapshot of a person's health. It provides the best interactive health tools on the Internet and millions of visitors have used its health risk assessment, body fat, and calories burned calculators.
Website: www.healthstatus.com/health_blog/sleep-2/anxiety-affect-sleep

How Sleep Works

How Stuff Works
HowStuffWorks creates great content that can live on just about any platform! It is a source of unbiased, reliable, and easy-to-understand answers and explanations of how the world actually works.
Website: science.howstuffworks.com/life/inside-the-mind/human-brain/sleep.htm

How to Cope with Sleep Problems

Mind
Mind has worked to improve the lives of all people with experience of mental-health problems. Through public campaigns, government lobbying, and more than 1,000 services, local Minds have delivered in communities across England and Wales, and have touched millions of lives.
Website: www.mind.org.uk/information-support/types-of-mental-health-problems/sleep- problems/#.WiFNlVV97IU

Mental Illness and Sleep Disorders

Tuck
Tuck aims to improve sleep hygiene, health, and wellness through the creation and dissemination of comprehensive, unbiased, free resources. Boasting the largest collection of aggregated data on sleep products on the web (more than 300,000 customer experiences from 1000 of unique sources), Tuck aims to power consumers, sleep professionals, and the troubled sleeper looking for answers.
Website: www.tuck.com/mental-illness-and-sleep

Sleep

NOVA ScienceNOW

NOVA is a science series on American television, reaching an average of five million viewers weekly. Now in its fourth decade of production, the series remains committed to producing in-depth science programming in the form of one-hour documentaries and long-form mini-series, from the latest breakthroughs in technology to the deepest mysteries of the natural world.
Website: www.pbs.org/wgbh/nova/body/sleep.html

HealthyWomen

HealthyWomen is an independent, nonprofit health information source for women and to educate and empower women to make informed health choices for themselves and their families.
Website: www.healthywomen.org/content/
article/4-most-common-sleep-disorders

Sleep Apnea

MedlinePlus

MedlinePlus is the National Institutes of Health's (NIH) website for patients and their families and friends. Produced by the U.S. National Library of Medicine (NLM), it brings you information about diseases, conditions, and wellness issues in language you can understand. MedlinePlus offers reliable, up-to-date health information, anytime, anywhere, for free.
Website: medlineplus.gov/sleepapnea.html

Sleep Disorders

American Psychiatric Association

American Psychiatric Association (APA) has more than 38,500 members involved in psychiatric practice, research, and academia representing the diversity of the patients for whom they care. As the leading psychiatric organization in the world, APA now encompasses members practicing in more than 100 countries.
Website: www.psychiatry.org/patients-families/sleep-disorders/
what-are-sleep-disorders

Infinity Sleep Solutions

Infinity Sleep Solutions provides patients with comprehensive sleep diagnostic testing and specializes in personalized care led by a board certified sleep physician and also will work hand-in-hand to diagnose and treat even the most complicated sleep disorders.
Website: www.infinitysleep.com/education-1.html

MedicineNet

MedicineNet is an online, healthcare media publishing company, which provides easy-to-read, in-depth, authoritative medical information for consumers via its robust, user-friendly, interactive website.
Website: www.medicinenet.com/sleep/article.htm

Sleep Disorders and Problems

Helpguide.org

HelpGuide provides mental-health education and support to a global audience. They provide empowering, evidence-based content that is easy to digest and focused on information you can use to help yourself and your loved ones.
Website: www.helpguide.org/articles/sleep/sleep-disorders-and-problems.htm

Sleep Disorders: Categories

American Academy of Sleep Medicine

The American Academy of Sleep Medicine (AASM) improves sleep health and promotes high quality, patient-centered care through advocacy, education, strategic research, and practice standards.
Website: www.sleepeducation.org/sleep-disorders-by-category

Sleep Disorders Center

Mayo Clinic

Mayo Clinic is a nonprofit organization that provides the best care to all patients through the integration of clinical practice, education, and research in order to instill hope and contribute to health and well being.
Website: www.mayoclinic.org/es-es/departments-centers/neurology/sleep-disorders-center-florida/overview

Sleep Disorders Health Center

WebMD
WebMD provides health information, tools for managing your health, and support to those who seek information.
Website: www.webmd.com/sleep-disorders

Sleep Disorders: Information, Diagnosis, and Treatment

Disabled World
Disabled-World.Com is an independent Health and Disability news source that offers subject areas covering seniors and disability news, assistive device reviews, and articles on everything from helpful tips to disability sports articles.
Website: www.disabled-world.com/health/neurology/sleepdisorders

Sleep Disorders: SSDI Eligibility Guidelines

Allsup
True Help is dedicated to simplifying the world of disability benefits for individuals and organizations with expertize in social security disability (SSDI) representation, return to work, veterans disability, and healthcare assistance.
Website: www.truehelp.com/understanding-ssdi/guidelines-by-disability/sleep-disorders- and-social-security-disability-insurance

Sleep for Kids

National Sleep Foundation
This website by the National Sleep Foundation provides easily readable information about the importance of sleep, sleep disorders, and tips for getting a good night's sleep to children ages 7 to 10, their parents, and their teachers.
Website: www.sleepforkids.org

American Psychological Association
American Psychological Association (APA) is a scientific and professional organization representing psychology in the United States, with more than 118,000 researchers, educators, clinicians, consultants, and students as its members.
Website: www.apa.org/monitor/feb04/sleep.aspx

490

Sleep Health

HealthyPeople.gov

HealthyPeople provides science-based, 10-year national objectives for improving the health of all Americans. HealthyPeople has established benchmarks and monitored progress over time in order to encourage collaborations across communities and sectors, empower individuals toward making informed health decisions, and to measure the impact of prevention activities.
Website: www.healthypeople.gov/2020/topics-objectives/topic/sleep-health

Sleep Problems

Caring.com

Caring.com is an online destination for those seeking information and support as they care for aging parents, spouses, and other loved ones. They equip family caregivers to make better decisions, save time and money, and feel less alone—and less stressed—as they face the many challenges of caregiving.
Website: www.caring.com/articles/sleep-problems

Sleep Problems in Teens

KidsHealth®

KidsHealth® provides information about health, behavior, and development from before birth through the teen years.
Website: kidshealth.org/en/parents/sleep-problems.html

The Sleep Doctor

Most people could improve their sleep and many others are dealing with disorders, such as insomnia. The Sleep Doctor has advice, news, and tools to help you.
Website: www.thesleepdoctor.com/2017/03/30/teens-need-sleep-think

Want to Sleep Better

Sound Sleep Health

Sound Sleep Health, founded by sleep medicine expert, Gandis Mazeika M.D., has been granted program accreditation from the American Academy of Sleep Medicine and fulfills the high standards required for receiving accreditation as a sleep disorder center.
Website: www.soundsleephealth.com

Chapter 65

Directory of Resources Providing Information about Sleep Disorders

General

American Academy of Dental Sleep Medicine (AADSM)
1001 Warrenville Rd., Ste. 175
Lisle, IL 60532
Phone: 630-686-9875
Fax: 630-686-9876
Website: www.aadsm.org
E-mail: info@aadsm.org

American Academy of Sleep Medicine (AASM)
2510 N. Frontage Rd.
Darien, IL 60561
Phone: 630-737-9700
Fax: 630-737-9790
Website: www.aasmnet.org
E-mail: contact@aasm.org

Resources in this chapter were compiled from several sources deemed reliable; all contact information was verified and updated in May 2019.

American Association of Sleep Technologists (AAST)
330 N. Wabash Ave., Ste. 2000
Chicago, IL 60611
Phone: 312-321-5191
Website: www.aastweb.org
E-mail: info@aastweb.org

American Sleep Association (ASA)
1002 Lititz Pike, Ste. 229
Lititz, PA 17543
Phone: 717-478-8556
Website: www.sleepassociation.org
E-mail: contactASA@sleepassociation.org

American Sleep Medicine
7900 Belfort Pkwy, Ste. 301
Jacksonville, FL 32256
Toll-Free: 855-U-SLEEP-2 (855-875-3372)
Phone: 904-517-5500
Fax: 904-517-5501
Website: www.americansleepmedicine.com
E-mail: info@americansleepmedicine.com

American Thoracic Society (ATS)
25 Bdwy.
New York, NY 10004
Phone: 212-315-8600
Fax: 212-315-6498
Website: www.thoracic.org
E-mail: atsinfo@thoracic.org

Better Sleep Council (BSC)
Website: bettersleep.org

The Center For Sleep & Wake Disorders
5454 Wisconsin Ave.
Ste. 1725
Chevy Chase, MD 20815
Phone: 301-654-1575
Fax: 301-654-5658
Website: www.sleepdoc.com
E-mail: mail@sleepdoc.com

Cleveland Clinic
9500 Euclid Ave.
Cleveland, OH 44195
Toll-Free: 800-223-2273
Phone: 216-444-2200
TTY: 216-444-0261
Website: my.clevelandclinic.org

Eastern Iowa Sleep Center (ESIC)
600 Seventh St. S.E.
Cedar Rapids, IA 52401
Toll-Free: 877-361-4433
Phone: 319-362-4433
Fax: 319-362-4466
Website: www.eisleep.com

Eunice Kennedy Shriver *National Institute of Child Health and Human Development (NICHD)*
Information Resource Center (IRC)
P.O. Box 3006
Rockville, MD 20847
Toll-Free: 800-370-2943
Toll-Free TTY: 888-320-6942
Toll-Free Fax: 866-760-5947
Website: www.nichd.nih.gov
E-mail: NICHDInformation
ResourceCenter@mail.nih.gov

Michigan Academy of Sleep Medicine (MASM)
3031 W. Grand Blvd.
Ste. 645
Detroit, MI 48202
Phone: 313-874-1360
Fax: 313-874-1366
Website: www.masm.wildapricot.org
E-mail: kcarter@wcmssm.org

National Center on Sleep Disorders Research (NCSDR)
National Heart, Lung, and Blood Institute (NHLBI)
6701 Rockledge Dr.
Bethesda, MD 20892
Phone: 301-435-0199
Fax: 301-480-3451
Website: www.nhlbi.nih.gov/about/divisions/division-lung-diseases/
national-center-sleep-disorders-research

National Fibromyalgia and Chronic Pain Association (NFMCPA)
31 Federal Ave.
Logan, UT 84321
Website: fibroandpain.org
E-mail: info.nfmcpa@gmail.com

National Heart, Lung, and Blood Institute (NHLBI)
Health Information Center
P.O. Box 30105
Bethesda, MD 20824-0105
Phone: 301-592-8573
Website: www.nhlbi.nih.gov
E-mail: nhlbiinfo@nhlbi.nih.gov

National Institute of Neurological Disorders and Stroke (NINDS)
NIH Neurological Institute
P.O. Box 5801
Bethesda, MD 20824
Toll-Free: 800-352-9424
Website: www.ninds.nih.gov

National Sleep Foundation (NSF)
Website: www.sleepfoundation.org
E-mail: nsf@sleepfoundation.org

The Nemours Foundation / KidsHealth®
Website: kidshealth.org

Nocturna Sleep Center, LLC.
Administration Office and Night Clinic
9077 S. Pecos Rd.
Ste. 3700
Henderson, NV 89074
Toll-Free: 866-990-8762
Phone: 702-896-7378
Website: www.nocturnasleep.com
E-mail: Scheduling@nocturnasleep.net

Ohio Sleep Medicine Institute (OSMI)
4975 Bradenton Ave.
Dublin, OH 43017
Phone: 614-766-0773
Fax: 614-766-2599
Website: www.sleepohio.com
E-mail: info@sleepmedicine.com

Sleep Research Society (SRS)
2510 N. Frontage Rd.
Darien, IL 60561
Phone: 630-737-9702
Fax: 630-737-9790
Website: www.sleepresearchsociety.org
E-mail: coordinator@srsnet.org

Sleep Services of America (SSA)
MedBridge Healthcare
890 Airport Park Rd., Ste. 119
Glen Burnie, MD 21061
Toll-Free: 800-340-9978
Website: www.medbridgehealthcare.com/sleep-services-of-america.
php
E-mail: info@medbridgegroup.com

Spectrum Health
100 Michigan St. N.E.
Grand Rapids, MI 49503
Toll-Free: 866-989-7999
Website: www.spectrumhealth.org

TalkAboutSleep.com
Website: www.talkaboutsleep.com
E-mail: info@talkaboutsleep.com

UT Sleep Disorders Center
1928 Alcoa Hwy
Ste. 119, Bldg. B
Knoxville, TN 37920
Phone: 865-305-8761
Website: www.utmedicalcenter.org/medical-care/specialty-practices/
ut-sleep-disorders-center

Valley Sleep Center
P.O. Box 30388
Mesa, AZ 85275-0388
Phone: 480-830-3900
Fax: 480-830-3901
Website: www.valleysleepcenter.com
E-mail: sleep@valleysleepcenter.com

Washington University Sleep Medicine Center
Washington University School of Medicine (WUSM)
1600 S. Brentwood Blvd.
Ste. 600
St. Louis, MO 63144
Phone: 314-362-4342
Fax: 314-747-3813
Website: sleep.wustl.edu

Circadian Rhythm Disorders

Circadian Sleep Disorders Network (CSD-N)
4619 Woodfield Rd.
Bethesda, MD 20814
Website: www.circadiansleepdisorders.org
E-mail: csd-n@csd-n.org

Hypersomnia

Hypersomnia Foundation
4514 Chamblee Dunwoody Rd.
Ste. 229
Atlanta, GA 30338
Phone: 678-842-3512
Website: www.hypersomniafoundation.org
E-mail: info@hypersomniafoundation.org

Kleine-Levin Syndrome

Kleine-Levin Syndrome (KLS) Foundation, Inc.
P.O. Box 5382
San Jose, CA 95150-5382
Phone: 408-265-1099
Website: klsfoundation.org
E-mail: info@klsfoundation.org

Narcolepsy

Narcolepsy Network
P.O. Box 2178
Lynnwood, WA 98036
Toll-Free: 888-292-6522
Phone: 401-667-2523
Fax: 401-633-6567
Website: www.narcolepsynetwork.org
E-mail: narnet@narcolepsynetwork.org

Wake Up Narcolepsy, Inc.
P.O. Box 60293
Worcester, MA 01606
Phone: 978-751-DOZE (978-751-3693)
Website: www.wakeupnarcolepsy.org

Other Disorders Affecting Sleep

Alzheimer's Association
225 N. Michigan Ave.
17th Fl.
Chicago, IL 60601
Toll-Free: 800-272-3900
Website: www.alz.org

American Gastroenterological Association (AGA)
4930 Del Ray Ave.
Bethesda, MD 20814
Toll-Free: 800-227-7888
Phone: 301-654-2055
Fax: 301-654-5920
Website: www.gastro.org
E-mail: member@gastro.org

American Parkinson Disease Association (APDA)
135 Parkinson Ave.
Staten Island, NY 10305
Toll-Free: 800-223-2732
Phone: 718-981-8001
Fax: 718-981-4399
Website: www.apdaparkinson.org
E-mail: apda@apdaparkinson.org

Anxiety and Depression Association of America (ADAA)
8701 Georgia Ave., Ste. 412
Silver Spring, MD 20910
Phone: 240-485-1001
Fax: 240-485-1035
Website: www.adaa.org
E-mail: information@adaa.org

COPD Foundation
Communications and Public Policy (COPP) Departments
1140 Third St. S.E.
Second Fl.
Washington, DC 20002
Toll-Free: 866-731-COPD (866-731-2673)
Website: www.copdfoundation.org
E-mail: info@copdfoundation.org

National Center for Posttraumatic Stress Disorder (NCPTSD)
Toll-Free: 800-273-8255
Phone: 802-296-6300
Website: www.ptsd.va.gov
E-mail: ncptsd@va.gov

National Institute of Mental Health (NIMH)
Office of Science Policy, Planning, and Communications (OSPPC)
6001 Executive Blvd.
Rm. 6200, MSC 9663
Bethesda, MD 20892-9663
Toll-Free: 866-615-6464
TTY: 301-443-8431
Toll-Free TTY: 866-415-8051
Fax: 301-443-4279
Website: www.nimh.nih.gov
E-mail: nimhinfo@nih.gov

National Multiple Sclerosis (MS) Society
733 Third Ave.
Third Fl.
New York, NY 10017
Toll-Free: 800-344-4867
Phone: 212-463-7787
Fax: 212-986-7981
Website: www.nationalmssociety.org
E-mail: INFO@MSNYC.ORG

Restless Legs Syndrome

Restless Legs Syndrome (RLS) Foundation
3006 Bee Caves Rd.
Ste. D206
Austin, TX 78746
Phone: 512-366-9109
Fax: 512-366-9189
Website: www.rls.org
E-mail: info@rls.org

Sleep Apnea

American Sleep Apnea Association (ASAA)
641 S. St. N.W.
Third Fl.
Washington, DC 20001-5196
Toll-Free: 888-293-3650
Toll-Free Fax: 888-293-3650
Website: www.sleepapnea.org
E-mail: asaa@sleepapnea.org

Infant and Children Sleep Apnea Awareness Foundation, Inc.
New Smyrna Beach, FL 32170
Phone: 386-426-5858
Website: www.kidssleepdisorders.org
E-mail: terrilynn@kidssleepdisorders.org

Nevada Sleep Diagnostics
8935 S. Pecos Rd.
Ste. 22D
Henderson, NV 89074-7336
Phone: 702-990-7660
Fax: 702-990-7665
Website: www.nevadasleep.com

Index

Index